HIV and AIDS: Strategies for Control

HIV and AIDS: Strategies for Control

Editor: Alison Swift

AMERICAN
MEDICAL PUBLISHERS
www.americanmedicalpublishers.com

AMERICAN
MEDICAL PUBLISHERS
www.americanmedicalpublishers.com

Cataloging-in-Publication Data

HIV and AIDS : strategies for control / edited by Alison Swift.
p. cm.
Includes bibliographical references and index.
ISBN 978-1-63927-204-4
1. HIV infections. 2. AIDS (Disease). 3. HIV infections--Prevention.
4. AIDS (Disease)--Prevention. I. Swift, Alison.
RC606.6 .H58 2022
616.979 2--dc23

American Medical Publishers,
41 Flatbush Avenue,
1st Floor, New York,
NY 11217, USA

ISBN 978-1-63927-204-4 (Hardback)

Contents

Preface

The human immunodeficiency virus (HIV) is a type of retrovirus that causes a spectrum of conditions called acquired immunodeficiency syndrome (AIDS). HIV damages the immune system and thus interferes with the body's ability to fight infection and disease. It is spread primarily through unprotected sex, but also by contaminated blood transfusions, hypodermic needles, and from mother to child during pregnancy, delivery, or breastfeeding. AIDS is a chronic, potentially life-threatening condition. HIV infection has become a manageable chronic health condition, owing to the increased access to effective HIV prevention, diagnosis, treatment and care. This book provides comprehensive insights about the strategies for controlling HIV and AIDS. Different approaches, evaluations, methodologies and advanced studies on HIV/AIDS have been included herein. This book will serve as a reference to a broad spectrum of readers.

The information shared in this book is based on empirical researches made by veterans in this field of study. The elaborative information provided in this book will help the readers further their scope of knowledge leading to advancements in this field.

Finally, I would like to thank my fellow researchers who gave constructive feedback and my family members who supported me at every step of my research.

Editor

1

Oral Neoplasms in HIV Positive Patient

Kelly Cristine Tarquinio Marinho,
Elcio Magdalena Giovani,
Camila Correia dos Santos and
Rodolfo Georgevich Neto

Abstract

Acquired immune deficiency syndrome (AIDS) is a disease that manifests itself after the human body is infected with human immunodeficiency virus (HIV). The virus destroys defense cells (T-CD4 lymphocytes) and an important increase identifier of immunosuppression and/or failure to an immune response, the early signs often appear in the oral cavity in the form of various lesions. With the advent of HAART, it was also observed that it is accompanied by medium- and long-term side effects, mainly metabolic and bone changes. Other clinical manifestations that may occur are the human papillomavirus (HPV) infections in the oral cavity; HPV infections show exophytic growth and are often confluent, showing a "cauliflower" appearance and may or may not correspond to keratinized or non-keratinized tissues. In recent studies on papillomavirus, the literature indicates that HPV 16 and 18 are considered risk factors in the etiology of oral cancer development. Several neoplasias can occur in the oral cavity of patients with AIDS or HIV, and often the oral cavity is the place where we have the first manifestation of the disease, but multidisciplinary follow-up is necessary, so that the patient has care and a better quality of life.

Keywords: neoplasm, HIV positive, oral

1. Introduction

Acquired immunodeficiency syndrome (AIDS) was recognized in 1981 by the Centers for Disease Control (CDC) in Atlanta, USA because of an explosion of unexplained cases of Kaposi Sarcoma and Pneumonia by *Pneumocystis carinii*, which is currently called as *Pneumocystis jirovecii*, in men who have sex with men (MSM), mainly in two major centers,

New York on the east coast and Los Angeles on the west coast of the USA. The first description of the clinical picture of AIDS was made by Gottlieb in Los Angeles and by Mansur in New York in 1981. In 1983 the HIV type 1 virus was discovered by Luc Montagnier at the Pasteur Institute in Paris and was identified later in 1984, as the etiological agent causing the disease, and in the same year, Robert Gallo in Bethesda (USA) established a cell culture system for the development and multiplication of HIV 1. In 1985, the laboratory test was started to prove the infection [1].

AIDS is a disease with a tendency to chronify, requiring follow-up, treatment and control. Acquired immunodeficiency syndrome (AIDS) is a disease that manifests itself after the human body is infected with the human immunodeficiency virus (HIV). This has received increased attention from researchers and health agencies because of its severity and seriousness. This is due to not only the mortality rate, but also the various economic, social and public health aspects associated with it. In order for the virus to reproduce, it must infect a cell, because viruses are not technically alive. As the human body is constantly producing new cells, each of them often makes new proteins to stay alive and reproduce [2, 3].

Since its clinical recognition in 1981, the human immunodeficiency virus and acquired immunodeficiency syndrome have been fatal even for people who administer highly potent antiretroviral therapy (HAART). In 1996, the "cocktail of drugs" = HAART was created. Currently, there are six groups of drugs that can be used in the treatment of HIV in individuals at the beginning of treatment or for those who have already started therapy, which is done by combining several drugs approved by the Brazilian Ministry of Health—Anvisa, belonging to six different classes, namely protease inhibitors, nucleoside reverse transcriptase inhibitors (NRTIs), fusion inhibitors (IF), integrase inhibitors (II), non-nucleoside reverse transcriptase inhibitors (NNRTIs) and CCR5 antagonist [4–6].

1. Protease inhibitors
2. Nucleoside reverse transcriptase inhibitors (NRTIs)
3. Fusion inhibitors (IF)
4. Integrase inhibitors (II)
5. Non-nucleoside reverse transcriptase inhibitors (NNRTIs)
6. CCR5 antagonist

1. Protease inhibitors. Protease inhibitors prevent new HIV from maturing and infecting other cells. Protease is essential for the production of infectious and mature viral particles. It breaks new viral multi-proteins into individual (central) internal structural proteins, and the action of protease is a key step in structuring these proteins, which occurs for the virus to become infectious.

2. Nucleoside reverse transcriptase inhibitors (NRTIs). NRTIs called "nucleoside analogs" or "nuclear weapons" contain defective versions of the building blocks (nucleotides) used by

reverse transcriptase to convert RNA to DNA. When reverse transcriptase uses these defective blocks, the new DNA cannot be properly constructed and the HIV genetic material cannot be incorporated into the healthy genetic material of the cell and prevents it from producing new viruses.

3. Fusion inhibitors (IF). Fusion inhibitors are a new type of compound that prevents the virus from binding to and entering human CD4 cells. They act at a stage in the life cycle of HIV, before the virus enters the cell, preventing the infection of new cells.

4. Integrase inhibitors (II). They prevent the insertion of HIV viral DNA into human DNA. It is a new mechanism of action, which inhibits the replication of the virus and its ability to infect new cells.

5. Non-nucleoside reverse transcriptase inhibitors (NNRTIs). NNRTIs bind to the reverse transcriptase at a specific site; after being bound to the enzyme, NNRTIs affect the activity of the enzyme, restricting its mobility at a critical point and rendering it incapable of functioning. The enzyme is now unable to interact properly with the viral RNA to produce the viral DNA. The production of the latter is discontinued, although the virus is not killed.

6. CCR5 antagonist. CCR5 is a co-receptor of the HIV virus. In other words, is, the virus needs beyond the CD4 receptor, this co-receptor, or some other, to penetrate the cell. CCR5 means chemokine (C-C motif) receptor 5.

People live longer because of the beneficial effects of antiretroviral treatment, which most of the time interferes positively in people's lives, improving the quality of life of this population. However, the number of AIDS-related deaths has fallen by more than 10% in the last 5 years, as more people have gained access to treatment, saving many lives. The UNAIDS and the WHO estimate that since 1996, when antiretroviral treatment became available, about 2.9 million lives were saved. As the progression of the disease is evidenced by association with high levels of HIV'S RNA in the blood (viral load), one of the important goals of antiretroviral therapy is to reduce viral load. Opportunistic diseases in HIV patients and quality of life have changed since the introduction of HAART, resulting in a significant reduction in viral load (VL) and an increase in T-CD4 lymphocyte count. However, access to HAART is still uneven and may vary depending on the public interest policies of each country [7, 8].

According to the WHO, there are currently more than 42 million infected 20–60% of those infected may present oral manifestations. Epidemiology has been delineated since the onset of the syndrome, predominantly in MSM (men who have sex with men), later in HET (heterosexual), followed by female partners of these HET/MSM, and consequently covered women of childbearing age, with vertical transmission occurring to children infected with HIV and older people. There is currently a stabilization in cases of women of childbearing age, but there is a marked increase in cases of young people starting sexually (12–16 years) and an increase in cases in the elderly, who are over 60 years of age.

The risk of vertical transmission is 25–30%, depending on CD4, viral load, STDs, nutritional status and previous pregnancies. With the use of zidovudine (AZT) medication, the risk of vertical transmission dropped to 8%.

The risk of infection of the fetus is greater when, during pregnancy, the woman shows signs of AIDS or has recently been infected. The baby is born with the antibodies of the mother, and every child born to women with AIDS has tested positive for HIV, and only 18 months after birth, the child begins to produce its own antibodies. Subsequently, the serological test with positive result indicates that the child is HIV positive.

There are several symptoms related to HIV infection. Depending on the stage of infection, such as an acute infection, occurs approximately 2-6 weeks after exposure to the virus.

In general, the most common constitutional signs and symptoms are fever, lymphadenopathy, pharyngitis, exanthema (= Rash), papular papular erythema and mucocutaneous ulcers (mouth, esophagus and genital organs).

In acute infection, there is a violent replication of HIV in the body, and only when a viral load (quantity of virus per ml in the blood) is reached, the body reacts, causing that viral load to decrease to a certain level, thus generally remaining from 8 to 10 years, when the body start to lose their ability to respond. The immune window is the space where the body cannot identify HIV. Only after severe infection by HIV, the virus can be identified, thus forming antibodies that, even so, are unable to contain the advancement of infection. For a period between 3 weeks to 6 months, the blood does not have antibodies to HIV; this means that an anti-HIV serological test can give a false-negative result.

The objective of this review is to guide the dental surgeon in the diagnosis and treatment of oral neoplasms that are common in patients with HIV/AIDS.

2. Oral neoplasms

Oral alterations in HIV patients are vast, comprising more than 40 manifestations, which many times appear as the first manifestations of the disease, or even today, as an important identifier of therapeutic failure. Early diagnosis of oral lesions due to HIV infection is important to define the stage of the disease or indicate the possibility of HIV infection in undiagnosed individuals, since oral manifestations are usually the first signs of infection. Oral exams are an essential component for the early recognition of disease progression and overall assessment of HIV-infected patients [9, 10].

The evaluation by the dental professional should include resolution of emergency problems such as pain, abscesses, ulcerated lesions and other acute infections, guidance on local procedures, resolution of chronic problems and resolution of traditional treatment. HIV patients are afflicted with multiple diseases and are medicated with several different drugs. The patient's medical history should be carefully considered, and important aspects should be noted [11, 12].

3. Human papillomavirus

The human papillomavirus appears in the oral mucosa of the white, vegetative, proliferative lesion, a wartlike appearance, similar to cauliflower. And its etiology is by Human papillomavirus (HPV) infection. It is presented as synonymy: cock crest, crested alligator, venereal wart, vulgar verruca, genital wart, and condyloma acuminata. HPV has more than 200 subtypes: pairs 6, 7, 11, 13, 16, 18, 32 are responsible for vegetative lesions in the oral cavity. Subtypes 16 and 18 are most related to induction for the development of malignant neoplasms [13].

Viruses belong to the papoviridase family that penetrates by absorption into microtraumatized regions, being highly infective. They present a high recurrence rate, with a tendency to reinfection. Incubation is generally 1–8 months for the onset of the first lesion, the active phase depends on the immune response. In the late phase, it is 9 months/years [14].

The main co-factors for HPV are smoking, alcohol, stress, low immunity (HIV/AIDS), sexual promiscuity and hygiene.

Diagnosis may be clinical (noting formations known as condyloma and/or papilloma), or subclinical by histopathological study, and latent biomolecular analyzes by in situ hybridization or PCR techniques [15].

The incidence in general is usually from 10 to 25% in the oral cavity [16].

4. Kaposi's sarcoma

Kaposi's sarcoma (KS) was first described in 1872 by Moritz Kaposi as "pigmented idiopathic sarcoma of the skin" before the advent of the AIDS epidemic. Kaposi's sarcoma was classified as: classic KS, involving men of European origin, mainly residents of eastern Europe and the Mediterranean Sea, with a preferential location in the lower limbs; African endemic KS occurring in black and young men in equatorial Africa; SK iatrogenic, related to immunosuppressive therapy in transplanted patients. But this epidemiological profile is altered with the first reports of AIDS, because there was an explosion of cases of KS, which was then called epidemic KS [17].

SK is the most common neoplasm in patients with AIDS. The incidence has been declining from 40% at the beginning of the epidemic to less than 15% today. The reason for this is not fully known, but it may be related to the greater preventive care, effectiveness of highly potent antiretroviral therapies and earlier diagnoses, as well as safer sexual practices in the community of men who have sex with men [18].

In some regions of Africa, the incidence of KS in women is much higher, occurring in 40% of all KS cases related to HIV infection. In these patients, SK tends to be more indolent, with a course similar to that observed in classic KS. The pathogenesis of KS is related to human herpes virus type 8 (HHV-8) or herpes virus associated with Kaposi's sarcoma (SK-HV). This virus is transmitted through sexual contact, which explains the prevalence in men who have sex with men in the US and in heterosexual women in Africa. The clinical characteristics are variable, usually beginning as erythematous, violet or brownish, asymptomatic macules that develop into papules, plaques, nodules or tumor lesions.

The manifestations of KS can compromise mucous membranes, such as the oral cavity and viscera, gastrointestinal tract, lungs and lymph nodes. Lesions in their evolution may grow, coalesce, form large plaques and envelop lymphatic vessels, leading to lymphoedema in the affected limb. KS can occur as the first manifestation of AIDS, concomitant with other manifestations or late in the course of the disease.

Initially they manifest themselves with enlarged and enlarged blood vessels in the dermis, with large endothelial cells, protruding into the lumen. There is perivascular infiltrate composed of lymphocytes, plasma cells and some macrophages, and groups of extravagant erythrocytes and hemosiderin deposits can be visualized. Several skin lesions, both inflammatory and neoplastic, should be included in the differential diagnosis: purpura, hemangiomas, bacillary angiomatosis, lichen planar dermatofibroma, pink pityriasis, fungal mycosis, nevi, malignant melanoma, cutaneous lymphoma and secondary syphilis were reported as SK simulators [19].

5. Non-Hodgkin lymphoma

Its etiology comes from the chronic stimulation of B cells and its incidence occurs with late manifestations, mainly located in the gingiva. For more than 30 years the relationship between immunodeficiency and non-Hodgkin's lymphoma is known, relating to AIDS. Non-Hodgkin's lymphoma is evidenced by polygamous hypergammaglobulinemia, cytokines, and growth factors: 11–6; 11–10. Since the beginning of the epidemic the CDC defines HIV+ patients with a diagnosis of non-Hodgkin's lymphoma as AIDS [17].

The diagnosis may be clinical, associated with biopsy, radiographs, CT scans, MRI [17].

6. Epidermal carcinoma

It is the most common malignant neoplasm of the oral cavity, corresponding to 95% of the tumors of the patients, of form. We highlight the growing prevalence of HIV/AIDS patients. According to the National Institute of Cancer (INCA)/Ministry of Health (MS), the estimate for 2018, regarding the number of cases of oral cancer in general in Brazil, is 14,700 new cases, considering the region as the seventh most frequently affected by malignant tumors in the Brazilian population.

Clinical features include ulcerated superficial, endophytic lesions (infiltrative ulcer and destructive ulcer), exophytic lesions (moriform vegetative, papilliferous vegetative and cauliflower vegetation), nodular (sub mucosa and deep) lesions. The most common clinical feature of squamous cell carcinoma is chronic ulcer. Due to this ulcerated clinical aspect, often granulomatous, we must associate in the differential diagnosis ulcerated lesions of long duration of infectious diseases such as tuberculosis, syphilis, histoplasmosis and paracoccidioidomycosis [20, 21].

Its prevalence and incidence is greatest in individuals over 40 years of age, smokers and alcoholics. The male gender is more affected than the female in the proportion of 3:1.

7. Discussion and recommendations

The relationship of the dentist to the patient's physician should result in knowledge of modifying factors that may interfere with dental treatment. See **Table 1**, which highlights these factors.

7.1. Evaluation of medical factors modifying the dental treatment

Treatment of human papilloma virus can be surgical (incisional biopsy) or cryotherapy, high-power laser therapy (CO^2), topical application of 25% podophylline alcoholic solution, topical application of 90% trichloroacetic acid (ATA) or medications such as Wartec®-Podofilotoxin and Aldara® Cream-Imiquimod Gel [8, 13–15, 22].

In relation to Kaposi's sarcoma, the biopsy is predominant to establish the diagnosis. Treatment of KS includes antiretroviral drugs, since the lesions usually regress with improved immune compromise. Localized destructive treatments may be indicated for isolated or sporadic injuries, such as cryotherapy with liquid nitrogen. Radiation therapy is effective for painful lesions of palms and plants and when there is edema. Intralesional injection of vinblastine may be effective if the patient has few lesions, but the method is associated with pain caused by the injection. The combination of traditional chemotherapeutic agents, such as vinblastine, etoposide (VP-16) and adriamycin, produces regression of SK lesions, but these drugs are myelosuppressive and potentially immunosuppressive. Vincristine and bleomycin, non-myelotoxic drugs, can be used with good results. Interferon can be used both intralesional and systemically. Doxorubicin and liposomal daunorubicin are also effective [17–19].

Treatment of Non-Hodgkin lymphoma may be via prophylaxis with infiltration into the central nervous system of cytarabine or methotrexate medications. Also noteworthy is the study of the use of antiviral, and growth factors should be observed, and the administration of prophylaxis for the treatment of *Pneumocystis carinii* (*jirovecii*) should be considered [17].

Epidermal carcinoma shows the main locations are the lower lip, tongue border, floor of mouth and gum. There are important factors and determinants of risks such as: heredity, sex,

Hematological status	Neutrophils and granulocytes (<300 mm^3)
Coagulation—platelets	(Thrombocytopenia <15,000 mm^3)
Drug interactions	Adverse effects of HAART
Opportunistic diseases	Related to immunosuppression

Table 1. Medical factors modifying dental treatment.

age and race. The treatment protocols and procedures go through surgical removal, chemotherapy and radiotherapy [20, 21].

8. Conclusion

This study evidences the early diagnosis, aiming mainly to guide the dental surgeon, regarding the evaluation and conduct of oral neoplasias that commonly affect patients with alterations in the immune system by HIV/AIDS, seeking to improve the quality of life of immunocompromised patients. It indicates the continuous study and deepening of the knowledge of the etiology, diagnosis and new treatments for oral neoplastic changes.

Author details

Kelly Cristine Tarquinio Marinho*, Elcio Magdalena Giovani, Camila Correia dos Santos and Rodolfo Georgevich Neto

*Address all correspondence to: kekeodonto@gmail.com

Paulista University, São Paulo, SP, Brazil

References

[1] Ferreira SS, et al. Assistência Odontológica a Pacientes Portadores do Vírus HIV- Grupo de Trabalho de Estomatologia/Rede CEDROS: Boletim Informativo. Ano II. N°3, 1993

[2] Burnett GW, Scherp HW, Schuster GS. Microbiologia Oral e Doenças Infecciosas. Rio de Janeiro: Guanabara Koogan; 1978

[3] Grassi M, Abb J, Hämmerle. Aids em odontologia. São Paulo: Revinter; 1994

[4] Gonçalves et al. Association of T CD4 lymphocyte levels and subgingival microbiota of chronic periodontitis in HIV-infected Brazilians under HAART. Oral Surgery, Oral Medicine, Oral Pathology, Oral Radiology, and Endodontology. 2004;**97**:196-203

[5] Greene WC et al. Novel targets for HIV therapy. Antiviral Research. 2008;**80**:251-265

[6] Greenspan D et al. Effect of highly active antiretroviral therapy on frequency of oral warts. The Lancet. 2001;**357**

[7] Aidsmeds. About HIV and AIDS. Disponível em: http://www.aidsmeds.com/ Acesso em 30 set 2010

[8] Giovani et al. The treatment of Hpv oral lesions: Report of 3 cases. International Journal of Current Research. 2017;**9**(12):62648-62652

[9] Jané-Salas E, Chimenos-Küstner E, López-López J, Roselló-Llabrés X, Ocaña-Rivera I. Efecto De Los Tratamientos Antirretrovirales En Las Manifestaciones Orales De Los Pacientes Vih+. Avances en Odontoestomatologia. 2006;**22**(6):315-326. Disponible En:

http://Scielo.Isciii.Es/Scielo.Php?Script=Sci_Arttext&Pid=S0213-12852006000600003&Lng=Es. DOI: 10.4321/S0213-12852006000600003

[10] Santos CC, Giovani EM. Xerostomy, caries and in black people with periodontal disease in black people periodontal disease risk studies HIV/AIDS. Landmark Research Journals of Medicine And Medical Sciences. 2017;**4**(2):025-030

[11] Bhayat A, Yengopal V, Rudolph M. Predictive value of group I oral lesions for HIV infection. Oral Surgery, Oral Medicine, Oral Pathology, Oral Radiology. 2010;**109**:720-723

[12] Filho AC, Abrão P. Alterações metabólicas do paciente infectado por HIV. Arquivos Brasileiros de Endocrinologia & Metabologia São Paulo. 2007;**1**:51

[13] Stoopler ET, Balasubramaniam R. Human papillomavirus lesions of the oral cavity. New England Journal of Medicine. 2011;**365**:E37

[14] Bouda M, Vg G, Ng K, et al. "High risk" Hpv types are frequently detected in potentially malignant oral lesions, but not in normal mucosa. Modern Pathology. 2000;**13**(6):644-653

[15] Giovani EM, Santos CC, Georgevich Neto R, Noro-Filho GA, Caputo BV. Diagnosis of bone changes in mandibles of aids patients who had administered haart and developed lipodistrophic syndrome. Landmark Research Journal of Medicine and Medical Sciences. 2017;**4**(5):058-067

[16] Chaturvedi AK, Engels EA, Pfeiffer RM, Hernandez BY, Xiao W, Kim E, Jiang B, Goodman MT, Sibug-Saber M, Cozen W, Liu L, Lynch CF, Wentzensen N, Jordan RC, Altekruse S, Anderson WF, Rosenberg PS, Gilisson ML. Human papillomavirus and rising oropharyngeal cancer incidence in the United States. Journal of Clinical Oncology. 2011;**29**(32):4294-4301

[17] Greenspan D et al. Incidence of oral lesions in HIV-1-infected women: Reduction with HAART. Journal of Dental Research. 2004;**83**(2):145-150

[18] Glick M et al. Oral manifestations associated with HIV-related disease as markers for immune suppression and aids. Oral Surgery Oral Medicine Oral Pathology. 1994;**77**(4):344-349

[19] Coogan MM, Greenspan J, Challacombe SJ. Oral lesions in infection with human immunodeficiency virus. Bulletin of the World Health Organization. 2005;**9**:83

[20] Brau N et al. Presentation and outcome of hepatocellular carcinoma in HIV-infected patients: A U.S.–Canadian multicenter study. Journal of Hepatology. 2007;**47**:527-537

[21] Hodgson TA, Greenspan D, Greespan JS. Oral lesion of disease and HAART in industrialized countries. Advances in Dental Research. 2006;**19**:57-62. Disponível em: http://www.spcd.org.br/prevencao01.htm [acessado em 14/07/10]

[22] Giovani EM, Martins RB, JAJ M, Tortamano N. Use of GaAlAs laser in the treatment of necrotizing ulcerative periodontitis in patients seropositive for HIV/AIDS. Journal of Oral Laser Applications. 2007;**07**(1):55-64

2

Vaginal Formulations for Prevention of Sexual Transmission of HIV

María-Dolores Veiga-Ochoa, Roberto Ruiz-Caro,
Raúl Cazorla-Luna, Araceli Martín-Illana and
Fernando Notario-Pérez

Abstract

According to UNAIDS, as there is still no effective vaccine against HIV, pre-exposure prophylasis (PrEP) is necessary to reduce its incidence. Sexual transmission rate is higher from men to women in developing countries and vertical transmission may also occur from mother to child. Hence, vaginal formulations are an interesting proposal for the protection of women, preventing the virus from infecting vagina through different mechanisms. Several drugs, such as Dapivirine, Tenofovir or Maraviroc, have been assessed and showed to be effective in this field. These microbicides are included in different dosage forms able to release the drug once in contact with the vaginal medium. Innovative excipients are being employed for the development of different systems trying to get an easier posology through control release and high comfortability, thus leading to a better compliance. In this line, several formulations have been developed and tested, such as rings, tablets, gels or films. Some of them are nowadays in clinical trials, such as a Tenofovir gel or a Dapivirine vaginal ring. The aim of this chapter is to synthetize the research and findings in the field of the development and assessment of vaginal formulations in the PrEP of HIV sexual transmission.

Keywords: HIV sexual transmission prevention, vaginal gels, vaginal tablets, vaginal films, vaginal rings

1. Introduction

It is well known that the human immunodeficiency virus (HIV) is one of the most serious epidemics facing humanity today, when 36.7 million people live with HIV. However, excellent progress has been made in access to antiretroviral therapy in the last decade, reducing acquired immunodeficiency disease syndrome (AIDS)-related deaths by 48% [1]. Prevention programmes have also succeeded in lowering the transmission of the virus in recent years, although it still continues to cause 1.8 million new infections per year.

One fact that gives pause for thought is that most of the people infected with HIV are women. The data is devastating, as AIDS-related diseases continue to be the leading cause of death among women of reproductive age, and it is also the second leading cause of death in Africa for women aged 15–24 [1]. The gender gap is much more pronounced among young people: in the 15–24 population group, new infections are 44% higher in women [1]. In light of these figures, there is no doubt that the risk of infection in young women is unacceptably high.

These already chilling figures are even more shocking in women living in sub-Saharan Africa, where 75% of new infections in the population aged 15–19 occur in girls [2]. This is also a population group where the incidence of new infections has barely diminished in recent years.

Although in theory their lower access to antiretroviral therapy might appear to be the main reason for the high prevalence of HIV among sub-Saharan women, a careful analysis of the living conditions in this area reveals that the high transmission rate of the virus cannot be attributed to a single reason. It is important to bear in mind that this is an area where rape and domestic violence are frequent. The World Health Organization (WHO) states that women living in these conditions are 50% more likely to acquire HIV [2].

However, the most important reason for this prevalence is undoubtedly women's lack of access to education and economic independence, which prevents them from negotiating the possibility of having safe sex with their partners. The stark reality is that 75% of young women do not have the final say over their own health [2]. To this must be added polygamy, which is still common in several sub-Saharan countries (Burkina Faso, Congo, Ivory Coast, Ethiopia, Gabon, Guyana, Rwanda, South Africa, Uganda, Tanzania and Zimbabwe) and the decrease in the use of condoms registered in Ivory Coast, Niger, Senegal and Uganda [3].

A cycle of HIV transmission has recently been described in sub-Saharan Africa to explain the negligible decline in the prevalence of AIDS in this area compared to the rest of the planet. Adult men typically infect young women (each year 15 million women are married before the age of 18). Later, when the women grow older, they tend to transmit the virus to men of their own age, who then start the cycle again [2].

This reflection points to the empowerment of women, especially in sub-Saharan Africa, as a fundamental milestone for halting the AIDS epidemic. It is essential to promote societies in which gender equality is achieved through adequate sexual and social education, and the aim of the United Nations (UN) is to ensure that young people have the skills, knowledge and tools to protect themselves from acquiring the virus [2]. However, this capacity for protection must be reinforced by empowering women and providing them with methods for preventing the sexual transmission of HIV that are not dependent on men, such as vaginal microbicides. This is the reason that research into vaginal microbicides has skyrocketed in recent decades, which, if they prove to be successful in preventing HIV, would represent an extraordinary step forward in the fight against AIDS.

Vaginal microbicides have been defined as "any agent included in a topical formulation designed to prevent the spread of sexually transmitted pathogens either through cell death, inactivation of cell mechanisms, inhibition of viral replication, the formation of a physical barrier between cells and pathogens, or by enhancing the natural protection mechanisms of the cervix and vagina" [4].

The strategies for developing an effective vaginal microbicide in recent decades have been so diverse that they require a preliminary classification to aid their understanding. They can initially be divided into two groups depending on whether the microbicides include antiretroviral drugs or not.

Microbicides that do not include drugs can be differentiated into surfactants, polyanions, acidifiers and glycoprotein 120 neutralizing monoclonal antibodies. The aim of these substances is to inactivate the virus before it meets the cells so the infection never occurs.

Microbicides that include antiretroviral drugs can be classified into entry inhibitors or viral enzyme inhibitors [4]. Of particular interest in this group is Tenofovir, an inhibitor of the reverse transcriptase of the virus, which was part of the first microbicide that proved its effectiveness in preventing the transmission of HIV, and has now become the most widely-studied drug for this purpose [3, 5]. Dapivirine, one of the most promising drugs for the development of vaginal microbicides against HIV, has subsequently also become very important [6].

The development of microbicides has evolved over the years. The initial conventional release formulations did not usually include antiretroviral drugs. Over time, the potential of useful antiretroviral drugs for preventing HIV infection use was assessed, and microbicides including different drugs gradually began to appear. The possibility of developing a microbicide that does not contain one of these antiretroviral drugs is now hardly contemplated, and the new trend in microbicides is to develop formulations for sustained drug release for more lasting protection [7].

Unfortunately, the vast majority of microbicide formulations developed to date have failed to afford protection due to their low efficacy or inadequate formulation [8]. This is often due to a failure to consider the characteristics of the vaginal route.

The main anatomical factor to bear in mind when developing a formulation for vaginal administration is the vaginal fluid, which can be both an ally and an enemy for our purpose. This aqueous fluid is produced from the mucous membranes of the endometrium and transudate serum, and accumulates inside the vagina and covers the vaginal epithelium [9]. The physical presence of this fluid and its high enzymatic activity has been identified as barriers to the release and absorption of drugs. It should also be noted that this fluid is generally the medium in which the drug must be dissolved, meaning that its components are highly likely to interfere in the drug's activity [10]. To make matters worse, it is also necessary to factor in dynamic changes in the volume and composition of this fluid, since the vaginal clearance of drugs administered by this route is also crucial for their efficacy [11].

pH also plays a significant role in the effectiveness of the formulations. The normal pH of vaginal fluid is between 4 and 4.5, while the pH of seminal fluid is around 7.9 [12]. Even if a formulation were to be developed that was effective in the pH of the vaginal environment, the microbicide could potentially lose its protective capacity in the presence of seminal fluid, when the medium undergoes alkalization.

Another similar example of failure due to the natural characteristics of the administration route is the collapse of certain microbicides (those that include polyanions) in *in vivo* trials, despite their success in blocking HIV *in vitro*. It was subsequently discovered that this inefficacy was due to the formation of a semen-derived enhancement of the virus infection that increased the infectious capacity of the virus in the presence of seminal fluid [13]. This study highlights the importance of evaluating the efficacy of microbicides in the presence of semen [4].

Another factor that must be considered when developing a microbicide is that the vaginal epithelium and the mucus layer covering it is already a barrier against infections. There is therefore an obvious need to maintain this natural barrier intact when seeking to prevent the acquisition of sexually transmitted diseases. A negative example of this is the microbicidal gel including Nonoxynol-9, a surfactant, which was shown in clinical trials to lead to an increase in vaginal ulcers [14].

Pharmaceutical form	Advantages	Drawbacks
Gels	• Widely studied and well known. • Easy and convenient for women to apply. • Low manufacturing cost and easy to mass produce.	• Unable to retain the drug and provide sustained release. • They require an applicator for administration • Possible local irritation and leakage. • Not particularly stable against adverse environmental conditions.
Tablets	• Easy and economical to manufacture on an industrial scale. • Easy to handle • Stable under different environmental conditions • Fast-dissolving or sustained-release tablets can be obtained depending on the excipients used in their development.	• Possible influence on sexual intercourse. • Possible local irritation.
Films	• Discreet use • No product leakage during use • No applicator required for insertion • Minimal packaging and reduced waste.	• Sustained release still not achieved • Possible local irritation • Mass production is currently unviable due to the underdevelopment of production resources.
Vaginal rings	• Sustained release of the drug. • Fewer applications. • The mass production of this dosage form is becoming increasingly advanced.	• They require a higher financial investment. • Higher manufacturing cost. • Possible influence on sexual intercourse.

Table 1. Advantages and disadvantages of pharmaceutical forms for vaginal administration of microbicides.

Another crucial factor is the vaginal microflora, which plays a very important role in establishing the microbicide's eventual environment. Special care should be taken with commensal bacteria, which are responsible for maintaining a healthy vaginal environment. Vaginal microbicides must therefore not be toxic to the vaginal microbiota [10].

The most common pharmaceutical dosage forms for the vaginal administration of drugs are gels, capsules, ovuli and tablets, although vaginal rings and films are rapidly gaining ground [4]. The first trials of vaginal microbicides mainly explored vaginal gels, but the current trend focuses more on vaginal rings and sustained-release tablets, which could prolong protection time. The advantages and drawbacks of each dosage form are summarized in **Table 1**.

Advanced drug delivery strategies are being incorporated for drug targeting, together with scientific methods to develop safer and more effective formulations [15]. Current research therefore gives cause for hope that within a few years women will be able to protect themselves from HIV acquisition through vaginal microbicides.

2. Main vaginal systems for HIV prevention

2.1. Vaginal gels

2.1.1. Overview

Gels are semisolid systems consisting of a liquid—generally water—and a solid component that acts as a gelling agent and traps the liquid within its three-dimensional structure, thus producing the characteristic consistency of these solid–liquid mixtures [16] (**Figure 1**). Vaginal gels can release drugs intended for local or systemic action [17]. However, the direct application of drugs onto the vaginal epithelium limits their systemic absorption, thus minimizing side effects and possible drug resistance [15, 18].

An ideal vaginal microbicide gel should be as spreadable as possible in order to cover the entire vaginal surface mucosa and thus protect effectively against the transmission of the virus. Several authors have pointed to an influence of the gel composition—which determines its viscosity and rheological properties—in its ability to form a stable coating layer. In addition to their composition, parameters such as the pH and osmolality of these gels must be suitable for the characteristics of the vaginal environment in order to achieve the microbicide effect without inducing side effects that could increase the risk of infection and/or result in the patients' loss of adherence [15, 19, 20].

One of the main problems associated with the vaginal administration of gels—especially those intended for the controlled release of drugs—is the low retention of the formulations at the site of action due to the effect of gravity and clearance by vaginal fluids. This causes a loss in the formulation and subsequent under-dosing, leading to low therapeutic efficacy—as more frequent administration is required—and low acceptability by patients [15, 21].

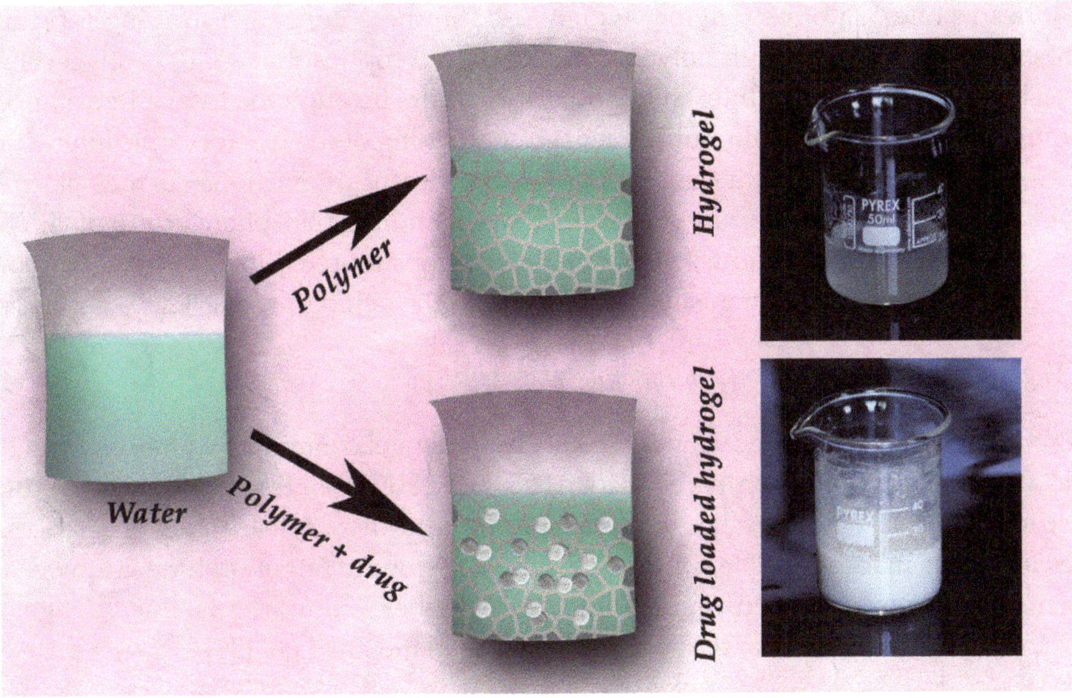

Figure 1. Process of obtaining a hydrogel and a drug-loaded hydrogel.

Two main approaches have been proposed to overcome this problem. One is to develop **mucoadhesive formulations** that remain attached to the vaginal surface for longer and allow a controlled release of the drugs they contain. These mucoadhesive properties are based on the interaction between the dosage form and either the secreted mucus or the mucosal membrane and are usually obtained by including polymers in the formulation. The mucoadhesive polymer chains create bonds—mainly van der Waals and hydrogen bonds or electrostatic interactions—with the mucins in the mucus. Polymers containing numerous functional groups, like hydroxyl or unionized carboxylate groups, are promising excipients for mucoadhesive formulations. Polyacrylic acid derivatives such as carbomer and polycarbophil, cellulose derivatives like hydroxyethyl cellulose (HEC), hydroxypropylmethyl cellulose (HPMC) and carboxymethyl cellulose (CMC), chitosan, hyaluronic acid, alginate, carrageenan and gums are therefore some of the most widely used mucoadhesive polymers in vaginal formulations [15, 19, 20, 22].

The second approach is the use of **thermogelling formulations**. These are *in situ* gel-forming systems which gel when the temperature exceeds a specific gelation value. Systems which gel between room temperature and physiological temperature are very useful in vaginal formulations. Their low viscosity before application means that thermogelling formulations offer a higher spreadability, resulting in the formation of a resistant gel layer in the vagina, a very important aspect for microbicide systems [15, 20]. Most vaginal thermogelling systems contain polymers that can gel at the physiological temperature and are also mucoadhesive. Poloxamers are a group of triblock copolymers composed of polyethylene oxide, polypropylene oxide and polyethylene oxide that are widely used in aqueous solutions in concentrations higher than a critical value for the manufacture of thermogelling systems. Gelation occurs when the poloxamer molecules aggregate to form micelles. However, poloxamer gel has low mucoadhesion properties, so thermogelling systems based on these polymers have been combined with mucoadhesive ones. Another polymer widely used in these *in situ* gel-forming formulations is chitosan, in combination with polyol salts like β-glycerophosphate (GP) or glyceryl monooleate. The thermogelling of chitosan/GP mixtures occurs through the loss of hydration water from the polymer chains and the subsequent strengthening of the hydrophobic interactions as the temperature increases. Other authors point to different interactions such as electrostatic attraction between the ammonium groups of chitosan and the phosphate group of GP, hydrogen bonds between chains, and hydrophobic interactions by reducing electrostatic repulsion of polymer chains, as the mechanisms responsible for the gelling process [20].

2.1.2. *Vaginal gels for HIV prevention under development*

Forbes *et al.* developed a non-aqueous silicone elastomer gel containing Maraviroc as a hydrophobic anti-HIV agent and compared it to a 2.2% w/w HEC gel. It was subjected to different assays, including *in vitro* placebo gel retention, *in vitro* drug release and pharmacokinetic studies in rhesus macaques. The silicone gel showed a longer retention time, a slower rate of Maraviroc release in simulated vaginal fluid and a higher and more sustained drug concentration in vaginal fluid, vaginal tissue and plasma than the HEC gel [23].

Li *et al.* proposed a thermosensitive hydrogel of methyl cellulose modified by stearic acid (MCS) in presence of sodium chloride and phosphates. The gelation process occurred at the physiological temperature and at an even lower value. *In vitro* cytotoxicity tests and *in vivo* evaluation of mucosal irritation attributed good biocompatibility properties to the MCS hydrogel, which also showed a sustained release of Tenofovir for 10 h without any burst effect [24].

In the field of nanotechnology, Lara *et al.* formulated polyvinylpyrrolidone-coated silver nanoparticles (PVP-coated AgNPs) in a concentration of 0.15 mg/mL in the non-spermicidal Replens gel [25]. These PVP-coated AgNPs had previously demonstrated anti-HIV activity [26]. The resulting gel containing the nanoparticles showed an inhibition of HIV-1 transmission after 1 min and offered prolonged protection for 48 h in human cervical cultures. This formulation was not found to be cytotoxic at the aforementioned concentration of PVP-coated AgNPs during the 48 h of protection [25]. Another example is the work of Date *et al.*, who developed a thermosensitive vaginal gel with poly(lactic-co-glycolic acid)—PLGA—nanoparticles loaded with Raltegravir and Efavirenz to prevent HIV infection. The mean encapsulation efficiency of the drugs was 55.5 and 98.2%, respectively. Two poloxamers (Pluronic® F127 and Pluronic® F68) were used to obtain the thermogelling system, which gelled at 32.5°C. The drug- loaded nanoparticles allowed the sustained intracellular release of Raltegravir and Efavirenz in HeLa cells and the cytotoxicity assays indicated that these particles or the blank gel were not toxic in these cells for the 14 days of the study, compared to control cells without treatment [27].

Some of the clinical trials currently underway on vaginal gels for HIV prevention are shown in **Table 2**.

2.2. Tablets

2.2.1. *Overview*

Vaginal tablets are solid monolithic matrix systems designed to be placed in the vagina and release the drug in this area. Since several vaginal tablets are already marketed in developed

Study	Phase	Formulation	Reference
MTN-004	I	3% w/w SPL7013 gel (VivaGelTM)	[28]
Population Council #558	I	PC-1005 (MIV-150/zinc acetate carrageenan gel)	[29]
CAPRISA 004	IIb	1% Tenofovir gel	[30]
Population Council #322	III	Carraguard®(PC 515) gel	[31]
C03-090	III	6% cellulose sulphate gel	[32]
FACTS 001	III	1% Tenofovir gel	[33]

Table 2. Vaginal gels for HIV prevention under clinical investigation.

and developing countries for the treatment of different diseases, such as vaginal atrophy, vulvovaginal candidiasis and bacterial vaginosis, tablets may represent a potential alternative for the formulation of microbicides [34].

The advantages of vaginal tablets include their higher dose accuracy and greater stability than semisolid dosage forms, and the fact that they are easy and cheap to manufacture [34, 35]. These formulations are also versatile as they can be used for immediate or controlled release, the first of which is achieved by rapid disintegration of the system using disintegrants such as crospovidone as excipients [36]. Nevertheless, controlled release systems must contain mucoadhesive polymers as the main excipients. These polymers need to interact with the vaginal surface through the interrelation of certain specific chemical groups in the polymers and biological tissues for the formulation to remain attached to the vaginal mucosa while the drug is being released, which is a critical factor [37]. The gelation process of these polymers in contact with aqueous media may be useful for controlling the release of the drug via diffusion through the gel layer (**Figure 2**). Some examples are cellulose derivatives, guar gum and chitosan [38].

However, the disadvantages of tablets include comfort issues such as difficulty in self-insertion and their slow rate of disintegration [39]. Contact between the mucosa and the solid formulation may provoke vaginal irritation. Vaginal hydration must also be increased to ensure the correct distribution of the drug over the whole vaginal surface [15].

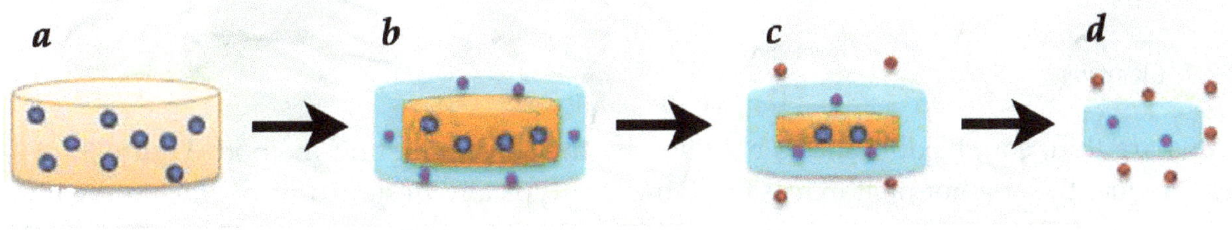

Figure 2. Drug release through tablets. Tablet after vaginal application (**a**). Formation of a drug-loaded gel in contact with the vaginal fluid (**b**). Drug diffusion through gel layer reaching vaginal environment. Erosion of external gel layers (**c**). Complete transformation of tablet into a gel; Total drug diffusion and gel erosion (**d**).

2.2.2. Vaginal tablets for HIV prevention under development

Immediate-release tablets containing Emtricitabine and Tenofovir as antiretroviral drugs were developed by Clark *et al.* Tablets containing disintegrants were prepared to produce immediate release in contact with vaginal fluid. Maximum concentrations in vaginal tissues and fluid were observed less than 1 h after administering the tablets to rabbits, so the drug distribution and release results were comparable to those observed in a clinical trial with a gel containing 1% TFV [34].

Immediate-release tablets have also been explored for the development of biotherapeutic assets, including MucoCept, the name for human vaginal *Lactobacillus jensenii* that has been genetically modified to express the HIV entry inhibitor, modified cyanovirin-N (mCV-N). These bacteria were mixed with various excipients and freeze-dried, obtaining fast-dissolving highly hydrophilic tablets. Samples were assessed *in vitro* and *in vivo* using macaques. The tablets showed complete disintegration in 2 min and the colonization of the vaginal mucosa occurred in up to 83% of the macaques in 21 days [40].

Some attempts have been made to achieve controlled drug release, but several factors must be improved to overcome vaginal leakage and obtain a more comfortable posology. McConville *et al.* developed multilayer tablets based on Kollidon® containing a combination of Acyclovir, Levonorgestrel and Dapivirine. These systems released the first two drugs immediately, and Dapivirine release was sustained for more than 8 h [36]. Nevertheless, daily administration would still be necessary.

Innovative formulations that have shown efficient controlled drug release are based on the addition of hydrophilic mucoadhesive polymers that form a gel in an aqueous medium such as the vaginal environment. The formulation remains attached to the mucosa and forms a strong gel that may lead to a the sustained diffusion of the drug, slowing its rate of release. This was demonstrated in research by Notario-Pérez *et al.*, where compacts based on a combination of chitosan and hypromellose proved their ability to gel in simulated vaginal fluid, and the gel obtained *in situ* produced the sustained release of Tenofovir in this medium, with high mucoadhesion [35]. These hydrophilic matrices have also been improved with the addition of hydrophobic granules of Eudragit® and zein containing the drug. This modification led to longer periods of release and mucoadhesion through complex release mechanisms, thus obtaining compacts suitable for the controlled release of Tenofovir over 6 days [7].

2.3. Films

2.3.1. Overview

Films are thin, soft, flexible sheets obtained by the solvent-casting method (**Figure 3**) or—less frequently—by hot-melt extrusion. Films are typically designed to disintegrate within a few minutes on contact with vaginal fluids, so the drugs are released promptly [41, 42]. Vaginal films are well accepted by women as they are discreet and easy to use and carry around due to their low weight and size, and suitable for the design of new microbicides [39]. They also have good physicochemical stability and resistance to microbial contamination.

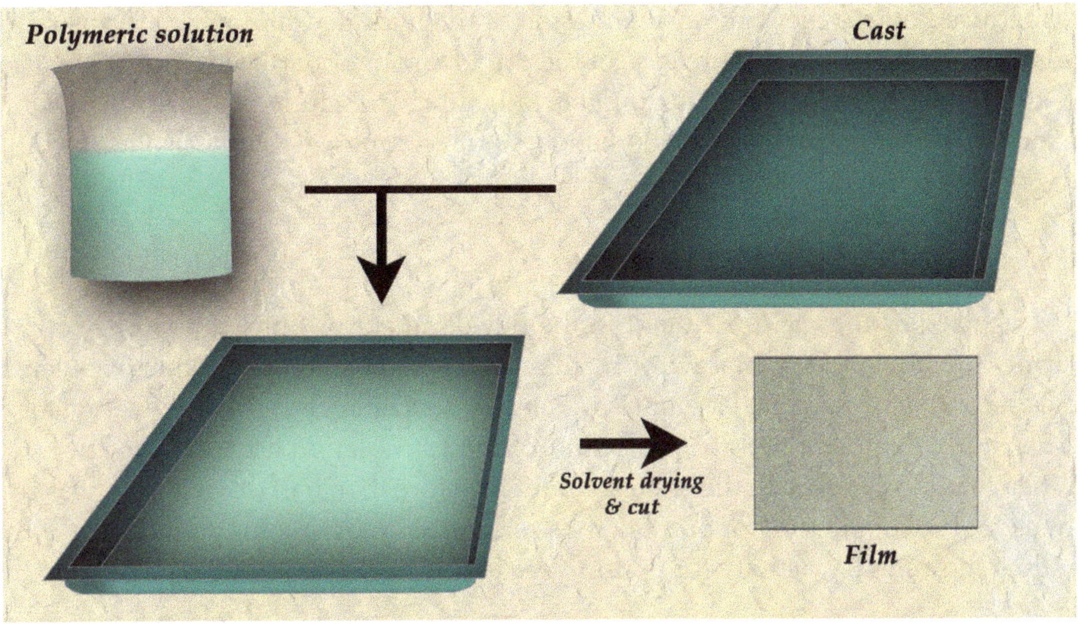

Figure 3. Solvent casting method for manufacturing films.

Matrix-forming polymers give the film mucoadhesive properties, which prevents vaginal leakage and improves drug release. Films are inexpensive to manufacture and can easily be reproduced, and their stable solid formulation makes them suitable for the release of drugs.

However, films also have some disadvantages that must be taken into account when developing these systems. Due to their small size and weight they can incorporate only a small amount of drug, generally less than 50% of the total weight of the formulation [42]. The limited volume of vaginal fluid may condition the disintegration process and hence the release of the drug. Another factor to consider is the wide variability in vaginal fluid secretion among different women and even at different times, making the release sometimes difficult to predict [43]. Administration may also be problematic, as the films start disintegrating immediately the come into contact with vaginal fluid [41]. Lastly, the mechanisms for regulating the manufacture and characterization of films are not yet sufficiently standardized [44].

Immediate-release films have been widely explored, and fast-dissolving products are generally used as matrix-forming polymers, which significantly influences the properties of the final product. These polymers cannot be toxic or irritant and must form films with good wetting properties and disintegration time and high tensile strength. Polyacrylates, polyethylene glycol, polyvinyl alcohol (PVA) and cellulose derivatives are currently the polymers of choice to formulate vaginal films. Plasticizers such as glycerol or polyethylene glycols are also included to give the film flexibility and facilitate handling and administration [44]. Other components are frequently included in addition to matrix-forming polymers and plasticizers; for example preservatives or disintegrants [42]. Work is currently underway to obtain controlled release and long-term efficacy and stability [45]. The inclusion of nanoparticles may also lead to promising drug delivery systems [46]; these thin polymer-based films could serve as platforms for the administration of nanosystems, as they overcome several of the disadvantages of other systems (nanoparticles alone or nanoparticles containing gels). For instance, the vaginal leakage observed in previous nanoparticle systems (free or contained in a gel) is reduced due to the high mucoadhesion of the hydrated film which forms polymers. They also prevent the premature release of the drug from nanoparticles to the aqueous phase of the gel that occurs during storage. Other advantages include reduced discomfort and easier incorporation and release of the nanosystems compared to other solid formulations (such as rings and tablets) [41].

2.3.2. Films for HIV prevention under development

HPMC was used as the main excipient in the development of films containing mixtures of Dapivirine, Tenofovir and/or Maraviroc by the solvent casting method. Other excipients were added as secondary polymers (PVA or CMC) and plasticizers (glycerol or polyethylene glycol 800). This study demonstrated the versatility of the formulation according to the polymers used when loading drugs with different solubilities. More than half of each drug was released within the first 30 minutes of application, thus serving as an option for pericoital prophylaxis. These films showed HIV activity for up to 1 year [47].

PVA -based films have also been used as formulations for the release of new drugs: Sassi *et al.* developed a fast-dissolving Retrocyclin-analogue film that showed *in vitro* and *ex vivo* activity against HIV [48].

HPMC has also been combined with sodium alginate for the development of Abacavir-based films containing glycerol as a plasticizer. The film gels in contact with vaginal fluid to obtain a highly bioadhesive formulation. More than half of the drug was released in the first 30 minutes, making this another interesting option for pericoital prevention [45].

Akil *et al.* combined HPMC with PVA and polyethylene glycol 8000 for the administration of Dapivirine. Again, an immediate-release formulation was obtained for the prevention of HIV, with no apparent toxicity for the vaginal microbiota. Good stability properties were also observed, and anti-HIV activity persisted for at least 18 months [49].

The use of antimicrobial products has also been proposed as film-forming agents. Garg *et al.* developed bioadhesive vaginal films of sodium polystyrene sulfonate. Their results suggested that these films could have interesting biological, pharmaceutical and esthetic properties and may offer substantial benefits for preventing the sexual transmission of HIV [50].

Lastly, films are currently an option for the incorporation of nanoparticles. Srinivasan *et al.* prepared vaginal films containing a novel non-nucleoside reverse transcriptase inhibitor—IQP0528—with and without PLGA-Eudragit® S 100 nanoparticle encapsulation of the drug. Both formulations released a higher amount than required to exceed IC50 and showed no toxicity or alterations in vaginal microbiota. The drug release profile from nanoparticle-based films was some orders of magnitude greater than for films containing the free drug [42].

Cunha-Reis *et al.* developed fast-dissolving HPMC/PVA-based films containing nanoencapsulated Efavirenz in PLGA nanoparticles and free TFV. They were characterized *in vitro* and *in vivo* and the results from mice revealed that concentrations of the drug in vaginal secretions decreased rapidly after administration, and were more pronounced for the free than for the encapsulated drug. However, AUCs for both drugs were some orders of magnitude higher than obtained when administering both drugs in an aqueous vehicle. Films therefore represent an option for drug administration due to their longer residence time in the vagina. It

Study	Phase	Formulation	Reference
FAME-02	Phase I	Dapivirine vaginal film and gel	[52]
FAME-05	Early Phase I	Tenofovir vaginal film and gel	[53]

Table 3. Vaginal films for HIV prevention under clinical investigation.

was also demonstrated that nanoparticles can prolong the release of the drug, indicating that nanoparticle-based films have potential for the development of controlled release systems [51].

Table 3 shows the vaginal films for HIV prevention currently under clinical investigation.

2.4. Vaginal rings

2.4.1. Overview

Vaginal or intravaginal rings are dosage forms placed closed to the cervix [54, 55] and designed to release drugs in a controlled or sustained manner over weeks or months to achieve either local or systemic action. From a physicochemical point of view, they are flexible toroidal devices with a polymeric structure. The first references to vaginal rings for drug delivery date from the late 1960s and 1970s with a patent from the Upjohn Company and the discovery that several drugs, including steroids, could be released through silicone elastomers [55–57]. The first clinical evaluation of a vaginal ring—for contraceptive purposes—took place in the 1970s [57]. The inclusion of microbicides against HIV in vaginal rings was proposed at a microbicide conference in 2002. The first article on microbicide vaginal rings for HIV prevention was published 1 year later, and described a matrix-type silicone elastomer vaginal ring with *in vitro* release of Nonoxynol-9 over 8 days. This drug subsequently ceased to be seen as a microbicidal candidate as its gel formulation increased the risk of HIV transmission due to the damage to the vaginal epithelium. In 2005, a core-type silicone elastomer vaginal ring was described which released Dapivirine (or TMC120) *in vitro* over the 71 days of the study, and was attributed a sustained release of the total dose for between 1 and 4 years [54–56].

Vaginal rings with microbicide formulations are well accepted by women as they can be inserted and removed by the patients themselves, they offer controlled release of the drugs—resulting in a convenient dosage regimen—and are compatible with the sexual act, all of which ensures greater therapeutic compliance and effectiveness [54–57].

Two main types of polymers are used in the development of vaginal rings: silicone and thermoplastic elastomers. Silicone elastomers are obtained by chemical crosslinking of functionalized, linear, polydimethylsiloxane [56]. Thermoplastic elastomers have rheological properties which alter during heating (flow) and cooling (harden). The most important elastomers for the manufacture of vaginal rings are polyurethanes (PUs) and ethylene and vinyl acetate (EVAs) copolymers [54, 55]. The vinyl acetate content (which ranges from 10–40% approximately) and the molecular weight of the EVAs influence the mechanical properties and the drug release rate of the final formulation. Although there are few cases of EVA vaginal rings for microbicide release [54, 56], the possibility of varying the vinyl acetate content of EVA materials offers a broader range of drug permeation properties than silicone elastomer materials, which are also more expensive. EVA polymers can also form rate-controlling membranes that are thinner than 100 μm. PUs are bi-phasic copolymers that constitute alternative biocompatible materials and are also under study for the development of microbicide vaginal rings. They are obtained by a polymerization reaction between diisocyanates, a low molecular weight diol and a high molecular weight diol. The combination of the diisocyanate with the low molecular weight diol leads to the formation of hard segments—responsible for the material's resilience—while combination with the high molecular weight diol produces soft segments which confer elasticity and elastomeric properties. By varying the proportion of hard and soft segments, hydrophobic and hydrophilic PUs can be obtained to allow the optimal release of different types of drugs [56].

Vaginal rings come in different designs (**Figure 4**). **Spring vaginal rings** were the first to appear and were formed by a metal spring over-molded by a silicone sheath. Despite offering good results in terms of their clinical efficacy, they were also rigid and had several adverse effects [56]. **Matrix or homogeneous vaginal rings** have the simplest design and consist of a polymeric matrix in which the drug is dispersed. Drug release occurs through a permeation mechanism involving the dissolution of the drug in the polymer and diffusion through the matrix. The delivery rate depends on the solubility of the drug in the polymer, the ability of the drug to diffuse through it, the drug content and the surface area of the ring [54, 55]. Until 2006, **reservoir vaginal rings** and matrix rings were the main microbicide vaginal ring designs. Also known as "core vaginal rings," they are formed by a polymer membrane which encapsulates one or more cores loaded with the drug. The possibility of including several cores in one reservoir ring ("multi-core ring") allows the formulation of different drugs in the same dosage form [55, 56]. The cores can also be inserted in a ring before sealing the ends [54]. Drug release also occurs through permeation and can be controlled by modifying the thickness of the membrane [55, 56]. **Segmented vaginal rings** are formed by two or more connected segments loaded with one or more drugs; they allow control over the release of each drug and avoid interactions between them [54, 55]; they may be either matrix- or reservoir-type systems [56]. **Sandwich or shell vaginal rings** are based on an outer membrane, a narrow drug-loaded

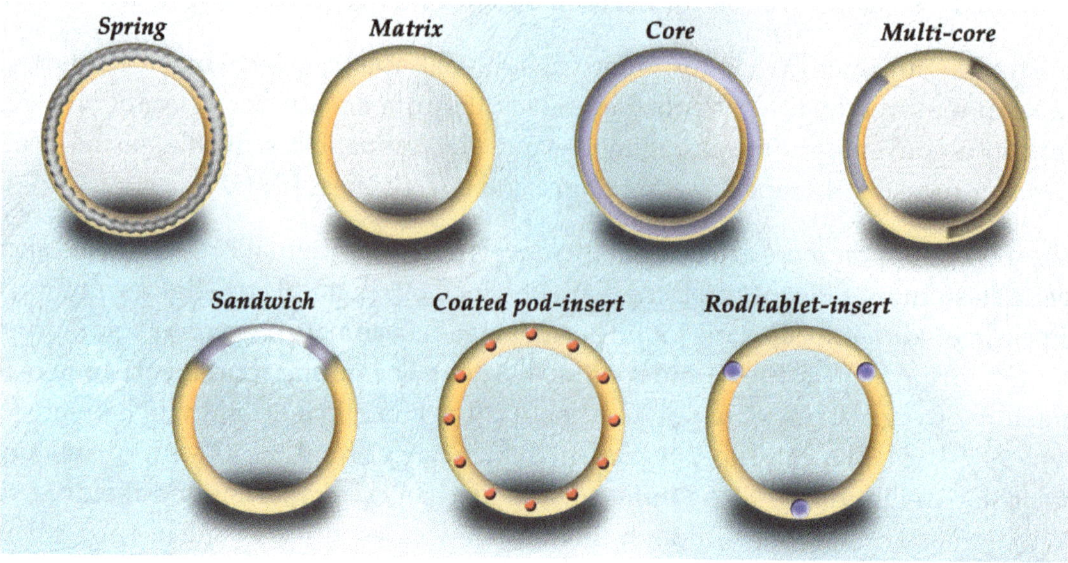

Figure 4. Vaginal ring designs.

polymer layer and an inner central core. As in the case of reservoir rings, the release rate depends on the thickness of the outer membrane [54, 55]. In order to overcome the problems of permeability when releasing hydrophilic and/or high molecular weight drugs from vaginal rings based on silicone or thermoplastic elastomers, several new designs of these dosage forms have been developed. **Coated pod-insert vaginal rings** are silicone elastomer rings containing drug cores or pods coated with layers of polymers such as semipermeable polylactic acid. The drug release rate depends on the size of the delivery window in the silicone ring, the number of cores and the amount and composition of the core coating. This ring design allows the release of drugs with different physicochemical properties from the same dosage form. **Rod and tablet-insert vaginal rings** are silicone elastomer rings containing freeze-dried polymer gel rods or compressed polymeric tablets with the drug/s. The gel reconstituted by vaginal fluid and the tablet both release the drug in a sustained manner. The lyophilized gel rods are interesting for the formulation of peptide- and protein-based microbicides, as the freeze-drying process stabilizes this kind of drug. **Biosoluble and hydrogel vaginal rings** are other new designs of vaginal rings. For instance, biosoluble acacia gum, nonbiodegradable hydrogels based on methacrylates and a nanoporous polydiol citrate elastomer hydrogel have been used to manufacture microbicide vaginal rings [54–56].

2.4.2. *Vaginal rings for HIV prevention under development*

Numerous vaginal rings are currently under development for preventing the sexual transmission of HIV. Some examples are described below.

Malcolm *et al.* developed matrix silicone elastomer vaginal rings containing Maraviroc and CMPD167. *In vitro* release tests showed a controlled release of both drugs over 28 days. Their concentrations in vaginal fluid in a 28-day study in rhesus macaques were around 10^6-fold higher than the 50% inhibitory concentrations for inhibiting a simian/human immunodeficiency virus in macaque lymphocytes *in vitro* [58].

A core-matrix vaginal ring for preventing HIV-1, HSV-2 (herpes simplex virus-2), HPV (human papilloma virus) and unwanted pregnancy was proposed by Ugaonkar *et al.* MIV-150 and zinc acetate (anti-HIV drugs), carrageenan (also for HPV) and Levonorgestrel (contraceptive) were included in this multipurpose dosage form. MIV-150 and Levonorgestrel diffused from the EVA hydrophobic matrix of the ring while zinc acetate and carrageenan diffused through a pore from the hydrophilic core. The drugs were released *in vitro* over 94 days, and up to 28 days of the study period in rhesus macaques, showing effectiveness for virus protection and contraception [59].

A segmented dual-reservoir PU vaginal ring containing Tenofovir and Levonorgestrel was formulated by Clark *et al.* to protect women against HIV and unwanted pregnancy. The rings comprised a 10- or 20 mm-long polyether urethane-based reservoir segment containing 1.3 wt% Levonorgestrel surrounded by a 100 μm thick rate-controlling membrane also of polyether urethane. Tenofovir was loaded as glycerol paste in a hydrophilic PU reservoir segment separated from the Levonorgestrel segment by PU caps to prevent it from diffusing into the Tenofovir reservoir. The rings formed by the 20 mm-long segment of Levonorgestrel released both drugs in vitro over 90 days [60].

Study	Phase	Formulation	Reference
MTN-013/IPM 026	I	Silicone elastomer matrix-type vaginal ring loaded with 25 mg Dapivirine and 100 mg Maraviroc	[65]
2013-329	I	Polyurethane Tenofovir Disoproxil Fumarate vaginal ring	[66]
The Ring Study/IPM 027	III	Silicone elastomer matrix-type vaginal ring containing 25 mg Dapivirine	[67]
ASPIRE/MTN-020	III	Silicone elastomer matrix-type vaginal ring containing 25 mg Dapivirine	[68]

Table 4. Vaginal rings for HIV prevention under clinical investigation.

Srinivasan *et al.* described a pod-vaginal ring containing 65 mg of Tenofovir Disoproxil Fumarate and 68 mg of Emtricitabine and tested it in female pigtailed macaques. The ring was made of silicon elastomer and included three poly(vinyl alcohol) coated-pods of each drug and one delivery channel per pod. All the animals treated with the ring were protected against the infection compared to the control group, despite the exposure to simian/human immunodeficiency virus. The drugs were also released in a sustained manner and maintained effective levels over 4 months [61, 62].

Murphy *et al.* formulated rod insert silicone elastomer vaginal rings to release the candidate antiretroviral peptides T-1249 and JNJ54310516-AFP (JNJ peptide). The drugs were contained in a hydrophilic excipient—sodium chloride, sodium glutamate, lactose or zinc acetate at different concentrations—to form the peptide-loaded rod inserts. *In vitro* release tests showed the sustained release profiles that could be achieved with these rings and which may be related to the type of hydrophilic excipient and its swelling properties [63].

Vaginal rings based on biosoluble acacia gum and a non-biodegradable hydrogel of 2-hydroxyethyl methacrylate (HEMA) to release one or two anti-HIV drugs were studied by Saxena *et al.* Five types of rings were formed, namely acacia gum rings with Dapivirine, Boc-lysinated-betulonic acid (Boc-LBA) or a combination of TMC120 (Dapivirine) and PMPA (Tenofovir), and HEMA rings with Zidovudine or Dapivirine and Tenofovir. The results of the drug release assays showed drug levels greater than the minimum dose required to inhibit the virus, which were sustained for at least 15 days for acacia gum and 28 days for HEMA rings [64].

Table 4 shows some of the clinical trials on vaginal rings for HIV prevention.

3. Authors' conclusions and future perspectives

HIV and AIDS are huge health problems today, and especially in women in developing countries. Current systems for preventing transmission are generally beyond their reach, so it is essential to develop new strategies, among which an interesting option is the use of topical vaginal formulations as prophylaxis .

The vaginal route of administration has various complexities, and intense research is underway around the world to find the formulation that best meet the requirements. Vaginal gels and tablets are easy to manufacture and administer, but patients report comfort issues such as substantial leakage after administration. Vaginal rings overcome this problem, but are more expensive and difficult to manufacture. Vaginal leakage is also reduced by vaginal films, which are cheap and easy to manufacture, but these tools are still fairly novel and require more knowledge and technical improvements in the production process.

We therefore consider that sustained-release formulations may represent the most attractive option, since greater compliance is crucial to ensure the effectiveness of the microbicide. Although vaginal rings are the most suitable formulation for sustained release, vaginal films and tablets are also being investigated to obtain longer protection times, and are seen as promising platforms for the inclusion of microbicides to prevent the sexual transmission of HIV.

Acknowledgements

This work was supported by the Spanish Ministry of Economy, Industry and Competitiveness [grant number MAT2012-34552]; and by the Spanish Research Agency and the European Regional Development Fund (AEI/FEDER, UE) [grant number MAT2016-76416-R].

Author details

María-Dolores Veiga-Ochoa*, Roberto Ruiz-Caro, Raúl Cazorla-Luna, Araceli Martín-Illana and Fernando Notario-Pérez

*Address all correspondence to: mdveiga@ucm.es

Department of Pharmaceutical Technology and Food Technology, Faculty of Pharmacy, Complutense University of Madrid, Madrid, Spain

References

[1] UNAIDS data 2017 [Internet]. 2017. Available from: http://www.unaids.org/sites/default/files/media_asset/20170720_Data_book_2017_en.pdf [Accessed: April 03, 2018]

[2] When women lead change happens [Internet]. 2017. Available from: http://www.unaids.org/sites/default/files/media_asset/when-women-lead-change-happens_en.pdf [Accessed: April 03, 2018]

[3] Global Report. UNAIDS report on the global AIDS epidemy 2013 [Internet]. 2013. Available from: http://www.unaids.org/sites/default/files/media_asset/UNAIDS_Global_Report_2013_en_1.pdf [Accessed: April 03, 2018]

[4] Notario-Pérez F, Ruiz-Caro R, Veiga-Ochoa MD. Historical development of vaginal microbicides to prevent sexual transmission of HIV in women: From past failures to future hopes. Drug Design, Development and Therapy. 2017;**11**:1767-1787. DOI: 10.2147/DDDT.S133170

[5] Abdool Karim Q, Abdool Karim SS, Frohlich JA, Grobler AC, Baxter C, Mansoor LE, Kharsany AB, Sibeko S, Mlisana KP, Omar Z, Gengiah TN, Maarschalk S, Arulappan N, Mlotshwa M, Morris L, Taylor D. Effectiveness and safety of tenofovir gel, an antiretroviral microbicide, for the prevention of HIV infection in women. Science. 2010;**329**(5996):1168-1174. DOI: 10.1126/science.1193748

[6] Nel AM, Smythe SC, Habibi S, Kaptur PE, Romano JW. Pharmacokinetics of 2 dapivirine vaginal microbicide gels and their safety vs. Hydroxyethyl cellulose-based universal placebo gel. Journal of Acquired Immune Deficiency Syndromes. 2010;**55**(2):161-169. DOI: 10.1097/QAI.0b013e3181e3293a

[7] Notario-Pérez F, Martín-Illana A, Cazorla-Luna R, Ruiz-Caro R, Peña J, Veiga MD. Improvement of Tenofovir vaginal release from hydrophilic matrices through drug granulation with hydrophobic polymers. European Journal of Pharmaceutical Sciences. 2018;**117**:204-215. DOI: 10.1016/j.ejps.2018.02.022

[8] Garg S, Tambwekar KR, Vermani K, Kandarapu R, Garg A, Waller DP, Zaneveld LJ. Development pharmaceutics of microbicide formulations. Part II: Formulation, evaluation, and challenges. AIDS Patient Care and STDs. 2003;**17**(8):377-399. DOI: 10.1089/108729103322277402

[9] Valore EV, Park CH, Igreti SL, Ganz T. Antimicrobial components of vaginal fluid. American Journal of Obstetrics and Gynecology. 2002;**187**(3):561-568. DOI: 10.1067/mob.2002.125280

[10] Rohan LC, Sassi AB. Vaginal drug delivery systems for HIV prevention. The AAPS Journal. 2009;**11**:78-87. DOI: 10.1208/s12248-009-9082-7

[11] Ferguson LM, Rohan LC. The importance of the vaginal delivery route for antiretrovirals in HIV prevention. Therapeutic Delivery. 2011;**2**(12):1535-1550. DOI: 10.4155/tde.11.126

[12] Woolfson AD, Malcolm RK, Gallagher R. Drug delivery by the intravaginal route. Critical Reviews in Therapeutic Drug Carrier Systems. 2000;**17**(5):509-555. DOI: 10.1615/CritRevTherDrugCarrierSyst.v17.i5.30

[13] Tan S, Lu L, Li L, Liu J, Oksov Y, Lu H, Jiang S, Liu S. Polyanionic candidate microbicides accelerate the formation of semen-derived amyloid fibrils to enhance HIV-1 infection. PLoS One. 2013;**8**(3):e59777. DOI: 10.1371/journal.pone.0059777

[14] Wilkinson D, Tholandi M, Ramjee G, Rutherford GW. Nonoxynol-9 spermicide for prevention of vaginally adquired HIV and other sexually transmitted infections: Systematic review and meta-analysis of randomised controlled trials including more than 5,000 women. The Lancet Infectious Diseases. 2002;**2**(10):613-617. DOI: 10.1016/S1473-3099(02)00396-1

[15] Antimisiaris SG, Mourtas S. Recent advances on anti-HIV vaginal delivery systems development. Advanced Drug Delivery Reviews. 2015;**92**:123-145. DOI: 10.1016/j.addr.2015.03.015

[16] Singh VK, Banerjee I, Agarwal T, Pramanik K, Bhattacharya MK, Pal K. Guar gum and sesame oil based novel bigels for controlled drug delivery. Colloids and Surfaces. B, Biointerfaces. 2014;**123**:582-592. DOI: 10.1016/j.colsurfb.2014.09.056

[17] Garg S, Goldman D, Krumme M, Rohan LC, Smoot S, Friend DR. Advances in development, scale-up and manufacturing of microbicide gels, films, and tablets. Antiviral Research. 2010;**88**(Suppl 1):S19-S29. DOI: 10.1016/j.antiviral.2010.09.010

[18] Adams JL, Kashuba AD. Formulation, pharmacokinetics and pharmacodynamics of topical microbicides. Best Practice & Research. Clinical Obstetrics & Gynaecology. 2012;**26**(4):451-462. DOI: 10.1016/j.bpobgyn.2012.01.004

[19] Agashe H, Hu M, Rohan L. Formulation and delivery of microbicides. Current HIV Research. 2012;**10**(1):88-96. DOI: 10.2174/157016212799304599

[20] Caramella CM, Rossi S, Ferrari F, Bonferoni MC, Sandri G. Mucoadhesive and thermogelling systems for vaginal drug delivery. Advanced Drug Delivery Reviews. 2015;**92**:39-52. DOI: 10.1016/j.addr.2015.02.001

[21] Campaña-Seoane M, Peleteiro A, Laguna R, Otero-Espinar FJ. Bioadhesive emulsions for control release of progesterone resistant to vaginal fluids clearance. International Journal of Pharmaceutics. 2014;**477**(1-2):495-505. DOI: 10.1016/j.ijpharm.2014.10.066

[22] Cook MT, Brown MB. Polymeric gels for intravaginal drug delivery. Journal of Controlled Release. 2018;**270**:145-157. DOI: 10.1016/j.jconrel.2017.12.004

[23] Forbes CJ, Lowry D, Geer L, Veazey RS, Shattock RJ, Klasse PJ, Mitchnick M, Goldman L, Doyle LA, Muldoon BC, Woolfson AD, Moore JP, Malcolm RK. Non-aqueous silicone elastomer gels as a vaginal microbicide delivery system for the HIV-1 entry inhibitor maraviroc. Journal of Controlled Release. 2011;**156**(2):161-169. DOI: 10.1016/j.jconrel.2011.08.006

[24] Li N, Yu M, Deng L, Yang J, Dong A. Thermosensitive hydrogel of hydrophobically-modified methylcellulose for intravaginal drug delivery. Journal of Materials Science. Materials in Medicine. 2012;**23**(8):1913-1919. DOI: 10.1007/s10856-012-4664-9

[25] Lara HH, Ixtepan-Turrent L, Garza-Treviño EN, Rodríguez-Padilla C. PVP-coated silver nanoparticles block the transmission of cell-free and cell-associated HIV-1 in human cervical culture. Journal of Nanobiotechnology. 2010;**8**:15. DOI: 10.1186/1477-3155-8-15

[26] Lara HH, Ayala-Nuñez NV, Ixtepan-Turrent L, Rodriguez-Padilla C. Mode of antiviral action of silver nanoparticles against HIV-1. Journal of Nanobiotechnology. 2010;**8**:1. DOI: 10.1186/1477-3155-8-1

[27] Date AA, Shibata A, Goede M, Sanford B, La Bruzzo K, Belshan M, Destache CJ. Development and evaluation of a thermosensitive vaginal gel containing raltegravir+efavirenz loaded nanoparticles for HIV prophylaxis. Antiviral Research. 2012;**96**(3):430-436. DOI: 10.1016/j.antiviral.2012.09.015

[28] McGowan I, Gomez K, Bruder K, Febo I, Chen BA, Richardson BA, Husnik M, Livant E, Price C, Jacobson C; MTN-004 Protocol Team. Phase 1 randomized trial of the vaginal safety and acceptability of SPL7013 gel (VivaGel) in sexually active young women (MTN-004). AIDS. 2011;**25**(8):1057-1064. DOI: 10.1097/QAD.0b013e328346bd3e

[29] Friedland BA, Hoesley CJ, Plagianos M, Hoskin E, Zhang S, Teleshova N, Alami M, Novak L, Kleinbeck KR, Katzen LL, Zydowsky TM, Fernández-Romero JA, Creasy GW. First-in-human trial of MIV-150 and zinc acetate Coformulated in a carrageenan gel: Safety, pharmacokinetics, acceptability, adherence, and pharmacodynamics. Journal of Acquired Immune Deficiency Syndromes. 2016;**73**(5):489-496. DOI: 10.1097/QAI.0000000000001136

[30] Matthews LT, Sibeko S, Mansoor LE, Yende-Zuma N, Bangsberg DR, Karim QA. Women with pregnancies had lower adherence to 1% tenofovir vaginal gel as HIV preexposure prophylaxis in CAPRISA 004, a phase IIB randomized-controlled trial. PLoS One. 2013;**8**(3):e56400. DOI: 10.1371/journal.pone.0056400

[31] Skoler-Karpoff S, Ramjee G, Ahmed K, Altini L, Plagianos MG, Friedland B, Govender S, De Kock A, Cassim N, Palanee T, Dozier G, Maguire R, Lahteenmaki P. Efficacy of carraguard for prevention of HIV infection in women in South Africa: A randomised, double-blind, placebo-controlled trial. Lancet. 2008;**372**(9654):1977-1987. DOI: 10.1016/S0140-6736(08)61842-5

[32] Crucitti T, Fransen K, Maharaj R, Tenywa T, Massinga Loembé M, Murugavel KG, Mendonca K, Abdellati S, Beelaert G, Van Damme L. Obtaining valid laboratory data in clinical trials conducted in resource diverse settings: Lessons learned from a microbicide phase III clinical trial. PLoS One. 2010;**5**(10):e13592. DOI: 10.1371/journal.pone.0013592

[33] Rees H, Delany-Moretlwe SA, Lombard C, Baron D, Panchia R, Myer L, Schwartz JL, Doncel GF, Gray G. FACTS 001 phase III trial of pericoital tenofovir 1% gel for HIV prevention in women. In: Proceedings of the Conference on Retroviruses and Opportunistic Infections (CROI). Seattle, WA: CROI; 23-26 February 2015. abstract 26LB

[34] Clark MR, Peet MM, Davis S, Doncel GF, Friend DR. Evaluation of rapidly disintegrating vaginal tablets of tenofovir, emtricitabine and their combination for HIV-1 prevention. Pharmaceutics. 2014;**6**(4):616-631. DOI: 10.3390/pharmaceutics6040616

[35] Notario-Pérez F, Cazorla-Luna R, Martín-Illana A, Ruiz-Caro R, Tamayo A, Rubio J, Veiga MD. Optimization of tenofovir release from mucoadhesive vaginal tablets by polymer combination to prevent sexual transmission of HIV. Carbohydrate Polymers. 2018;**179**:305-316. DOI: 10.1016/j.carbpol.2017.10.001

[36] McConville C, Major I, Devlin B, Brimer A. Development of a multi-layered vaginal tablet containing dapivirine, levonorgestrel and acyclovir for use as a multipurpose prevention technology. European Journal of Pharmaceutics and Biopharmaceutics. 2016;**104**:171-179. DOI: 10.1016/j.ejpb.2016.05.003

[37] Valenta C. The use of mucoadhesive polymers in vaginal delivery. Advanced Drug Delivery Reviews. 2005;**57**(11):1692-1712. DOI: 10.1016/j.addr.2005.07.004

[38] Notario-Pérez F, Martín-Illana A, Cazorla-Luna R, Ruiz-Caro R, Bedoya LM, Tamayo A, Rubio J, Veiga MD. Influence of chitosan swelling behaviour on controlled release of tenofovir from mucoadhesive vaginal systems for prevention of sexual transmission of HIV. Marine Drugs. 2017;**15**(2):50. DOI: 10.3390/md15020050

[39] Fan MD, Kramzer LF, Hillier SL, Chang JC, Meyn LA, Rohan LC. Preferred physical characteristics of vaginal film microbicides for HIV prevention in Pittsburgh women. Archives of Sexual Behavior. 2017;**46**(4):1111-1119. DOI: 10.1007/s10508-016-0816-1

[40] Lagenaur LA, Swedek I, Lee PP, Parks TP. Robust vaginal colonization of macaques with a novel vaginally disintegrating tablet containing a live biotherapeutic product to prevent HIV infection in women. PLoS One. 2015;**10**(4):e0122730. DOI: 10.1371/journal.pone.0122730

[41] das Neves J, Sarmento B. Antiretroviral drug-loaded nanoparticles-in-films: A new option for developing vaginal microbicides? Expert Opinion on Drug Delivery. 2017;**14**(4):449-452. DOI: 10.1080/17425247.2017.1270938

[42] Srinivasan P, Zhang J, Martin A, Kelley K, McNicholl JM, Buckheit RW Jr, Smith JM, Ham AS. Safety and pharmacokinetics of quick-dissolving polymeric vaginal films delivering the antiretroviral IQP-0528 for preexposure prophylaxis. Antimicrobial Agents and Chemotherapy. 2016;**60**(7):4140-4150. DOI: 10.1128/AAC.00082-16

[43] das Neves J, Martins JP, Sarmento B. Will dapivirine redeem the promises of anti-HIV microbicides? Overview of product design and clinical testing. Advanced Drug Delivery Reviews. 2016;**103**:20-32. DOI: 10.1016/j.addr.2015.12.015

[44] Machado RM, Palmeira-de-Oliveira A, Martinez-De-Oliveira J, Palmeira-de-Oliveira R. Vaginal films for drug delivery. Journal of Pharmaceutical Sciences. 2013;**102**(7):2069-2081. DOI: 10.1002/jps.23577

[45] Ghosal K, Ranjan A, Bhowmik BB. A novel vaginal drug delivery system: Anti-HIV bioadhesive film containing abacavir. Journal of Materials Science. Materials in Medicine. 2014;**25**(7):1679-1689. DOI: 10.1007/s10856-014-5204-6

[46] Cautela MP, Moshe H, Sosnik A, Sarmento B, das Neves J. Composite films for vaginal delivery of tenofovir disoproxil fumarate and emtricitabine. European Journal of Pharmaceutics and Biopharmaceutics. 2018. DOI: 10.1016/j.ejpb.2018.02.001

[47] Akil A, Agashe H, Dezzutti CS, Moncla BJ, Hillier SL, Devlin B, Shi Y, Uranker K, Rohan LC. Formulation and characterization of polymeric films containing combinations of antiretrovirals (ARVs) for HIV prevention. Pharmaceutical Research. 2015;**32**(2):458-468. DOI: 10.1007/s11095-014-1474-4

[48] Sassi AB, Cost MR, Cole AL, Cole AM, Patton DL, Gupta P, Rohan LC. Formulation development of retrocyclin 1 analog RC-101 as an anti-HIV vaginal microbicide product. Antimicrobial Agents and Chemotherapy. 2011;**55**(5):2282-2289. DOI: 10.1128/AAC.01190-10

[49] Akil A, Parniak MA, Dezzutti CS, Moncla BJ, Cost MR, Li M, Rohan LC. Development and characterization of a vaginal film containing dapivirine, a non- nucleoside reverse transcriptase inhibitor (NNRTI), for prevention of HIV-1 sexual transmission. Drug Delivery and Translational Research. 2011;**1**(3):209-222. DOI: 10.1007/s13346-011-0022-6

[50] Garg S, Vermani K, Garg A, Anderson RA, Rencher WB, Zaneveld LJ. Development and characterization of bioadhesive vaginal films of sodium polystyrene sulfonate (PSS), a novel contraceptive antimicrobial agent. Pharmaceutical Research. 2005;**22**(4):584-595. DOI: 10.1007/s11095-005-2490-1

[51] Cunha-Reis C, Machado A, Barreiros L, Araújo F, Nunes R, Seabra V, Ferreira D, Segundo MA, Sarmento B, das Neves J. Nanoparticles-in-film for the combined vaginal delivery of anti-HIV microbicide drugs. Journal of Controlled Release. 2016;**243**:43-53. DOI: 10.1016/j.jconrel.2016.09.020

[52] Robinson JA, Marzinke MA, Bakshi RP, Fuchs EJ, Radebaugh CL, Aung W, Spiegel HM, Coleman JS, Rohan LC, Hendrix CW. Comparison of dapivirine vaginal gel and film formulation pharmacokinetics and pharmacodynamics (FAME 02B). AIDS Research and Human Retroviruses. 2017;**33**(4):339-346. DOI: 10.1089/AID.2016.0040

[53] Robinson JA, Marzinke MA, Fuchs EJ, Bakshi RP, Spiegel HML, Coleman JS, Rohan LC, Hendrix CW. Comparison of the pharmacokinetics and pharmacodynamics of single-dose tenofovir vaginal film and gel formulation (FAME 05). Journal of Acquired Immune Deficiency Syndromes. 2018;**77**(2):175-182. DOI: 10.1097/QAI.0000000000001587

[54] Malcolm RK, Fetherston SM, McCoy CF, Boyd P, Major I. Vaginal rings for delivery of HIV microbicides. International Journal of Women's Health. 2012;**4**:595-605. DOI: 10.2147/IJWH.S36282

[55] Malcolm RK, Edwards KL, Kiser P, Romano J, Smith TJ. Advances in microbicide vaginal rings. Antiviral Research. 2010;**88**(Suppl 1):S30-S39. DOI: 10.1016/j.antiviral.2010.09.003

[56] Malcolm RK, Boyd PJ, McCoy CF, Murphy DJ. Microbicide vaginal rings: Technological challenges and clinical development. Advanced Drug Delivery Reviews. 2016;**103**:33-56. DOI: 10.1016/j.addr.2016.01.015

[57] Thurman AR, Clark MR, Hurlburt JA, Doncel GF. Intravaginal rings as delivery systems for microbicides and multipurpose prevention technologies. International Journal of Women's Health. 2013;**5**:695-708. DOI: 10.2147/IJWH.S34030

[58] Malcolm RK, Veazey RS, Geer L, Lowry D, Fetherston SM, Murphy DJ, Boyd P, Major I, Shattock RJ, Klasse PJ, Doyle LA, Rasmussen KK, Goldman L, Ketas TJ, Moore JP. Sustained release of the CCR5 inhibitors CMPD167 and maraviroc from vaginal rings in rhesus macaques. Antimicrobial Agents and Chemotherapy. 2012;**56**(5):2251-2258. DOI: 10.1128/AAC.05810-11

[59] Ugaonkar SR, Wesenberg A, Wilk J, Seidor S, Mizenina O, Kizima L, Rodriguez A, Zhang S, Levendosky K, Kenney J, Aravantinou M, Derby N, Grasperge B, Gettie A, Blanchard J, Kumar N, Roberts K, Robbiani M, Fernández-Romero JA, Zydowsky TM. A novel intravaginal ring to prevent HIV-1, HSV-2, HPV, and unintended pregnancy. Journal of Controlled Release. 2015;**213**:57-68. DOI: 10.1016/j.jconrel.2015.06.018

[60] Clark JT, Clark MR, Shelke NB, Johnson TJ, Smith EM, Andreasen AK, Nebeker JS, Fabian J, Friend DR, Kiser PF. Engineering a segmented dual-reservoir polyurethane intravaginal ring for simultaneous prevention of HIV transmission and unwanted pregnancy. PLoS One. 2014;**9**(3):e88509. DOI: 10.1371/journal.pone.0088509

[61] Srinivasan P, Moss JA, Gunawardana M, Churchman SA, Yang F, Dinh CT, Mitchell JM, Zhang J, Fanter R, Miller CS, Butkyavichene I, McNicholl JM, Smith TJ, Baum MM, Smith JM. Topical delivery of tenofovir disoproxil fumarate and emtricitabine from pod-intravaginal rings protects macaques from multiple SHIV exposures. PLoS One. 2016;**11**(6):e0157061. DOI: 10.1371/journal.pone.0157061

[62] Moss JA, Srinivasan P, Smith TJ, Butkyavichene I, Lopez G, Brooks AA, Martin A, Dinh CT, Smith JM, Baum MM. Pharmacokinetics and preliminary safety study of pod-intravaginal rings delivering antiretroviral combinations for HIV prophylaxis in a macaque model. Antimicrobial Agents and Chemotherapy. 2014;**58**(9):5125-5135. DOI: 10.1128/AAC.02871-14

[63] Murphy DJ, Amssoms K, Pille G, Clarke A, O'Hara M, van Roey J, Malcolm RK. Sustained release of the candidate antiretroviral peptides T-1249 and JNJ54310516-AFP from a rod insert vaginal ring. Drug Delivery and Translational Research. 2016;**6**(3):234-242. DOI: 10.1007/s13346-015-0273-8

[64] Saxena BB, Han YA, Fu D, Rathnam P, Singh M, Laurence J, Lerner S. Sustained release of microbicides by newly engineered vaginal rings. AIDS. 2009;**23**(8):917-922. DOI: 10.1097/QAD.0b013e32832af57c

[65] Chen BA, Panther L, Marzinke MA, Hendrix CW, Hoesley CJ, van der Straten A, Husnik MJ, Soto-Torres L, Nel A, Johnson S, Richardson-Harman N, Rabe LK, Dezzutti CS. Phase 1 safety, pharmacokinetics, and pharmacodynamics of dapivirine and maraviroc vaginal rings: A double-blind randomized trial. Journal of Acquired Immune Deficiency Syndromes. 2015;**70**(3):242-249. DOI: 10.1097/QAI.0000000000000702

[66] Keller MJ, Mesquita PM, Marzinke MA, Teller R, Espinoza L, Atrio JM, Lo Y, Frank B, Srinivasan S, Fredricks DN, Rabe L, Anderson PL, Hendrix CW, Kiser PF, Herold BC. A phase 1 randomized placebo-controlled safety and pharmacokinetic trial of a tenofovir disoproxil fumarate vaginal ring. AIDS. 2016;**30**(5):743-751. DOI: 10.1097/QAD.0000000000000979

[67] Nel A, van Niekerk N, Kapiga S, Bekker LG, Gama C, Gill K, Kamali A, Kotze P, Louw C, Mabude Z, Miti N, Kusemererwa S, Tempelman H, Carstens H, Devlin B, Isaacs M, Malherbe M, Mans W, Nuttall J, Russell M, Ntshele S, Smit M, Solai L, Spence P, Steytler J, Windle K, Borremans M, Resseler S, Van Roey J, Parys W, Vangeneugden T, Van Baelen B, Rosenberg Z. Ring study team. Safety and efficacy of a dapivirine vaginal ring for HIV prevention in women. The New England Journal of Medicine. 2016;**375**(22):2133-2143. DOI: 10.1056/NEJMoa1602046

[68] Montgomery ET, van der Straten A, Chitukuta M, Reddy K, Woeber K, Atujuna M, Bekker LG, Etima J, Nakyanzi T, Mayo AJ, Katz A, Laborde N, Grossman CI, Soto-Torres L, Palanee-Phillips T, Baeten JM, MTN-020/ASPIRE Study. Acceptability and use of a dapivirine vaginal ring in a phase III trial. AIDS. 2017;**31**(8):1159-1167. DOI: 10.1097/QAD.0000000000001452

3

Latent Tuberculosis Infection: Pathobiology and Treatment

Rajneesh Thakur and
Vangal Krishnaswamy Sashindran

Abstract

Tuberculosis continues to be an epidemic disease worldwide especially in the developing countries. One of the main reasons behind the continuation of this epidemic is latent tuberculosis infection. Globally, 2–3 billion people have latent TB infection. Prevention of reactivation TB is now considered as one of the important strategies of TB prevention and is one of the main pillars for the WHO "End TB Strategy." Biostatistical modeling has shown that protecting 8% of persons with latent tuberculosis every year can bring down the global incidence rate by 14 times by 2050 as compared to that in 2013 without any other intervention. One of the most effective strategies recommended by WHO has been Isoniazid preventive therapy for 6–9 months. Chemoprophylaxis for LTBI can prevent 60–90% of reactivation TB. Isoniazid preventive therapy is considered safe; however, it can occasionally result in significant adverse effects like hepatitis and rarely mortality. In conclusion, chemoprophylaxis of LTBI can be considered an important intervention being done to curb the epidemic of TB especially in high-risk group and reduce the morbidity and mortality associated with active TB disease.

Keywords: latent tuberculosis infection, World Health Organization, chemoprophylaxis, isoniazid therapy

1. Introduction

The medical, economic and social impact of the dual epidemics of human immunodeficiency virus (HIV) and tuberculosis (TB) will continue to remain one of the biggest public health challenges of the twenty-first century. According to the World Health Organization (WHO) Global Status Report, 11% of 10.4 million new cases of TB in 2015 were HIV-positive [1]. This is an increase in the number of new TB cases from 9.2 million in 2014 [1]. Sixty percent of the new TB cases are reported from India, Indonesia, China, Nigeria, Pakistan and South Africa [1]. It has been difficult to rein in the TB epidemic, and there are many reasons for it. One of the main reasons for spread of TB in low TB/HIV burden countries is the reactivation of latent tuberculosis. In high TB/HIV burden countries, the main factors are lack of accessible health facilities where timely and effective treatment of TB can be given and the burgeoning numbers of drug-resistant TB cases. Another significant factor in the failure of TB control programmes in the developing countries has been the ongoing HIV epidemic. HIV-infected patients are at increased risk of new TB infection as well as reactivation of latent TB infection (LTBI). Prevention of reactivation TB in those with LTBI is now considered as one of the key strategies of TB prevention and is one of the pillars for the WHO "End TB Strategy" [1]. The WHO aims to implement LTBI detection and treatment in the 30 high-TB burden countries first. In these countries, it has set out an ambitious target of bringing 90% of children under 5 years who are TB contacts and PLHA under the chemoprophylaxis programme by 2025 [1]. Biostatistical modeling shows that if 8% of persons with latent tuberculosis could be permanently protected each year, the global incidence in 2050 would be 14 times lower than incidence in 2013, with no other intervention needed [2].

2. LTBI

Latent tuberculosis infection (LTBI) is a state of persistent immune response to *Mycobacterium tuberculosis* (Mtb) antigens without evidence of clinically manifested active TB [3]. In simpler terms, LTBI is infection with viable bacilli of Mtb complex but without symptoms of the disease. LTBI has great public health significance because a significant proportion of these people can develop active TB and contribute to spread and persistence of TB in the population. About 2–3 billion people, that is, one-third of the world's population, has TB infection but no TB disease. Among the people with LTBI, the lifetime risk of developing TB disease is 5–15% [4–6]. In HIV-infected, the annual risk of developing reactivation TB is 5–15% [7]. The risk is similar in people on anti-TNF-α therapy, patients on dialysis and those undergoing solid organ or hematological transplant [3]. Another similar high-risk group is that of children under 5 years of age who are household contacts of pulmonary TB cases [3].

Operational constraints and unfounded fears of increased incidence of drug-resistant TB have been the two main reasons for the poor implementation of LTBI programme in high-TB burden countries. Only 87,236 children under 5 years age who were household contacts of TB cases were initiated on TB chemoprophylaxis in 2015 [1]. The best chemoprophylaxis coverage was from the Americas (67%, range 63–71%) and European Region (42%, range 40–44%). In high TB or HIV/TB burden countries, the figures ranged from 2.6% in Cameroon to 41% in Malawi. These numbers belie the actual magnitude of the problem. The total number of children on TB chemoprophylaxis (87236) is only 7.1% (range 6.9–7.4%) of the 1.2 million children who are eligible for treatment. PLHA have a higher coverage with TB chemoprophylaxis, especially in the African region. In 2015, TB chemoprophylaxis was being offered to PLHA enrolling for HIV care in 57 countries. These countries represent 61% of the global TB burden. These data are encouraging because in 2014 there were only 49 countries where TB preventive treatment was available. South Africa, Malawi, Mozambique and Kenya have the largest number of PLHA on TB chemoprophylaxis. Much more needs to be done. Of the 30 high TB/HIV burden countries, no preventive treatment was available in 21 countries. Even in nine that did report so, coverage of people newly enrolled in HIV care varied from 2% in Indonesia to 79% in Malawi. The National AIDS Control Organization (NACO) in India issued new TB management guidelines in 2016 [8]. TB care has now been integrated into the services provided by the ART centres and isoniazid preventive therapy (IPT) has also been included in it [8].

3. Pathobiology of LTBI

Ninety percent of people infected with Mtb are able to successfully contain the microbe and ward of clinical disease. It should be realized that Mtb infection cannot be eradicated but only contained even in healthy immune-competent people and a key pathological mechanism in this is formation of tubercular granuloma.

Mtb infection occurs via the respiratory tract and on entry, mycobacteria encounter alveolar macrophages in the airways and immediately infect them. Macrophages can provide an intracellular sanctuary for mycobacteria, and Mtb has evolved numerous mechanisms to survive within macrophages. A characteristic set of pro-inflammatory cytokines and chemotactic factors for macrophages are released and cause granuloma formation. The granuloma is composed of various cells including macrophages, lymphocytes, dendritic cells, neutrophils, and sometimes fibroblasts, often with a necrotic centre. This structure serves to contain the bacilli and acts as an immune microenvironment that limits *M tuberculosis* replication. However, formation of a granuloma is not enough to control infection, as it has been seen that persons with active TB can have multiple granulomas in the lungs and possibly other tissues. Instead, granulomata must have optimal immunologic function to contain or eliminate the bacilli [9]. When they fail to do so, they release anti-inflammatory cytokines which aim to prevent tissue destruction but at the same time trigger fibrosis.

Structural or functional disruption of the granuloma is likely to lead to reactivation of latent *M. tuberculosis* infection, dissemination, and active disease [9]. Research in HIV-TB has given insight into some of the mechanisms involved in reactivation of TB [10]. The cause of disruption can be understood as general and overlapping processes, including increase in the HIV viral load within involved tissue, a reduced number of CD4 T cells, a defective macrophage function, and perturbation of Mtb-specific T-cell function [9]. They can all lead to detrimental changes within granulomas.

Depletion of CD4 cell population leads to an inability to mount an effective cell-mediated immune response against Mtb. Studies on macaques infected with simian immunodeficiency virus (SIV) have shown that reactivation of LTBI is directly associated with depletion of CD4+ T cells [10–12]. Critical decline in the number of CD4+ T cells is associated with a decrease in the number of memory CD4+ T cells (CD27+ CDRO45+) that can recognize Mtb antigens, decrease in polyfunctional antigen-specific CD4+ T cells and a relative increase in interferon gamma + CD 8+ T cells [10–12]. Other mechanisms include suppression of cell-mediated responses of regulatory T cells (Tregs) and impairment of TNF-α- mediated apoptosis of Mtb-infected cells [13].

4. Diagnosis of LTBI

Prior to putting people on chemoprophylaxis for LTBI, active TB has to be first excluded by standard case finding methods. Latent tuberculosis infection (LTBI) is most often diagnosed by the tuberculin skin test (TST), and the Mantoux TST is the standard method of determining *Mycobacterium tuberculosis* infection. This test is performed by injecting 0.1 ml of tuberculin purified protein derivative (PPD) (equivalent to 1 TU of PPD RT 23 or 2.5 TU of PPD- S) into the inner surface of the forearm. In India, PPD-RT 23 with Tween 80 of strength 1 TU and 2 TU are standardized tuberculins available which is supplied by the Bacillus Calmette-Guérin (BCG) vaccine Laboratory, Guindy, Chennai. CDC recommended strength is 5 TU of PPD-S. The injection is given intradermally with a tuberculin syringe, with the needle bevel facing upward. The injection should produce a pale wheal 6–10 mm in diameter and the skin test reaction should be read between 48 and 72 hours after administration. The reaction should be measured in millimeters of the induration (palpable, raised, hardened area or swelling) across the forearm (perpendicular to the long axis) and not the erythema (redness).

Classification of positive TST results

Induration size/Patient profile	**≥5 mm**	**≥10 mm**	**≥15 mm**
	HIV-infected persons • A recent contact of a person with TB disease • Persons with fibrotic changes on chest radiograph consistent with prior TB • Patients with organ transplants • Persons who are immunosuppressed for other reasons (e.g., taking the equivalent of >15 mg/day of prednisone for 1 month or longer, taking TNF- alpha antagonists)	• Recent immigrants (<5 years) from high-prevalence countries • Injection drug users • Residents and employees of high-risk congregate settings • Mycobacteriology laboratory personnel • Persons with clinical conditions that place them at high risk • Children <4 years of age • Infants, children, and adolescents exposed to adults in high-risk categories	Any person, including persons with no known risk factors for TB

In interpreting a positive TST, it is important to consider much more than only the size of the induration. Rather, the TST should be considered according to three dimensions: size of induration, pre-test probability of infection and risk of disease if the person were truly infected [14].

There are two important causes of false-positive results: nontuberculous mycobacterial (NTM) infection and prior BCG vaccination [15]. NTMs are not a clinically important cause of false-positive TST results, except in populations with a high prevalence of NTM sensitization and a very low prevalence of TB infection [15]. The impact of BCG on TST specificity depends on when BCG is given and on how many doses are administered. If BCG is administered at birth or infancy and not repeated, then its impact on TST specificity is minimal and can be ignored while interpreting the results [15]. In contrast, if BCG is given after infancy (e.g., school entry) and/or given multiple times (i.e., booster shots), then TST specificity is compromised [15].

Tuberculin skin tests are subject to variability when repeated tuberculin tests are given. Chance variation should result in differences of less than 6 mm (representing two standard deviations) in 95% of subjects. This supports the adoption of 6 mm as a criterion to distinguish increases in reaction size due to random variation alone from true biologic phenomena, which could be either conversion or boosting [16]. Boosting is best distinguished from conversion on clinical grounds. One can attribute an increase in reaction size to boosting when the increase in reaction is seen after an interval of 1–5 weeks during which there has been no possibility of exposure, such as pre-employment testing of a health care worker [16]. Conversion can be confidently stated to have occurred when a previously tuberculin-negative individual becomes tuberculin test positive after receiving BCG vaccination, or following significant exposure such as during an outbreak or as a result of close contact with a highly contagious index case [17, 18]. Among subjects vaccinated in infancy, and tested after an interval of 5 years or more, prevalence of initial tuberculin reactions is the same in vaccinated and unvaccinated reference populations but prevalence of boosting was 7% higher in vaccinated than unvaccinated [19].

The other method of detecting LTBI is based on IFNγ release assays (IGRA). These tests detect a set of Mtb genes that are present in Mtb complex but not present in BCG immunized or in a setting of NTM infection. In this test, the sera of patients is incubated with Mtb specific T lymphocytes. The T cells respond to Mtb-specific gene products by secretion of pro-inflammatory cytokines that are detected. Two IGRAs are commercially available today. QuantiFERON-Gold In Tube test (QFT; Germany) uses whole blood and is ELISA based. The T-SPOT.TB test (Oxford Immunotec, Abingdon, UK) uses peripheral blood mononucleated cell (PBMC) and ELISPOT technique. Both IGRAs incorporate the region of difference 1 (RD1)-encoded 6 kDa early secretory antigenic target (ESAT-6) and 10 kDa culture filtrate protein (CFP10) antigens, whereas an additional single peptide from TB7.7, encoded in RD11, is added to the QFT [20]. The selections of antigens for these tests are critical. Natural immunity to *M. tuberculosis* is highly individual, multi-epitopic and multiantigenic, and more than 80 antigens are necessary to capture 80% of the MTB-specific T-cell response [21]. The currently used antigens ESAT-6, CFP10 and TB7.7 were selected for their high immunogenicity and specificity for *M. tuberculosis* infection, not for their predictive potential. ESAT-6 is considered among the most immunogenic proteins, but it has a drawback when used to detect LTBI. It is secreted through the entire spectrum of latency and also in active stages of the infection. Therefore, disease stage-specific diagnosis is impossible using ESAT-6 [22].

Various studies have evaluated the utility of IGRAs and TST. A study from Turkey published in 2007 seems relevant to countries like India as Turkey is also a country with high prevalence of TB and high BCG vaccination coverage [23]. The workers compared TST with QuantiFERON®-TB in three population groups: household contacts of smear-positive TB cases, community members who had been exposed to index smear-positive TB cases and healthcare workers dealing with TB cases or handling TB specimens. They did a Kappa analysis to look for agreement between the tests. They found that QuantiFERON®-TB values were higher in the first group of patients when compared to the other two groups. In case of TST, there was no difference among the three groups. Evaluation for agreement rates between the groups showed poor agreement in all three groups. The authors concluded that while Quantiferon Gold was more objective, practical and gave quantitative values, it was more expensive and required a well-equipped laboratory and thus did not have a programmatic role in detection of LTBI in a country will high TB prevalence and high BCG coverage [23].

In a Japanese study, the specificity of IGRA was studied in healthy low-risk individuals with history of BCG vaccination [24]. It was seen that TST was positive (≥ 10 mm) in 64.6% (specificity 35.4%) while QuantiFERON®-TB test was positive in 1.9% (specificity 98.1%,) [24]. Similar results were obtained in another study done in Korea [25].In this study, 273 participants were included, 220 (95.7%) had received BCG vaccine. Participants were grouped according to their risk of infection: group 1, no identifiable risk of *M. tuberculosis* infection (n = 99); group 2, recent casual contacts (n = 72); group 3, recent close contacts (n = 48); group 4, bacteriologically or pathologically confirmed TB patients (n = 54). They studied the levels of agreement between the TST and the IFN-gamma assay and the likelihood of infection in the various groups and found out that the overall agreement between the TST and the IFN-gamma assay in healthy volunteers was a kappa value of 0.16. The odds of a positive test result per unit increase in exposure across the four groups increased by a factor of 5.31 (95% confidence interval [CI], 3.62–7.79) for the IFN-gamma assay and by a factor of 1.52 (95% CI, 1.20–1.91) for the TST (P < .001). In another study of 590 HIV-infected patients, QuantiFERON® -TB Gold test correlated with known risk factors for LTBI or past history of TB [26].

Both TST and IGRAs are acceptable but imperfect LTBI tests, with advantages and disadvantages [27]. In some situations, neither test is appropriate (e.g., active TB diagnosis in adults) and in some situations, both the tests may be necessary to detect *M. tuberculosis* infection (e.g., immunocompromised populations), and there are situations where one test may be preferable to another. For example, IGRAs may be preferable to the TST in populations where BCG is given after infancy or given multiple times. In contrast, TST may be preferable to the IGRAs for serial testing of health care workers. Both TST and IGRAs have reproducibility challenges, and dichotomous cut-offs are inadequate for interpretation [27]. The ability of tuberculin skin tests and IGRAs to identify persons at highest risk of progressing to active tuberculosis is poor. Neither test reliably predicts future disease among persons with positive tests nor do strongly positive tests mean a higher risk. In one meta-analysis, the pooled positive predictive value for progression to active tuberculosis was 2.7% (95% confidence interval [CI], 2.3–3.2) for IGRAs and 1.5% (95% CI, 1.2–1.7) for the tuberculin skin test [28]. A meta-analysis of only longitudinal studies of IGRAs, with a median follow-up of 4 years, showed a moderate association between positive tests and subsequent tuberculosis (unadjusted incidence ratio, 2.10 [95% CI, 1.42–3.08]) [29]. The other limitations of these tests are inability to distinguish reactivation from reinfection, reduced accuracy in immunocompromised patients, and inability to discriminate the various stages within the spectrum of LTBI [30]. To maximize the positive predictive value of existing LTBI tests, LTBI screening should be reserved only for those who are at sufficiently high risk of progressing to disease. The recommendations for systematic testing for LTBI as per WHO 2015 guidelines are as follows [31]:

Population groups	Test	Quality of recommendation
PLHA, child contacts of TB cases, patients being initiated on anti-TNF treatment, patients receiving dialysis, patients preparing for organ/haemotologic transplant and patients of silicosis	IGRA/TST	Strong recommendation, low/very low quality evidence
Prisoners, health-care workers, immigrants from high TB-burden countries, homeless persons and illicit drug users	IGRA/TST	Conditional recommendation, low/very low quality evidence

In the long term, highly predictive biomarkers need to be identified. This is an active area of research, and future generations of LTBI tests should overcome the limitations of current assays. A great endeavor is on to discover reliable, low-cost biomarkers. Gene signatures can distinguish between active and latent TB [32]. A lot of works have been done to identify differential expression of cytokines and chemokines in active TB and LTBI. It has been shown that plasma levels of the CXC chemokine IP-10 and soluble TNF receptor type 2 (sTNFr2) can significantly differentiate active TB from the LTBI group, irrespective of HIV status [33]. Another study showed that serum IL-2, IL-9, IL-13, IL-17, TNF-α, sCD40L and VEGF-A levels may be adjunctive biomarkers for differential diagnosis of active TB, LTBI, and NTM disease [34]. Assessment of serum sCD40L and Mtb antigen-specific IFN-γ, TNF-α, and IL-2 levels could also help predict successful anti-TB treatment in conjunction with Mtb clearance [31]. Achkar et al. looked at biomarkers to distinguish active TB and LTBI from no TB infection in HIV positive and negative populations [35]. They did so because inflammatory response and repair are both blunted in PLHA. They identified a set of biomarkers which reliably predict active TB. The biomarkers identified are shown in **Table 1** [32]:

Functional category	HIV-Positive TB	HIV-Negative TB
Immune response	CD14, SEPP1, SELL	CD14, SEPP1, PGL YR P2
Tissue development & repair	TNXB, LUM, PEPD, QSOX1, COMP	PFN1, VASN
Lipid metabolism	APOC1	
Other	GP1BA	CPN2, TAGLN2, IGFBP6

SEPP, selenoprotein P; SELL, selectin L; TNXB, tenascin XB; LUM, lumican; PEPD-peptidase D; QSOX1, quiescin sulfhydryl oxidase 1; COMP, cartilage oligomeric matrix protein; APOC1, apolipoprotein C-I; GP1 BA-glycoprotein 1 BA; VASN, vasorin; PFN 1, profilin1; CPN 2, chaperon 2; TAGLN2, transgelin 2; IGFBP 6, insulin-like growth factor binding protein 6; PGLYRP2, peptidoglycan recognition protein 2.

Table 1. Newer biomarkers for diagnosis of active TB.

5. Treatment of LTBI

Treatment of LTBI reduces the risk for active disease and hence various authorities have recommended treatment for this entity. Chemoprophylaxis for LTBI can prevent 60–90% of reactivation TB [36]. But chemoprophylaxis cannot be considered as a universal approach due to the inherent toxicity of all TB drugs. However, in vulnerable populations, the benefits far outweigh the risks [33].

The International Union against Tuberculosis (IUAT) trial, conducted in Eastern Europe, randomized approximately 28,000 individuals with positive tuberculin skin tests (TST) and fibronodular changes on chest X-ray [37]. Approximately 7000 participants each were randomized to placebo, 3, 6 or 12 months of INH. Compared to participants who took placebo, participants who completed 3 months INH had 31% reduction in TB; those who completed 6 months INH (6INH) 69% reduction and the subjects who completed 12 months INH (12INH) had 93% reduction in TB. The efficacy of 6INH and 12INH waned during 5 years of follow-up but remained significantly better than the placebo. It is to be noted that fewer people completed 12 INH regimens as compared to 6INH [34].

Concerns regarding the relatively low efficacy of 6INH, and equally serious concerns regarding the poor completion of 12INH resulted in recommendations for 9 months INH by the American Thoracic Society in 2000 [38]. The optimal duration of INH was recommended as 9 months, with estimated efficacy of 90% and no significant gain with extension to 12 months [35].

In another trial, in Hong Kong, people who had pulmonary silicosis with a positive TST were randomized to placebo, 6INH, 3 m INH + Rifampin, or 3 m Rifampin alone [39]. During 5 years of follow-up, 27% of those randomized to placebo arm developed active TB, compared to 16, 13, and 10% for the three regimens respectively [36]. The estimated effectiveness of 3-months rifampin was approximately 65%; this was better than the other regimens although the differences between active regimens were not significant, and all were significantly better than placebo [36].

A series of randomized trials have demonstrated that the efficacy of 3-4INH + RIF to be equivalent to that of 6INH (four studies) or 9INH (one study) although adverse events are significantly more frequent [40, 41].

For adults, the recommended duration of treatment is at least 6, and preferably 9, months. Children younger than 18 years and persons with HIV infection should be treated for 9 months [42]. In HIV TB setting, IPT has been shown to slow the progression to active disease. A Cochrane systematic review of 12 trials, published in 2010 among 8578 patients showed that IPT reduced the risk of active TB by 64% among TST positive HIV-infected participants [43]. WHO has recommended that in resource-limited countries and other middle-income countries, people living with HIV and children below 5 years of age who are household or close contacts of people with TB and who, after an appropriate clinical evaluation, are found not to have active TB but have LTBI should be treated. WHO has recommended the following regimens for the treatment of LTBI which are similar to current CDC guidelines [26, 44–46].

The 9-month regimen with isoniazid is preferred because it is more efficacious. However, treatment of LTBI for 6 months rather than 9 months may be more cost-effective and result in greater adherence by patients.

Regimen	Dose isoniazid	Dose rifapentine or rifampicin	Maximum dose
6 m or 9 m isoniazid daily	Adults = 5 mg/kg Children = 10 mg/kg		isoniazid - 300 mg
3 m rifapentine + isoniazid weekly	Adults & children isoniazid - 15 mg/kg	Rifapentine (wt band): 10.0–14.0 kg = 300 mg; 14.1–25.0 kg = 450 mg; 25.1–32.0 kg = 600 mg; 32.1–49.9 kg = 750 mg; ≥50.0 kg = 900 mg	isoniazid - 900 mg Rifapentine - 900 mg
3 or 4 m isoniazid + rifampicin daily	Isoniazid: Adults - 5 mg/kg Children - 10 mg/kg	Rifampicin: Adults & children - 10 mg/kg	isoniazid-300 mg Rifampicin - 600 mg
3 or 4 m rifampicin alone daily	Adults & children 10 mg/kg		Rifampicin - 600 mg

Directly observed once-weekly regimen of isoniazid and rifapentine is recommended as an option equal to the standard INH 9-month daily regimen for treating LTBI. The regimen may be used in otherwise healthy HIV-infected persons, 12 years of age and older, who are not on antiretroviral medications. It may also be considered for children aged 2–11 years if completion of 9 months of INH is unlikely and hazard of TB disease is great.

The regimen using 4 months of rifampicin can be considered for persons who cannot tolerate INH or who have been exposed to INH-resistant TB. It should also not be used to treat HIV-infected persons taking some combinations of ART especially protease inhibitors.

The National Aids Control Organization guidelines for LTBI in PLHA published in 2016 recommends the following strategy [8]

- Adults and adolescents living with HIV should be screened for TB with a clinical algorithm and those who do not report any one of the symptoms of current cough, fever, weight loss or night sweats are unlikely to have active TB and should be offered Isoniazid Preventive Therapy (IPT).
- Children living with HIV (more than 12 months of age) who do not report poor weight gain, fever, current cough or history of contact with a TB case, are unlikely to have active TB and should be offered IPT.
- Additional investigations will help in ruling out active TB (X-ray chest and tuberculin skin test) but are not mandatory.
- The treatment recommended in adult and adolescent is Isoniazid 300 mg + Pyridoxine 50 mg (Vitamin B6) per day for 6 months and for children above 12 months is Isoniazid 10 mg/kg + Pyridoxine 25 mg (Vitamin B6) per day for 6 months.

6. Chemoprophylaxis after contact with MDR-TB

Treatment of close contacts of drug-resistant active TB cases is difficult and yet is an increasingly common clinical problem. For contacts of INH-resistant index cases, INH will be ineffective, so 4RIF is recommended [47, 48].

In a prospective study, two of 41 children receiving tailored preventive therapy developed TB (confirmed and probable TB) compared to 13 of 64 children not receiving preventive treatment (OR 0.2, 95% CI 0.04–0.94) [49]. However, WHO has not recommended any form of preventive therapy for MDR contact cases. Based on the available evidence and the probability of increased likelihood to develop active TB disease following recent infection, strict clinical observation and close monitoring for the development of active TB disease for at least 2 years is preferred over the provision of preventive treatment for contacts of MDR-TB cases [1].

Clinical management of latent tuberculosis infection should also address such concomitant risk factors as illicit-drug use, alcohol abuse, and smoking through opioid-substitution treatment and counseling about alcohol and smoking cessation, respectively. Acceptance of and adherence to the full course of latent tuberculosis treatment must be encouraged. In a study conducted in the United States and Canada, 17% of persons who were offered treatment for latent infection refused it [1]. Treatment completion varies widely (from 19 to 96%), and the reasons for non-completion need to be fully assessed [1]. The use of various incentives to promote treatment initiation and adherence, depending on the specific need of the person being treated, should be considered. Peer education, counseling, people-friendly services, and properly trained service providers boost confidence and may improve adherence to treatment [1].

7. Adverse effects of LTBI treatment

The lengthy duration of treatment reduces patient compliance, while the potential occurrence of serious adverse events such as hepatitis, further discourages patients' and providers' acceptance of this therapy [50–52].

INH has the major disadvantage of potential serious adverse events. Of particular concern is hepatotoxicity, as this is difficult to detect, and can be fatal. Surveillance studies have confirmed that hepatotoxicity is quite common in patients taking INH and can be severe resulting in up to 1 per cent mortality in older patients [53].The relative risk for developing hepatotoxicity associated with isoniazid compared with placebo were 3.45 (95% CI, 1.49–7.99) for 12 weeks of treatment, 4.59 (95% CI, 2.03–10.39) for 24 weeks of treatment, and 6.21 (95% CI, 2.79–13.79) for 52 weeks of treatment in the IUAT trial [34].

In another randomized trial, rates of grade 3 and 4 adverse events were significantly lower with 4RIF than 9INH [54]. Grade 3–4 hepatotoxicity occurred in 4% of patients taking 9INH compared to less than 1% in those taking 4RIF [54].

Comparison of drug toxicity of INH and Rifampicin has been studied in many trials. Rates of hepatotoxicity among patients receiving isoniazid were 5.2, 3.7, 34 and 11.4% compared to rates among patients treated with rifampicin (0.0, 0.7 and 4.4%, respectively) [55, 56].

In PREVENT TB study, rates of grade 3 and 4 hepatotoxicity were 4.9 and 1.0% in the rifapentine plus isoniazid arm and 5.5 and 1.1% in the isoniazid-only arm, respectively [57]. The RR for grade 3 or 4 hepatotoxicity was 0.90 (95% CI, 0.75–1.08). Mortality from hepatotoxicity was reported to be 1.0% among patients on isoniazid and 0.8% on those on isoniazid plus rifapentine (RR, 0.83 [95% CI, 0.51–1.35]) [57]. Therefore, unless the index TB case has INH-resistant TB or an abbreviated regimen is required in a special situation, there is no reason not to use INH for LTBI chemoprophylaxis.

8. Conclusion

Identification and early chemoprophylaxis for LTBI can prevent reactivation TB and thus reduce both TB morbidity and transmission of TB in the community. In low TB-burden countries LTBI detection and IPT are important strategies for TB eradication. Diagnosis of LTBI is based on either TST or TB IGRA. The test preferred usually depends on the financial support available for public health programmes. In high TB- burden countries, LTBI detection and treatment can contribute to decreasing TB burden and transmission and also emergence of drug resistant TB. Here the guidelines are pretty straightforward and IPT should be offered to all children less than 5 years who have contact with pulmonary TB cases or HIV-positive individuals. INH is the preferred drug for LTBI and a 9-month regimen is considered optimal. However, careful clinical monitoring is required to detect drug induced liver injury early and also to ensure adherence to therapy. Clinical trials in different parts of the world have shown that this effort is worth it.

Author details

Rajneesh Thakur* and Vangal Krishnaswamy Sashindran

*Address all correspondence to: rajneesh2207@gmail.com

Armed Forces Medical College, Pune, India

References

[1] WHO. Global Tuberculosis Report 2016. Geneva: WHO; 2016

[2] Dye C, Glaziou P, Floyd K, Raviglione M. Prospects for tuberculosis elimination. Annual Review of Public Health. 2013;**34**:271-286

[3] Mack U, Migliori GB, Sester M, Rieder HL, Ehlers S. Goletti D, et al and TBNET. LTBI: Latent tuberculosis infection or lasting immune responses to *M. tuberculosis*? A TBNET consensus statement. The European Respiratory Journal. 2009;**33**:956-973

[4] Comstock GW, Livesay VT, Woolpert SF. The prognosis of a positive tuberculin reaction in childhood and adolescence. American Journal of Epidemiology. 1974;**99**:131-138

[5] Dye C, Scheele S, Dolin P, Pathania V, Raviglione MC. Consensus statement. Global burden of tuberculosis: Estimated incidence, prevalence, and mortality by country. WHO global surveillance and monitoring project. JAMA. 1999;**282**(7):677-686

[6] Vynnycky E, Fine PE. Lifetime risks, incubation period, and serial interval of tuberculosis. American Journal of Epidemiology. 2000;**152**(3):247-263

[7] Pawlowski A, Jansson M, Skold M, Rottenberg ME, Kallenius G. Tuberculosis and HIV coinfection. PLOS Pathogens. 2012;**8**:e1002464

[8] NACO 2016. National Framework for HIV TB in India 2013, Integrated HIVTB module 2016, NACO-CTD, MoHFW GOI and Vihaan program guidelines

[9] Diedrich CR, Flynn JL. HIV-1/*Mycobacterium tuberculosis* co infection immunology: How does HIV-1 exacerbate tuberculosis? Infection and Immunity. 2011;**79**(4):1407-1417

[10] Geldmacher C et al. Early depletion of *Mycobacterium tuberculosis*-specific T helper 1 cell responses after HIV-1 infection. The Journal of Infectious Diseases. 2008;**198**:1590-1598

[11] Preferential infection and depletion of *Mycobacterium tuberculosis*-specific CD4 T cells after HIV-1 infection. The Journal of Experimental Medicine. 2010;**207**:2869-2881. [PubMed: 21115690]

[12] Sutherland JS et al. PolyfunctionalCD4(+) and CD8(+) T cell responses to tuberculosis antigens in HIV-1-infected patients before and after anti-retroviral treatment. Journal of Immunology. 2010;**184**:6537-6544. [PubMed: 20435929]

[13] Patel NR et al. HIV impairs TNF-alpha mediated macrophage apoptotic response to *Mycobacterium tuberculosis*. Journal of Immunology. 2007;**179**:6973-6980. [PubMed: 17982088]

[14] Menzies D, Gardiner G, Farhat M, Greenaway C, Pai M. Thinking in three dimensions: A web-based algorithm to aid the interpretation of tuberculin skin test results. The International Journal of Tuberculosis and Lung Disease. 2008;**12**:498-505

[15] Farhat M, Greenaway C, Pai M, Menzies D. False-positive tuberculin skin tests: What is the absolute effect of BCG and nontuberculous mycobacteria? The International Journal of Tuberculosis and Lung Disease. 2006;**10**:1192-1204

[16] Menzis D. Interpretation of repeated tuberculin testing, boosting,conversion and reversions. AJRCCM. 1999;**159**:15-21

[17] Menzies RI, Vissandjee B. Effect of Bacille Calmette-Guerin vaccination on tuberculin reactivity. The American Review of Respiratory Disease. 1992;**145**:621-625

[18] Johnson H, Lee B, Doherty E, Kelly E, McDonnell T. Tuberculin sensitivity and the BCG scar in tuberculosis contacts. Tubercle and Lung Disease. 1995;**76**:122-125

[19] Menzies RI, Vissandjee B, Rocher I, St. Germain Y. The booster effect in two-step tuberculin testing among young adults in Montreal. Annals of Internal Medicine. 1994;**120**:190-198

[20] Sorensen AL, Nagai S, Houen G, Andersen P, Andersen AB. Purification and characterization of a low-molecular-mass T-cell antigen secreted by *Mycobacterium tuberculosis*. Infection and Immunity. 1995;**63**:1710-1717

[21] Lindestam Arlehamn CS, Gerasimova A, Mele F, et al. Memory T cells in latent *Mycobacterium tuberculosis* infection are directed against three antigenic islands and largely contained in a CXCR3+CCR6+ Th1 subset. PLOS Pathogens. 2013;**9**:e1003130

[22] Andersen P, Askgaard D, Ljungqvist L, et al. Proteins released from *Mycobacterium tuberculosis* during growth. Infection and Immunity. 1991;**59**:1905-1910

[23] Oztürk N, Sürücüoğlu S, Ozkütük N, Gazi H, Akçali S, Köroğlu G, Ciçek C. Comparison of interferon-gamma whole blood assay with tuberculin skin test for the diagnosis of tuberculosis infection in tuberculosis contacts. Mikrobiyoloji Bülteni. 2007; **41**(2):193-202

[24] Mori T, Sakatani M, Yamagishi F, Takashima T, Kawabe Y, Nagao K, et al. Specific detection of tuberculosis infection: An interferon-gamma-based assay using new antigens. American Journal of Respiratory and Critical Care Medicine. 2004 Jul 1;**170**(1):59-64

[25] Kang YA, Lee HW, Yoon HI, Cho B, Han SK, Shim YS, et al. Discrepancy between the tuberculin skin test and the whole-blood interferon gamma assay for the diagnosis of latent tuberculosis infection in an intermediate tuberculosis-burden country. Journal of the American Medical Association. 2005;**293**(22):2756-2761

[26] Brock I, Ruhwald M, Lundgren B, Westh H, Mathiesen LR, Ravn P. Latent tuberculosis in HIV positive, diagnosed by the *M. tuberculosis* specific interferon-gamma test. Respiratory Research. 2006;**7**:56

[27] LoBue PA, Castro KG. Is it time to replace the tuberculin skin test with a blood test? JAMA. 2012;**308**:241-242. DOI: 10.1001/jama .2012.7511

[28] Diel R, Loddenkemper R, Nienhaus A. Predictive value of interferon-γ release assays and tuberculin skin testing for progressionfrom latent TB infection to disease state: A meta-analysis. Chest. 2012;**142**:63-75

[29] Rangaka MX, Wilkinson KA, Glynn JR, et al. Predictive value of interferon-γ release assays for incident active tuberculosis: A systematic review and meta-analysis. The Lancet Infectious Diseases. 2012;**12**:45-55

[30] Pai M. Spectrum of latent tuberculosis— Existing tests cannot resolve the underlying phenotypes. Nature Reviews. Microbiology. 2010;**8**:242. DOI: 10.1038/nrmicro2236-c1

[31] WHO Guidelines for management of latent TB infection; 2015

[32] Lu JW, Wang H, Wang S, Diao N, Wang F, et al. Novel biomarkers distinguishing active tuberculosis from latent infection identified by gene expression profile of peripheral blood mononuclear cells. PLoS One. 2011;**6**:e2429

[33] Wergeland I, Pullar N, Assmus J, Ueland T, Tonby K, Feruglio S, et al. IP-10 differentiates between active and latent tuberculosis irrespective of HIV status and declines during therapy. The Journal of Infection. 2015 Apr;**70**(4):381-391

[34] Hur YG, Kang YA, Jang SH, Hong JY, Kim A, Lee SA, et al. Adjunctive biomarkers for

improving diagnosis of tuberculosis and monitoring therapeutic effects. The Journal of Infection. 2015 Apr;**70**(4):346-355

[35] Achkar JM, Cortes L, Croteau P, Yanofsky C, Mentinova M, Rajotte I, Schirm M, Zhou Y, Junqueira-Kipnis AP, Kasprowicz VO, Larsen M, Allard R, Hunter J, Paramthiotis E. Host protein biomarkers identify active TB in HIV uninfected and co-infected individuals. EBio Medicine. 2015;**2**:1160-1168 Published online 30 Jul 2015

[36] Lobue P, Menzies D. Treatment of latent tuberculosis infection: An update. Respirology. 2010;**15**:603-622

[37] International Union against Tuberculosis Committee on Prophylaxis. Efficacy of various durations of isoniazid preventive therapy for tuberculosis: Five years of follow-up in the IUAT trial. Bulletin of the World Health Organization. 1982;**60**:555-564

[38] American Thoracic Society. Targeted tuberculin testing and treatment of latent tuberculosis infection. American Journal of Respiratory and Critical Care Medicine. 2000;**161**:S221-S247

[39] Hong Kong Chest Service Tuberculosis Research Centre MBMRC. A double-blind placebo-controlled clinical trial of three antituberculosis chemoprophylaxis regimens in patients with silicosis in Hong Kong. The American Review of Respiratory Disease. 1992; **145**:36-41

[40] Ena J, Valls V. Short-course therapy with rifampin plus isoniazid, compared with standard therapy with isoniazid, for latent tuberculosis infection: A meta-analysis. Clinical Infectious Diseases. 2005;**40**:670-676

[41] Kunst H, Khan KS. Age-related risk of hepatotoxicity in treatment of latent tuberculosis infection; a systematic review. The International Journal of Tuberculosis and Lung Disease. 2010;**14**:1374-1381

[42] American Thoracic Society, Centers for Disease Control and Prevention. Targeted tuberculin testing and treatment of latent tuberculosis infection. American Journal of Respiratory and Critical Care Medicine. 2000;**161**(4 pt 2):S221-S247

[43] Akolo C, Adetifa I, Shepperd S, Volmink J. Treatment of latent tuberculosis infection in HIV infected persons. Cochrane Database of Systematic Reviews. 2010;**1**:CD000171

[44] CDC. Targeted tuberculin testing and treatment of latent TB infection. MMWR. 2000;**49** (No. RR-6)

[45] CDC. Recommendations for use of an isoniazid-rifapentine regimen with direct observation to treat latent *Mycobacterium tuberculosis* infection. MMWR. 2011;**60**(48):1650-1653

[46] CDC. Updated guidelines for the use of rifamycins for the treatment of tuberculosis among HIV-infected patients taking protease inhibitors or nonnucleoside reverse transcriptase inhibitors. MMWR. 2004;**53**(2):37

[47] American Thoracic Society. Targeted tuberculin testing and treatment of latent tuberculosis infection. American Journal of Respiratory and Critical Care Medicine. 2000;**161**:S221-S247

[48] Long RL, Ellis E. Canadian Tuberculosis Standards. 6th ed. Toronto: Canadian Lung Association, Public Health Agency of Canada, Tuberculosis Prevention and Control; 2007

[49] Schaaf HS, Gie RP, Kennedy M, et al. Evaluation of young children in contact with adult multidrug-resistant pulmonary tuberculosis: A 30-month follow-up. Pediatrics. 2002;**109**: 765-771

[50] Sumartojo E. When tuberculosis treatment fails: A social behavioural account of patient adherence. The American Review of Respiratory Disease. 1993;**147**:1311-1320

[51] Dosanjh DPS, Hinks T, Innes JA, Deeks JJ, Pasvol G, Hackforth S, et al. Improved diagnostic evaluation of suspected tuberculosis in routine practice. Annals of Internal Medicine. 2008;**148**:325-333

[52] Dash LA, Comstock GW, Flynn JPG. Isoniazid preventive therapy. The American Review of Respiratory Disease. 1980;**121**:1039-1044

[53] Kopanoff DE, Snider D, Caras GJ. Isoniazid-related hepatitis. The American Review of Respiratory Disease. 1978;**117**:991-1001

[54] Menzies D, Long R, Trajman A, Dion MJ, Yang J, Al-Jahdali H, et al. Adverse events with 4 months rifampin or 9 months isoniazid as therapy for latent TB infection: Results of a randomized trial. Annals of Internal Medicine. 2008;**149**:689-697

[55] Menzies D, Dion MJ, Rabinovitch B, et al. Treatment completion and costs of a randomized trial of rifampin for 4 months versus isoniazid for 9 months. American Journal of Respiratory and Critical Care Medicine. 2004;**170**(4):445-449. PMID: 15172892

[56] White MC, Tulsky JP, Lee JR, et al. Isoniazid vs. rifampin for latent tuberculosis infection in jail inmates: Toxicity and adherence. Journal of Correctional Health Care. 2012;**18**(2): 131-142. PMID: 22419641

[57] Sterling TR, Villarino ME, Borisov AS, et al. Three months of rifapentine and isoniazid for latent tuberculosis infection. The New England Journal of Medicine. 2011;**365**(23):2155-2166. PMID: 22150035

4

Drug-Resistant Bacterial Infections in HIV Patients

Marimuthu Ragavan Rameshkumar and
Narasingam Arunagirinathan

Abstract

The human immunodeficiency virus (HIV) was first detected in 1982 among homosexual men, and subsequently, it was further detected in various regions of world. In 2016, WHO estimated that 36.7 million people were living with HIV, 1.9 million were newly infected HIV patients and approximately 1 million people died worldwide. HIV attacks CD4 T cells and causes immunodeficiency. Weakened immune system of HIV patients increases the opportunity to acquire various infections caused by fungi, bacteria, parasites and other viruses. Bacterial infections that cause huge threats to HIV patients are tuberculosis, syphilis, bacterial enteric diseases and bacterial pneumonia. Important bacterial etiologies are *Streptococcus pneumoniae*, *Salmonella* spp. *Haemophilus influenzae*, *Staphylococcus aureus*, *Citrobacter freundii*, *Escherichia coli*, *Klebsiella pneumoniae*, *Morganella morganii*, *Pseudomonas aeruginosa* and *Mycobacterium tuberculosis*. Frequent bacterial infections in HIV patients increase the usage and also highly expose bacteria to antibiotics. Most problematic multidrug-resistant bacteria are extended-spectrum β-lactamases producing *P. aeruginosa*, *Acinetobacter baumannii*, *E. coli* and *K. pneumoniae*; vancomycin-resistant enterococci; methicillin-resistant *S. aureus* and multidrug-resistant and extensively drug-resistant *M. tuberculosis*. These antibiotic-resistant bacteria complicate the treatment of infections in HIV patients with available antibiotics and sometimes cause death. It also causes higher medical costs, prolonged hospital stays, increased mortality and economic burden on families and societies.

Keywords: HIV patients, multidrug resistant, vancomycin-resistant enterococci, methicillin-resistant *Staphylococcus aureus*, antibiotic resistance

1. Introduction

Human immunodeficiency virus (HIV) is a lentivirus belongs to the family of Retroviridae and it causes Acquired Immunodeficiency Syndrome (AIDS) in an advanced stage of HIV infection. HIV was first detected in 1981 among homosexual men in the New York City who had unusual clusters of *Pneumocystis jirovecii* pneumonia and Kaposi sarcoma [1, 2]. After that, HIV positivity was detected in the various regions globally and actively spread in the community with increased rate of HIV infection. In 2016, the World Health Organization (WHO) has reported that HIV continues to be a major global public health issue, having claimed more than 35 million lives so far. One million people died from HIV-related causes; furthermore, approximately 36.7 million people are living with HIV and 1.8 million people becoming newly infected worldwide. African region is the most affected area with 25.6 million people living with HIV in 2016. It accounts for almost two-thirds of the global total number of new HIV infections [3, 4].

HIV spreads from one person to another by sexual contact such as vaginal sex, anal sex and oral sex and also spreads by sharing injection equipment, getting tattoos or body piercings with unsterilized needles, accidental needle sticks, contaminated blood transfusions and splashing blood in eyes. HIV can pass from HIV-positive pregnant women to their babies in the womb and during birth. It can also be transferred to other persons through certain body fluids such as blood, semen, vaginal fluid and breast milk [5]. After entry into the human body system, HIV infects vital immune cells such as helper T cells (specifically CD4+ T cells), macrophages and dendritic cells [6]. Hence, HIV infection leads to low level of CD4+ T cells through three important mechanisms. First mechanism is direct viral killing of the infected cells; second is increased rate of apoptosis in infected cells; and third is killing of infected CD4+ cells by CD8 cytotoxic lymphocytes. Virus multiplication declines the number of CD4+ cells below a critical level; therefore, the cell mediated immunity is lost and the weaken immune system signal to various opportunistic infections (OIs) and cancers [6–9]. Compromised immune system of HIV patients increases the chances of acquiring various OIs caused by fungi, bacteria, parasites and other viruses based on the CD4 cell counts. Tuberculosis (TB) generally develops at CD4 count of 200–500 cells/mm^3, as does *Candida albicans* infection *Pneumocystis jirovecii* pneumonia (PCP, earlier known as *Pneumocystis carinii*) occurs at CD4 count <200 cells/mm^3 and cytomegalovirus (CMV) infection occurs when the CD4 count falls below 100 cells/mm^3 [10]. As compared to other microbes, bacteria cause high rate of infections such as tuberculosis, syphilis, bacterial enteric diseases, pneumonia and bartonellosis. Bacteria causing various infections associated with HIV patients include *Streptococcus pneumoniae*, *Salmonella* spp., *Haemophilus influenzae*, *Staphylococcus aureus*, *Citrobacter freundii*, *Escherichia coli*, *Klebsiella pneumoniae*, *Morganella morganii*, *Pseudomonas aeruginosa*, *Mycobacterium tuberculosis* and *Mycobacterium avium* complex, and they have emerged as an important cause of morbidity and mortality in HIV individuals [11, 12].

High frequency of bacterial infections in HIV patients increases the chance of consumption of high level of antibiotics. Over usage and mishandling of antibiotics develop various resistance mechanisms among bacteria. The dramatic increase in the incidence of multidrug-resistant (MDR) bacteria and transfer of resistance from one organism to another make bacterial infections more difficult to treat with current antibiotics, so the treatment options are often extremely limited [13]. This chapter describes about various bacterial diseases and antibiotic-resistant bacteria from HIV patients.

2. Bacterial infections among HIV patients

2.1. Respiratory tract infections

Respiratory tract infection (RTI) is defined as infectious disease of upper or lower respiratory tract of human body system. RTI is classified as an upper respiratory tract infection and a lower respiratory tract infection. Pneumonia is an infection in one or both side of lungs causing inflammation in the air sacs (alveoli). In this condition, alveoli fill with phlegm (mucus) or pus making difficult to breathe. Bacterial pneumonia is a common cause of HIV-related morbidity with the symptoms of body chills, rigors, pleuritic chest pain and purulent sputum, fever, tachypnea, tachycardia, rales or rhonchi and other signs. Incidence of bacterial respiratory infections among HIV-positive population has been reported approximately 90 cases per 1000 per year, which is higher than noninfected population [14]. Bacterial pneumonia among HIV infection was 7.8 times more likely to develop bacterial pneumonia than HIV sero-negative persons. The count of CD4+ T lymphocyte is the most consistent predictor of bacterial infections and other factors are also involved that include qualitative B-cell defects (reduced ability to produce antibody), impaired neutrophil function or both and non-HIV related factors such as cigarette smoking, use of crack cocaine, IDU, alcoholism, or liver diseases [15, 16]. The causative of bacterial pneumonia among persons with HIV has been relative prominence of *Streptococcus pneumoniae* followed by *Haemophilus influenzae, Pseudomonas aeruginosa* and *Staphylococcus aureus.* Some studies encountered *Legionella pneumophila, Mycoplasma pneumoniae* and *Chlamydia pneumoniae* that are causative organisms for atypical pneumonia. *S. pneumoniae* infection is 15–300 times more common among HIV individuals than among age-matched non-HIV individuals and also rate of recurrent pneumococcal pneumonia is 8–25% within 6 months. The second most common cause of bacterial pneumonia is *H. influenza* and in an advanced immunosuppression, *S. aureus* and *P. aeruginosa* can cause invasive pneumonias, sometimes associated with bacteremia. HIV patients ill over a period of weeks to months are more likely to have *Pneumocystis jirovecii* pneumonia, tuberculosis (caused by *Mycobacterium tuberculosis*) or chronic fungal infection.

2.2. Enteric infections

Rates of Gram-negative bacterial enteric infections are at least 10 fold higher among HIV infected persons than in the general population. Risk of bacterial enteric infections varies according to CD4 T-cell with the count of <200CD4 cells/mm^3. The common causes of bacterial diarrhea among persons with HIV are Salmonella (*Salmonella enterica* serotypes Typhimurium and Enteritidis), *Campylobacter* and *Shigella* species. Patients with HIV are at increased risk for developing salmonellosis and they have the incidence rates of salmonellosis as 20–100 folders higher than the non-HIV patients. *Campylobacter jejuni* has been reported among HIV patients particularly men who have sex with men (MSM) with the incidence rate of 39 times higher than general population. Other than these infections, *Shigella* bacteremia is more common among HIV patients and might occur in both mild and severe cases of clinical shigellosis.

The major clinical syndromes of salmonellosis among person with HIV infection include a self-limited gastroenteritis; a more severe and prolonged diarrheal disease, associated with fever, bloody diarrhea and weight loss and *Salmonella* septicemia, which might present with or without gastrointestinal symptoms. Sometimes, bacteremia can occur with each of these syndromes and is more likely to occur among those with advanced immunosuppression. Diarrheagenic *E. coli*, particularly enteroaggregative *E. coli* also contribute to the burden of diarrheal disease. The lower CD4 cell count of <50 cells/mm^3 is an independent risk factor for *Clostridium difficile* associated infection (CDI) among HIV population [15].

2.3. Urinary tract infections

The urinary tract system of human is divided into two major divisions such as upper urinary tract (kidneys, renal pelves and ureters) and lower urinary tract (urinary bladder and urethra). Urinary tract infections (UTIs) are an infection in any part of urinary system, but most UTIs occur in lower urinary tract especially bladder (cystitis). Women are at high risk of developing a UTIs then men. UTIs occur when bacteria enter and infect the urinary tract and sometimes spread to the kidneys (pyelonephritis) [17]. UTIs are one of the significant illnesses that cause clinical burden among HIV individuals. It is the most common nosocomial infection [7] and cause high rate of morbidity [18]. HIV disease is associated with a variety of renal syndromes in patients with low CD4+ cell counts, causing neurologic complications such as bladder areflexia and hyporeflexia, which lead to urinary stasis and ultimately infection [19, 20]. Once a patient's CD4+ T-cell count falls below 200 cell/mm^3, the individual is then at risk of a variety of opportunistic infection. The most predominant causative organisms are encapsulated bacteria which include *Streptococcus pneumoniae* and *Haemophilus influenzae*, but non-typhoidal *Salmonella, Staphylococcus aureus* and *Pseudomonas aeruginosa* have also been implicated. Among opportunistic infections, UTI accounts for 60% of AIDS defining illness [21]. Signs and symptoms of UTIs are pain or burning while urinating, frequent urination, feeling urinate even having an empty bladder, fever (less than 101°F), cloudy and bloody urine and pressure or cramping in the groin or lower abdomen [22].

2.4. Bloodstream infections

Even reduction of AIDS-related deaths and opportunistic infections after introduction of combined antiretroviral therapy (cART), infection with HIV causes the increased risk of bloodstream infection (BSI). It is a frequent complication found in HIV-infected patients and is usually associated with a poor prognosis, responsible for the immediate cause of death up to 32% of HIV-infected patients, especially under particular conditions (e.g., intravenous drug abuse, use of a central venous catheter (CVC), neutropenia, and a low CD4 T-cell count) [23]. BSI is associated with increased mortality rate, length of hospital stay and intensive care unit (ICU) admission rate, and it is more frequent cause of ICU admission than *Pneumocystis jirovecii* pneumonia in HIV-infected patients. In majority of cases, the BSI is due to bacterial pathogens. The infectious agents begin infecting almost any part of any organ (from skin, lung [pneumonia], gastrointestinal tract [bacterial penetration or ruptured intestine from trauma]) or through implanted devices (surgical instruments, intravenous catheter, etc.).

The infecting microorganisms or their toxins spread directly or indirectly into the bloodstream that allows spreading from infection site to any other organ system. Common bacterial causes of BSI are nontyphoidal salmonella, *Streptococcus pneumoniae*, *Escherichia coli* and *Staphylococcus aureus* are the most important pathogens of BSI. Fungal and mycobacterial infections are less frequent but have considerable clinical and economic impact. Among the pathogens responsible for BSI, *Mycobacteria* spp., *Cryptococcus neoformans* and recurrent nontyphoidal salmonella constitute AIDS-defining conditions [24]. Symptoms of BSI are altered mental status (altered consciousness, mental confusion or delirium), fast respiratory rate, low blood pressure, elevated heart rate (tachycardia), fever, body chills, dizziness, fatigue, shivering, facial flushing, skin discoloration, shock and sleepiness.

2.5. Syphilis

Syphilis is a bacterial infection caused by *Treponema pallidum* which is usually spread by sexual contact and associated with an increased risk of sexual acquisition and transmission of HIV. The disease starts as a painless sore-typically on genitalis, rectum and mouth. Direct contact with sores would spread syphilis from person to person, and the bacteria enter through minor cuts and abrasions in the skin or mucous membrane. It is contagious during its primary and secondary and early syphilis can be cured sometimes with a single dose of penicillin. Clinical manifestations of syphilis are similar to persons without HIV infection, difference is genital lesions may be more apparent and accelerated progression of disease seen in HIV population. Syphilis has various stages like primary syphilis, secondary syphilis and latent syphilis. The symptoms are small bumps or tumors called gummas, which develop on skin, bones, liver or any other organ in the late stage of syphilis. It also causes some neurological problems such as stroke, meningitis, hearing loss, visual problems, dementia, loss of pain and temperature sensations and sexual dysfunction in men, bladder incontinence and sudden lightning like pains along with fever, malaise, anorexia, arthralgias and headache. It may also cause inflammation of the aorta and miscarriage, can transfer from mother to fetus [15].

2.6. Tuberculosis

Tuberculosis (TB) is a potentially serious infectious disease mainly affects lungs. TB is mainly caused by *Mycobacterium tuberculosis* (MTB) and also caused by other organisms of *Mycobacterium tuberculosis* complex—*M. bovis*, *M. africanum*, *M. canetti*, and *M. microti* [25]. TB can also attack any part of the body including kidneys, spine and brain. TB is spread from person having lung TB to another person through the air, while cough, sneeze or spit. Transmission of TB occurs when a person inhales droplet nuclei containing *M. tuberculosis*, the droplet nuclei traverse the mouth or nasal passages, upper respiratory tract and bronchi to reach the alveoli of the lungs. In 2010, there were 8.8 (8.5–9.2 million) incident cases of TB, 1.1 million (0.9–1.2 million) deaths from TB among HIV-negative people and other 0.35 million deaths from HIV associated TB. In 2016, there were an estimated 10.4 million new cases of tuberculosis (TB) worldwide. Seven countries accounted for 64% of the total, with India leading the count, followed by Indonesia, China, Philippines, Nigeria, Pakistan and South Africa. A total of 1.7 million people died from TB in 2016 (0.4 million people with HIV) [26].

Two types of TB conditions exist: latent TB infection and TB disease. (1) Latent TB infection: Among persons with latent TB infection (LTBI), bacteria present in the body in an inactive state and cause no symptoms. It is also called inactive TB or TB infection; it has positive reaction to tuberculin skin rest or TB blood test. Persons with LTBI are not infectious and do not spread TB infection to others. Chest X-ray would be normal and negative sputum test, they do not feel sick. (2) TB disease: The symptoms of TB disease include feel of sickness or weakness, weight loss, fever and night swears, coughing, chest pain, and coughing up of blood. The signs and symptoms of active TB include coughing (lasts three or more weeks), coughing up blood, chest pain or pain with breathing or coughing, unintentional weight loss, fatigue, fever, night sweats, body chills and loss of appetite. Tuberculosis in spine may develop back pain and in kidneys might cause blood in urine.

3. Bacterial resistance to antibiotics

Antibiotics are natural microbial drugs used for the treatment and control of bacterial infections. First time the antibiotic penicillin was discovered by Fleming [27] while examining some colonies of *Staphylococcus aureus*. He observed that *Staphylococcus* colonies became transparent and undergo lysis around a large colony of mold. Finally, he identified that mold as penicillium and concluded that certain types of penicillium produced a powerful antibacterial substance that acts against pyogenic cocci and the diphtheria bacilli. Since the discovery of penicillin, many other antibiotics have been discovered or developed. Antibiotics may either kill or inhibit the growth of the bacteria and they are commonly classified based on their mechanism of action, chemical structure and spectrum of activity. Penicillins, cephalosporins and carbapenems are cell wall synthesis inhibitors, polymyxins are cell membrane synthesis inhibitors, rifamycins, lipiarmycins, quinolones, and sulfonamides interfere with the activity of essential bacterial enzymes and macrolides, lincosamides and tetracyclines are protein synthesis inhibitors [28]. The time line of antibiotic discovery was given in **Table 1**.

Antibiotic resistance is the ability of bacteria to resist the effects of drugs previously used to treat them [13]. Resistant bacteria are more difficult to treat, requiring alternative medications or higher doses, both of which may be more expensive or more toxic. Microbes resistant to multiple antimicrobials are called multidrug resistant (MDR); those extensively drug resistant (XDR) or totally drug resistant (TDR) are sometimes called "superbugs." Bacteria have various drug-resistant mechanisms contributing toward inactivation of antibiotics [30, 31] following as

- novel penicillin-binding proteins (PBPs),
- enzymatic mechanisms of drug modification,
- mutated drug targets,
- enhanced efflux pump expression and
- altered membrane permeability.

Timeline	Antibiotics	Resistance
>1910	Salvarsan	–
1921–1930	Penicillin; Prontosil	–
1940–1050	Gramicidin; Neomycin; Streptomycin; Bacitracin; Nitrofurans; Chloramphenicol; Polymyxin; Chlortetracycline; Cephalosporin	Sulfonamide; Penicillin; Spectinomycin; Bacitracin; Chloramphenicol; Streptomycin
1950–1960	Erythromycin; Isoniazid; Vancomycin; Virginiamycin; Cycloserine; Novobiocin; Kanamycin; Rifamycin; Metronidazole	Macrolide; Tetracycline; Neomycin; Nalidixic acid
1960–1970	Methicillin; Ampicillin; Nalidixic acid; Trimethoprim; Fusidic acid, Fosfomycin; Actinomycin D; Lincomycin	Methicillin; Cephalosporin; Polymyxin; Rifamycin; Vancomycin; Erythromycin; Kanamycin
1970–1990	Gentamicin; Mupirocin; Azithromycin; Carbapenem; Imipenem; Ciprofloxacin; Oxazolidinone	Metronidazole; Ampicillin; Gentamycin; Carbapenem
1990–2010	Linezolid; Telithromycin; Daptomycin; Tigecycline; Retapamulin; Garenoxacin; Telavancin; Besifloxacin; Ce-aroline fosamil	Imipenem; Ciprofloxacin; Mupirocin; Azithromycin; Linezolid; Daptomycin; Tigecycline
2010–2016	Fidaxomicin; Bedaquiline; Teixobactin	–

Table 1. Timeline of antibiotic discovery and emergence of antimicrobial resistance [29].

3.1. Factors influencing emergence of drug resistance

Various factors are involved in the emergence of antibiotic drug-resistant bacteria, the factors are inappropriate usage of antibiotics, patient movement within and between medical institutions, infection control measures, travel of people and food stuffs, antibiotic residues in the environment, dose duration and treatment, cross selection, gene transfer and clonal spread and socioeconomic factors [31]. The time line of development of antibiotic resistance was presented in **Table 2**.

3.2. β-Lactamases

The production of β-lactamase enzymes is the most common mechanism of bacterial resistance to β-lactam antibiotics such as the penicillins and cephalosporins. These enzymes catalyze the hydrolysis of the β-lactam ring to create ineffective antimicrobials. β-Lactamases were first identified in *Staphylococcus aureus* strains in the late 1940s, prior to the introduction of penicillin into the clinical setting [46]. Some β-lactamases are having substrate specificities relatively narrow and these are often traditionally referred as penicillinases or cephalosporinases. Over 400 β-lactamases have been reported to date, and new β-lactamases continue to

Infections, Reference/ Country	Isolated bacteria	Drug resistance
RTI (Peru) [32]	*M. tuberculosis*	MDR-TB -43% Isoniazid resistance – 4%; Isoniazid, rifampicin and pyrazinamide – 32%; Isoniazid, rifampicin, ethambutol, streptomycin and pyrazinamide – 14%
UTI (India) [33]	*Escherichia coli, 10.3%* *S. aureus, 5%* *K. pneumoniae, 4%* *E. faecalis, 2%,* *P. aeruginosa 1%* *Proteus* spp *.1%* *S. epidermidis, 1%*	Amp, ctx, cip, sxt-33.3%; amp, ctx, cip, nit, sxt- 27.8%
BSI (Combodia) [34]	*Escherichia coli, 30.7%* *S. choleraesuis, 11.4%* *Nontyphoidal* *Salmonella* spp. *6.8%* *S. typhi, 2.3%* *Klebsiella* spp. *5.7%* *Enterobacter* spp *3.4%* *B. pseudomallei, 2.3%* *Pseudomonas* sp. *3.4%* *Acinetobacter* sp.2. *9%* *S. aureus, 19.3%* *Streptococcus suis, 1.1%* *Enterococci, 1.1%*	*E. coli:* amx-96%; cot-80%; cip-61%; amc-57%; ctr-46%; gen-57% S. typhi: cip-100%; amx and cot-50% Nontyphoidal *Salmonella* spp.: amx-80%; cot-60%; cip-40% *S. aureus:* oxa-28%; cot-28%
UTI (India) [35]	*E. coli, 100%*	*FQ resistance: 77.6%; ESBL and AmpC-71.1%* *ESBL-3.9%*
RTI (India) [36]	*M. tuberculosis*	MDR-TB – 38%;XDR-TB- 6%; Mono-resistant TB - 21%; Poly-resistant TB – 12%; Extremely drug-resistant TB – 2%
UTI and WI (Tanzania) [37]	*E. coli, 56%;* *K. pneumoniae, 37%* *S. aureus, 72%* *Proteus* spp. *43%* *P. aeruginosa, 38%*	Cot-75%; amc-34%; cip-33.3%; amp-86.4%; cro-66.7%; tet-81.3%; ery-27.3%

Infections, Reference/ Country	Isolated bacteria	Drug resistance
UTI (Nigeria) [38]	*E. coli, 30%* *K. pneumoniae, 14.2%* *P. aeruginosa, 27.6%* *S. aureus, 28.3%*	*E. coli: caz-95.2%; oxa-92.8%; amp-88%; chl-73.8%; cro-69%; tet-50%; nit-45.2%; cot & ery-42.9%*
UTI & BSI (India) [39]	*E. coli, 51%* *K. pneumoniae, 14.6%* *K. oxytoca, 12.6%* *P. aeruginosa, 11.2%* *Proteus mirabilis, 7.3%* *P. vulgaris, 2.6%*	Ery-99%; amp-94%; cpd-91%; atm-90%; cfp & fox-89.4%; pip-85.4%; caz-84.8%; cro-74.2%; ipm-73.5%; tzp-72.4%; tet-66.9%; cip-66.2%; dox-58.2%
Nasopharynx colonization (Ghana) [40]	*M. catarrhalis*, 39.8%; Coagulase negative *staphylococci*, 33.1%; *S. pneumoniae*, 30.5%; Diphtheroids, 29.7%; Viridian streptococci, 27.1%; *S. aureus*, 22%; *Citrobacter* spp. 4.2%;	*M. catarrhalis*: amp-80%; CoT-60%; mrp-42.6%; chl-23% *S. aureus*: pcn-100%; tet-80%; cfx-73%; ery-38% *S. pneumoniae:* cot-58%; tet-33%; ery-33%; oxa-27%
EI(Cameroon) [41]	*E. coli*, 85.3% *Klebsiella* spp. 29.4% *Enterobacter* spp. & *Citrobacter* spp. 23.5% *Salmonella* sp. 5.9% *Serratia* sp. 1.5% *Proteus* sp. 2.9%	*E. coli*: amx-60.3%; amc-62%; cro-39.6%; chl-32.7%; dox-91.3% *Klebsiella* spp: amx, amc – 100%; dox-70%; tet-50%; chl-35 *Enterobacter* spp: amx, amc-93.7%; dox-87.5%; tet-63.8%; chl and cip-37.5% *Citrobacter* sp.: amx, amc, cro-43.7%; dox-68.7%; tet-30% *Salmonella* spp.: dox & chl-75% *Serratia* spp: amx, amc, chl & dox- 100%
UTI (India) [42]	*E. coli*, 50.7% *K. pneumoniae, 13.2%* *K. oxytoca, 11.8%* *P. mirabilis, 6.3%* *P. vulgaris, 1.4%* *P. aeruginosa, 5.5%*	Azt-94.6%; cpd-93.8%; cefoperazone-91.3%, fox-90.3%; ctx-89%, amp-89%, ipm-72% Enterobacteriaceae- ESBL-52.5%; MBL & AmpC- 62.5% *P. aeruginosa*- ESBL-50%; MBL and AmpC-62.5%

Infections, Reference/ Country	Isolated bacteria	Drug resistance
UTI (Tanzania)	*E. coli, 57.7%*	*E. coli*: amp-93.3%; sxt-90%; amc-43.3%;
[43]	*K. pneumoniae, 23.1%*	*K. pneumoniae*: amp-100%; sxt-72.7%; nit-33.3%; amc-54.5%
	C. freundii, 3.9%	
	S. aureus, 3.9%	
	P. agglomerans, 1.9%	
	S. agalactiae, 1.9%	
RTI (China)	*P. aeruginosa, 24.1%*	MRSA-3%; VRE-1%; ESBL-62%;
[44]	*E. coli, 16%*	Multidrug resistant TB-22%
	A. baumannii, 15.1%	Extensively drug-resistant TB-3.5%
	K. pneumoniae, 13.4%	
	Stenotrophomonas maltophilia, 11.6%	
	S. aureus, 4.4%	
	S. pneumoniae, 1.8%	
	Tuberculosis-19.3%	
OM (Tanzania)	*P. aeruginosa, 6.4%*	*P. aeruginosa:* amp-73.3%; amc-53.3%; ery-40%
[45]	*E. coli, 5.3%*	*E. coli*: amp & fox- 51.4%; ery-45.9%
	K. oxytoca, 5%	*K. oxytoca*: ery-62.5%; fox-50%; amp-43.8%
	K. pneumoniae, 12.4%	*K. pneumoniae*: amp-51.2%; amc-48.6%
	S. aureus, 45.7%	*S. aureus*: amp-46.5%; fox-42.7%; ery-37.4%
	M. catarrhalis, 3.2%	*M. catarrhalis:* amk & amp-55.6%
	P. mirabilis, 1.1%	*P. mirabilis*: ery-100%; amc & amp- 66.7%
	S. epidermidis, 5.0%	*S. epidermidis:* ery-64.3%; fox-55.5%; amp-50%
	S. pneumoniae, 2.5%	*S. pneumoniae:* ery-71.4%; fox-42.9%
		S. pyogenes: amp-48.7%; ery-42.1%

RTI: respiratory tract infections; BSI: blood stream infection; UTI: urinary tract infection; WI: wound infection; EI: enteric infection; OM: Otitis Media; amk – amikacin; amx – amoxicillin; amc - amoxicillin-clavulanic acid; amp – ampicillin; ctx – cefotaxime; fox – cefoxitin; cpd – cefpodoxime; caz – ceftazidime; cro – ceftriaxone; chl – chloramphenicol; cip – ciprofloxacin; dox – doxycycline; ery – erythromycin; gen – gentamicin; ipm – imipenemmem – meropenem; nit – nitrofurantoin; oxa – oxacillin; pen – penicillin; pip – piperacillin; tzp - piperacillin-tazobactam; tmp – trimethoprim; sxt - trimethoprim-sulfamethoxazole.

Table 2. Bacterial infections and drug resistance in HIV patients.

emerge rapidly worldwide [47, 48]. β-Lactamase producing organisms pose a major problem for clinical therapeutics. The incidence of β- lactamase producing strains among clinical has been steadily increasing over the past few years resulting in limitation of therapeutic options. β-Lactamases are classified based on the molecules (Ambler Classification) and functions (Bush-Jacoby-Medeiros classification) of the enzymes [49]. Most important β-lactamase enzymes are extended spectrum β-lactamases (ESBLs), AmpC β- lactamase (AmpC) and Metallo β-lactamase (MBL).

4. Drug-resistant bacteria from HIV patients

Human immunodeficiency virus (HIV)-infected individuals are highly vulnerable to a various opportunistic infections (OIs) due to their compromised immune system. For the prophylaxis of OIs, HIV patients are frequently exposed to high level of antimicrobial agents which leads to the emergence of multidrug-resistant bacteria. MDR bacteria become a major problem in the clinical management of HIV disease. Treatment of common bacterial infections like acute respiratory tract infections, urinary tract infections, wound infections, meningitis, and blood stream infections are very difficult when they are associated with MDR bacteria leading to increased morbidity and mortality. Multidrug resistant (MDR) pathogens are relentlessly multiplying in HIV patients and thus become an important circulating source of infection in the community. Globally, very few scientific data are available on the drug-resistant bacteria from HIV population.

Co-trimoxazole (also called as trimethoprim-sulfamethoxazole (TMP-SMX)) is a broad-spectrum antibiotic, used as a prophylactic agent against opportunistic infections among HIV/AIDS patients. Especially, TMP-SMX is an active drug against Pneumocystis pneumonia (PCP) caused by *Pneumocystis jirovecii* among HIV-infected patients [50, 51]. World Health Organization and Joined Nations Programme on HIV/AIDS have recommended TMP-SMX prophylaxis for immunosuppressed adults and children born to HIV-infected women [52–54]. Long-term receiving of TMP-SMX prophylaxis has lead to increase in the development of TMP-SMX-resistant bacteria, which spreading in the bacterial community and cause therapeutic problems for bacterial infections in HIV population. In Enterobacteriaceae, sulfonamide drug resistance genes such as *sul1*, *sul2*, and *sul3* are responsible for dihydropteroate synthases, and more than 20 dihydrofolate reductase (*dfr*) genes conferring resistance to trimethoprim [55] (**Table 2**).

UTI accounts for consumption of large proportion of anti-bacterial drugs [18]. Resistance to commonly prescribed antibiotics for UTI is an expanding global problem both in developed as well as developing countries [56]. UTI became quite alarming as isolated uropathogens exhibit high percentage resistance to almost all antibiotics [57]. The pattern of antibacterial susceptibility of UTI causing pathogen has been changing over the years, and the drug resistant of the bacteria is influenced by the extensive and misuse of antibiotics and changing patient population, especially among immunocompromised patients. β-Lactam antibiotics such as penicillins, cephalosporins and carbapenems are the most commonly used antibacterial drugs. The predominant drug resistance mechanisms against β-lactam antibiotics among Gram-negative bacteria are the production of Extended Spectrum β-lactamases (ESBLs) and AmpC β-lactamases [58] and they are associated with increased morbidity and mortality with immunocompromised individuals. The frequency of *Pseudomonas aeruginosa* and *Staphylococcus aureus* as community-acquired pathogens is higher in HIV-infected individuals than in those not HIV infected. Methicillin-resistant *Staphylococcus aureus* (MRSA) infection should be considered as a potential etiology for pneumonia, given that community outbreaks of MRSA have been seen in men who have sex with men and nasal carriage of MRSA is more common in HIV-infected individuals, particularly at lower CD4 cell counts. Multidrug resistance (MDR) bacteria like ESBL producers and MRSA are a major public health concern worldwide [21, 39] (**Table 2**).

WHO has documented that MDR-TB is emerging as a major challenge for tuberculosis control programs and is becoming extensively widespread today throughout the world, even in high-income countries with low TB incidence. Resistance to anti-TB drugs occurs due to misuse of drugs such as patients do not compete full course of treatment, wrong treatment provide by physicians, wrong dose or length of time for taking the drugs and supply of poor quality drugs. Multidrug-resistant TB is caused by *Mycobacterium tuberculosis* that is resistant to at least to two most potent TB drugs such as isoniazid and rifampicin. Extensively drug-resistant TB (XDR-TB) is MTB resistant to isoniazid and rifampicin along with any fluoroquinolone and at least one of three injectable second-line drugs includes amikacin, kanamycin or capreomycin. Treatment options for XDR-TB have more side effects, and they are more expensive. XDR-TB can weaken the immune system, and persons are more likely to develop TB disease and they are at high risk of death.

In 2010, about 650,000 cases have MDR-TB, which account for 5% of all newly diagnosed TB patients, and more than 150,000 MDR-TB deaths are estimated to occur worldwide each year with case fatality rate of 30 per 100 individuals [59]. The proportion of MDR-TB reported globally ranges from 0 to 28.3% and 0 to 61.6% among new TB cases and among previously treated TB cases respectively [60]. People living with HIV are at a higher risk of developing MDR and XDR tuberculosis associated with increased mortality, and greatly reduced survival time of patients [61] (**Table 2**).

5. Future impact of antimicrobial resistance

The two multidisciplinary research teams such as RAND Europe and KPMG, have provided their own high-level assessments of the future impact of antimicrobial resistance, based on scenarios for rising drug resistance and economic growth to 2050. The studies estimate 300 million people are expected to die prematurely due to drug resistance over the next 35 years and the world's Gross Domestic Product (GDP) will be 2% to 3.5% lower than it otherwise would be in 2050. This means that between now and 2050, the world can expect to lose between 60 and 100 trillion USD worth of economic output if antimicrobial drug resistance is not tackled. This is equivalent to the loss of around 1 year's total global output over the period, and will create significant and widespread human suffering. Furthermore, in the nearer term, they expect the world's GDP to be 0.5% smaller by 2020 and 1.4% smaller by 2030 with more than 100 million people having died prematurely [62].

6. Tackle of antimicrobial resistance

WHO developed a global priority of pathogens list (global PPL) of antibiotic-resistant bacteria to help in prioritizing the research and development (R&D) of new and effective antibiotic treatments. Drug-resistant bacteria were categorized into critical priority, high priority and medium priority pathogens (**Table 3**) [63].

Type of priority	List of drug-resistant pathogens
Critical priority	Carbapenem-resistant *Acinetobacter baumannii;* Carbapenem-resistant *Pseudomonas aeruginosa;* Carbapenem-resistant, 3rd generation cephalosporin-resistant *Enterobacteriaceae*
Medium priority	Penicillin-non-susceptible *Streptococcus pneumonia;* Ampicillin-resistant *Haemophilus influenza;* Fluoroquinolone-resistant *Shigella* spp.
High priority	Vancomycin-resistant *Enterococcus faecium;* Methicillin-resistant, Vancomycin-intermediate and resistant *Staphylococcus aureus*
	Clarithromycin -resistant *Helicobacter pylori;* Fluoroquinolone-resistant *Campylobacter;* Fluoroquinolone-resistant *Salmonella* spp.
	3rd generation cephalosporin-resistant, fluoroquinolone-resistant *Neisseria gonorrhoeae*

Table 3. Global priority of pathogens list by World Health Organization.

7. Global action plan, WHO

WHO developed the global action plan with five strategic objectives to achieve the goal of ensuring continuity of successful treatment and prevention of infectious diseases with effective and safe medicines [64]. They (1) improve the awareness and understanding of antimicrobial resistance through effective communication, education and training, (2) strengthen the knowledge and evidence base through surveillance and research, (3) reduce the incidence of infection through effective sanitation, hygiene and infection prevention measures, (4) optimize the use of antimicrobial medicines in human and animal health and (5) develop the economic case for sustainable investment that takes account of the needs of all countries, and increase investment in new medicines, diagnostic tools, vaccines and other interventions.

7.1. Examples for global impact of antimicrobial resistance research and interventions

Examples of global research into antimicrobial resistance and its impact are given below [29]:

- Chinese Ministry of Health in 2011, reduced unnecessary prescription of antimicrobials by 10–12%.
- The Swedish Strategic Programme against Antibiotic Resistance (STRAMA): decrease in antibiotic use for outpatients from 15.7 to 12.6 daily doses per 1000 inhabitants and from 536 to 410 prescriptions per 1000 inhabitants per year from 1995 to 2004. The decrease was most evident for macrolides (65%).
- WHO essential medicines policies: reductions in antibiotic use of ≥20% in upper respiratory tract infections and 30% of reduction in the use of antibiotics in acute diarrheal illness.
- Antimicrobial stewardship programme (2009–2014) in 47 South African hospitals: reduction of antibiotic doses daily per 100 patient days from 101.4 to 83.04.

- Antimicrobial Resistance Monitoring and Research Programme (United States): Infections with carbapenem-resistant Enterobacteriaceae declined and there were no further reports of outbreaks of colistin-resistant *Acinetobacter* spp.
- In the Netherlands, a decrease of CTX-M^{-1}-1-like ESBL genes (from 44 to 25%) in livestock was seen during 2010–2014 due to >60% reduction in antibiotic use in livestock.

8. Conclusion(s)

Spread of antibiotic-resistant bacteria is leading to untreatable infections causing a major public health threat. Handling of new approaches such as combination therapeutics, organism specific drugs and repurposing of antibiotics might helpful in the treatment of drug-resistant bacterial infections on stipulated time and reduce the burden in clinical settings. Effective global investments are needed to improve the way prevent, control and monitor the emergence and global spread of drug resistance.

Conflict of interest

There is no conflict of interest to declare.

Author details

Marimuthu Ragavan Rameshkumar[1] and Narasingam Arunagirinathan[2,3*]

*Address all correspondence to: n_arunagiri@yahoo.co.in

1 Infectious Diseases Laboratory, Y. R. Gaitonde Centre for AIDS Research and Education, Voluntary Health Service Hospital, Chennai, India

2 Department of Microbiology, Presidency College (Autonomous), Chennai, India

3 Faculty of Humanities and Science, Meenakshi Academy of Higher Education and Research, Chennai, India

References

[1] Centers for Disease Control and Prevention. Kaposi's sarcoma and *Pneumocystis pneumonia* among homosexual men—New York City and California. MMWR. 1981;**30**:305-308

[2] Centers for Disease Control and Prevention. *Pneumocystis pneumonia*—Los Angeles. MMWR. 1981;**30**:250-252

[3] World Health Organization. HIV and AIDS. 2018. Available from: http://www.who.int/news-room/fact-sheets/detail/hiv-aids [Accessed: April 05, 2018]

[4] US Department of Veteran Affairs. HIV and AIDS. 2018. Available from: https://www.hiv.va.gov/patient/basics/how-HIV-spread.asp [Accessed: April 05, 2018]

[5] Centers for Disease Control and Prevention. HIV transmission. Available from: https://t.cdc.gov/synd.aspx?js=0&rid=cs_3605&url=http://t.cdc.gov/VIK [Accessed: May 05, 2018]

[6] Doitsh G, Galloway NL, Geng X, Yang Z, Monroe KM, Zepeda O, Hunt PW, Hatano H, Sowinski S, Muñoz-Arias I, Greene WC. Cell death by pyroptosis drives CD4 T-cell depletion in HIV-1 infection. Nature. 2014;**505**:509. DOI: 10.1038/nature12940

[7] Deokar S, Badhankar MG. Studies on emergence of drug resistance in HIV associated bacterial urinary tract infections. American Journal of Infectious Diseases. 2009;**5**:183-187

[8] Cunningham AL, Donaghy H, Harman AN, Kim M, Turville SG. Manipulation of dendritic cell function by viruses. Current Opinion in Microbiology. 2010;**13**:524-529. DOI: 10.1016/j.mib.2010.06.002

[9] Garg H, Mohl J, Joshi A. HIV-1 induced bystander apoptosis. Viruses. 2012;**4**:3020-3043. DOI: 10.3390/v4113020

[10] National AIDS Control Organisation. Guidelines for Prevention and Management of Common Opportunistic Infections/Malignancies Among HIV-Infected Adult and Adolescent. New Delhi: NACO, Government of India; 2007. p. 2

[11] Jaspan HB, Huang LC, Cotton MF, Whitelaw A, Myer L. Bacterial disease and antimicrobial susceptibility patterns in HIV-infected, hospitalized children: A retrospective cohort study. PLoS One. 2008;**3**:1-6. DOI: 10.1371/journal.pone.0003260

[12] Abraham M, De N, Sudi IY, Ma'ori L. Isolation of methicillin resistant *Staphylococcus aureus* (MRSA) from AIDS patients attending the state specialist hospital, Yola and Federal Medical Centre, Yola, Adamawa State, Nigeria. Report and Opinion. 2009;**1**:103-107

[13] Siegel JD, Rhinehart E, Jackson M, Chiarell L. Management of multidrug resistant organisms in healthcare settings. CDC. 2006;**2006**:1-74. DOI: 10.1016/j.ajic.2007.10.006

[14] Feikin DR, Feldman C, Schuchat A, Janoff EN. Global strategies to prevent bacterial pneumonia in adults with HIV disease. The Lancet Infectious Diseases. 2004;**4**:445-455. DOI: 10.1016/S1473-3099(04)01060-6

[15] Department of Health and Human Services. AIDS Info. HIV and Opportunistic Infections, Coinfections, and Conditions. 2017. Available from: https://aidsinfo.nih.gov/understanding-hiv-aids/fact-sheets/26/86/what-is-an-opportunistic-infection [Accessed: April 12, 2018]

[16] Mayo Clinic. Pneumonia. 2018. Available from: https://www.mayoclinic.org/diseases-conditions/pneumonia/symptoms-causes/syc-20354204 [Accessed: April 12, 2018]

[17] Lane DR, Takhar SS. Diagnosis and management of urinary tract infection and pyelonephritis. Emergency Medicine Clinics of North America. 2011;**29**:539-552. DOI: 10.1016/j.emc.2011.04.001

[18] Iweriebor BC, Obi CL, Akinyemi O, Ramalivhana NJ, Hattori T, Okoh AI. Uropathogens isolated from HIV-infected patients from Limpopo province, South Africa. African Journal of Biotechnology. 2012;**11**:10598-10604. DOI: 10.5897/AJB10.2413

[19] Rashmi KS, Ravi Kumar KI, Rhagyashree HN. Asymptomatic bacteriuria in HIV/AIDS patients occurrence and risk associated with low CD4 counts. JEMDS. 2013;**2**:3358-3360. DOI: 10.14260/jemds/705

[20] Staiman VR, Lowe FC. Urologic problems in patients with acquired immunodeficiency syndrome. Scientific World Journal. 2004;**4**:427-437. DOI: 10.1100/tsw.2004.84

[21] Hidron AI, Kempker R, Moanna A, Rimland D. Methicillin-resistant *Staphylococcus aureus* in HIV-infected patients. Infection and Drug Resistance. 2010;**3**:73-86

[22] Mayo Clinic. Urinary Tract Infection. 2017. Available from: https://www.mayoclinic.org/diseases-conditions/urinary-tract-infection/diagnosis-treatment/drc-20353453 [Accessed: April 14, 2018]

[23] Tumbarello M, Tacconelli E, Caponera S, Cauda R, Ortona L. The impact of bacteremia on HIV infection. Nine years experience in a large Italian university hospital. The Journal of Infection. 1995;**31**:123-131. DOI: 10.1016/S0163-4453(95)92110-9

[24] Taramasso L, Tatarelli P, Di Biagio A. Bloodstream infections in HIV-infected patients. Virulence. 2016;**7**(3):320-328. DOI: 10.1080/21505594.2016.1158359

[25] van Ingen J, Rahim Z, Mulder A, Boeree MJ, Simeone R, Brosch R, van Soolingen D. Characterization of *Mycobacterium orygis* as *M. tuberculosis* complex subspecies. Emerging Infectious Diseases. 2012;**18**(4):653. DOI: 10.3201/eid1804.110888

[26] World Health Organization. Tuberculosis. 2017. Available from: http://www.afro.who.int/health-topics/tuberculosis-tb [Accessed: April 15, 2018]

[27] Fleming A. On the antibacterial action of cultures of a penicillium, with special reference to their use in the isolation of *B. influenzae*. British Journal of Experimental Pathology. 1929;**10**:226-236

[28] Finberg RW, Moellering RC, Tally FP, Craig WA, Pankey GA, Dellinger EP, West MA, Joshi M, Linden PK, Rolston KV, Rotschafer JC. The importance of bactericidal drugs: Future directions in infectious disease. Clinical Infectious Diseases. 2004;**39**:1314-1320. DOI: 10.1086/425009

[29] Das B, Chaudhuri S, Srivastava R, Nair GB, Ramamurthy T. Fostering research into antimicrobial resistance in India. BMJ. 2017;**358**:j3535. DOI: 10.1136/bmj.j3535

[30] Alekshun MN, Levy SB. Molecular mechanisms of antibacterial multidrug resistance. Cell. 2007;**128**:1037-1050. DOI: 10.1016/j.cell.2007.03.004

[31] Levy SB. Factors impacting on the problem of antibiotic resistance. The Journal of Antimicrobial Chemotherapy. 2002;**49**:25-30. DOI: 10.1093/jac/49.1.25

[32] Campos PE, Suarez PG, Sanchez J, Zavala D, Arevalo J, Ticona E, Nolan CM, Hooton TM, Holmes KK. Multidrug-resistant *Mycobacterium tuberculosis* in HIV-infected persons, Peru. Emerging Infectious Diseases. 2003;**9**:1571. DOI: 10.3201/eid0912.020731

[33] Vignesh R, Shankar EM, Murugavel KG, Kumarasamy N, Sekar R, Irene P, Solomon S, Balakrishnan P. Urinary infections due to multi-drug-resistant *Escherichia coli* among persons with HIV disease at a tertiary AIDS care Centre in South India. Nephron. Clinical Practice. 2008;**110**:c55-c57. DOI: 10.1159/000151533

[34] Phe T, Vlieghe E, Reid T, Harries AD, Lim K, Thai S, Smet B, Veng C, Kham C, Ieng S, Griensven J. Does HIV status affect the aetiology, bacterial resistance patterns and recommended empiric antibiotic treatment in adult patients with bloodstream infection in Cambodia? Tropical Medicine & International Health. 2013;**18**:485-494. DOI: 10.1111/tmi.12060

[35] Padmavathy K, Padma K, Rajasekaran S. Extended-spectrum β-lactamase/AmpC-producing uropathogenic *Escherichia coli* from HIV patients: Do they have a low virulence score? Journal of Medical Microbiology. 2013;**62**(3):345-351. DOI: 10.1099/jmm.0.050013-0

[36] Isaakidis P, Das M, Kumar AM, Peskett C, Khetarpal M, Bamne A, Adsul B, Manglani M, Sachdeva KS, Parmar M, Kanchar A. Alarming levels of drug-resistant tuberculosis in HIV-infected patients in metropolitan Mumbai, India. PLoS One. 2014;**21**(9):e110461. DOI: 10.1371/journal.pone.0110461

[37] Marwa KJ, Mushi MF, Konje E, Alele PE, Kidola J, Mirambo MM. Resistance to cotrimoxazole and other antimicrobials among isolates from HIV/AIDS and non-HIV/AIDS patients at Bugando Medical Centre, Mwanza, Tanzania. AIDS Research and Treatment. 2015;**2015**:1-8. DOI: 10.1155/2015/103874

[38] Kemajou TS, Ajugwo AO, Oshoma CE, Enabulele OI. Antibiotic resistance of bacterial isolates from HIV positive patients with Urinary Tract Infection (UTI) in Portharcourt, Nigeria. Journal of AIDS and Clinical Research. 2016;7:594. DOI: 10.4172/2155-6113.1000594

[39] Ramesh Kumar MR, Arunagirinathan N, Srivani S, Dhanasezhian A, Vijaykanth N, Manikandan N, Balakrishnan S, Vignesh R, Balakrishnan P, Solomon S, Solomon SS. Dissemination of trimethoprim–sulfamethoxazole drug resistance genes associated with class 1 and class 2 integrons among gram-negative bacteria from HIV patients in South India. Microbial Drug Resistance. 2016;**23**:602-608. DOI: 10.1089/mdr.2016.0034

[40] Sampane-Donkor E, Badoe EV, Annan JA, Nii-Trebi N. Colonisation of antibiotic resistant bacteria in a cohort of HIV infected children in Ghana. The Pan African Medical Journal. 2017;**26**:60. DOI: 10.11604/pamj.2017.26.60.10981

[41] Marbou WJ, Kuete V. Bacterial resistance and immunological profiles in HIV-infected and non-infected patients at Mbouda AD LUCEM Hospital in Cameroon. Journal of Infection and Public Health. 2017;**10**:269-276. DOI: 10.1016/j.jiph.2016.04.009

[42] Kumar MR, Arunagirinathan N, Vignesh R, Balakrishnan P, Solomon S, Sunil SS. Ertapenem for multiple β-lactamases producing Gram-negative bacteria causing urinary tract infections in HIV patients. Journal of Research in Medical Sciences. 2017;**22**:69. DOI: 10.4103/jrms.JRMS_884_16

[43] Chaula T, Seni J, Ng'walida N, Kajura A, Mirambo MM, DeVinney R, Mshana SE. Urinary

tract infections among HIV-positive pregnant women in Mwanza City, Tanzania, are high and predicted by low CD4. International Journal of Microbiology. 2017;**2017**:4042686. DOI: 10.1155/2017/4042686

[44] Pang W, Shang P, Li Q, Xu J, Bi L, Zhong J, Pei X. Prevalence of opportunistic infections and causes of death among hospitalized HIV-infected patients in Sichuan, China. The Tohoku Journal of Experimental Medicine. 2018;**244**(3):231-242. DOI: 10.1620/tjem.244.231

[45] Mwambete KD, Eulambius M. High prevalence of antibiotic-resistant otitis media–associated bacterial flora of asymptomatic people living with HIV at Morogoro Hospital, Tanzania. JIAPAC. 2018;**13**:2325958218759761. DOI: 10.1177/2325958218759761

[46] Abraham EP, Chain E. An enzyme from bacteria able to destroy penicillin. Nature. 1940;**146**:837

[47] Jacoby GA, Munoz-Price LS. The new β-lactamases. The New England Journal of Medicine. 2005;**352**:380-391. DOI: 10.1056/NEJMra041359

[48] Miriagou V, Tassios PT, Legakis NJ, Tzouvelekis LS. Expanded-spectrum cephalosporin resistance in non-typhoid *Salmonella*. International Journal of Antimicrobial Agents. 2004;**23**:547-555. DOI: 10.1016/j.ijantimicag.2004.03.006

[49] Török E, Moran ED, Cooke F. Oxford Handbook of Infectious Diseases and Microbiology. New York: Oxford University Press; 2010. pp. 29-126

[50] Hardy WD, Feinberg J, Finkelstein DM, Power ME, He W, Kaczka C, Frame PT, Holmes M, Waskin H, Fass RJ, Powderly WG. A controlled trial of trimethoprim–sulfamethoxazole or aerosolized pentamidine for secondary prophylaxis of *Pneumocystis carinii* pneumonia in patients with the acquired immunodeficiency syndrome: AIDS Clinical Trials Group protocol 021. The New England Journal of Medicine. 1992;**327**:1842-1848. DOI: 10.1056/NEJM199212243272604

[51] Chintu C, Bhat GJ, Walker AS, Mulenga V, Sinyinza F, Lishimpi K, Farrelly L, Kaganson N, Zumla A, Gillespie SH, Nunn AJ, Gibb DM, trial team CHAP. Co-trimoxazole as prophylaxis against opportunistic infections in HIV-infected Zambian children (CHAP): A double-blind randomized placebo-controlled trial. Lancet. 2004;**364**:1865-1871. DOI: 10.1016/S0140-6736(04)17442-4

[52] World Health Organization. Provisional WHO/ UNAIDS Secretariat Recommendations on the Use of Cotrimoxazole Prophylaxis in Adults and Children Living with HIV/AIDS in Africa. Geneva, Switzerland: WHO/UNAIDS; 2000

[53] World Health Organization. Guidelines on Cotrimoxazole Prophylaxis for HIV Related Infections. Geneva, Switzerland: WHO; 2006

[54] Bpharm MS, Chimzizi R, Chotpitayasunondh T, Crowley S, Duncombe C. Guidelines on co-trimoxazole prophylaxis for HIV-related infections among children adolescents and adults. Recommendations for a public health approach. Geneca, Switzerland: WHO/UNAIDS; 2006

[55] Mazel D. Integrons: Agents of bacterial evolution. Nature Reviews. Microbiology. 2006;**4**: 608. DOI: 10.1038/nrmicro1462

[56] Biradar SK, Doddamani S, PK. Prevalence and anti-biogram of uropathogens in a tertiary care hospital. World Journal of Pharmaceutical Research. 2013;**2**:1534-1543. DOI: 10.3329/jsr.v9i3.31677

[57] Murugan K, Savitha T, Vasanthi S. Retrospective study of antibiotic resistance among Uropathogens from rural teaching hospital, Tamilnadu, India. Asian Pacific Journal of Tropical Disease. 2012;**2**:375-380. DOI: 10.1016/s2222-1808 (12) 60082-6

[58] Paterson DL, Bonomo RA. Extended-spectrum β-lactamases: A clinical update. Clinical Microbiology Reviews. 2005;**18**:657-686. DOI: 10.1128/CMR.18.4.657-686.2005

[59] World Health Organization. Global Tuberculosis Control. Surveillance, Planning, Financing. 2008. Available from: http://apps.who.int/iris/handle/10665/43831 [Accessed: April 25, 2018]

[60] World Health Organization. Global Report on Surveillance and Response on Multidrug and Extensively Drug-Resistant TB (M/XDR-TB). 2010. Available from: http://apps.who.int/iris/handle/10665/44286 [Accessed: April 26, 2018]

[61] Joshua F. MDR-TB and HIV: The perfect storm; University of California. The American Journal of Tropical Medicine and Hygiene. 2006;**75**:1025-1026

[62] O'Neill J. Tackling drug-resistant infections globally: Final report and recommendations. The review on antimicrobial resistance; London: HM Government and the Wellcome Trust; 2016

[63] World Health Organization. Global Priority List of Antibiotic-Resistant Bacteria to Guide Research, Discovery and Development of New Antibiotics. 2017. Available from: http://apps.who.int/medicinedocs/documents/s23171en/s23171en.pdf [Accessed: April 24, 2018]

[64] World Health Organization. Global Action Plan on Antimicrobial Resistance. Available from: http://www.who.int/antimicrobial-resistance/global-action-plan/en/ [Accessed: April 24, 2018]

5

The Process of Adherence to Treatment in People Living with HIV

Ariagor Manuel Almanza Avendaño,
Martha Patricia Romero Mendoza and
Anel Hortensia Gómez San Luis

Abstract

The purpose of this chapter is to review the concept of adherence and analyze its implications for the social construction of the patient as a subject, since this affects the relationship established with the health services for the maintenance of care. The facilitators and barriers to adherence reported in the literature are presented, based on studies focused on the perspective of people living with HIV. At the end of the chapter, the individual elements that promote adherence to treatment are shown, according to the experience of highly adherent patients. In addition, individual and contextual barriers to the adherence process are identified in the pharmacological and nonpharmacological dimensions.

Keywords: adherence, medical treatment, lifestyle, facilitators, barriers

1. Introduction

The development of highly active antiretroviral treatment (HAART) has allowed HIV infection to become a chronic condition. This historic event has transformed the experience of people living with HIV, since it has allowed them to extend their survival time and increase their quality of life [1]. However, this biomedical breakthrough has generated important challenges for public health. One of them is universal access to treatment. Social inequality in terms of the intersection between gender, social class, ethnic group, sexual orientation, or geographical region places patients at different levels of vulnerability regarding access to treatment. Likewise, social inequality affects the continuity of long-term treatment, as patients differ in access to services that allow maintaining care over time as food, education, health, housing, employment, and transportation, among others. For this reason, public health cannot be limited to a "pharmaceuticalization" or exclusive emphasis on access to medication, but it requires considering the social and economic conditions that affect the possibilities of patients to maintain a long-term pharmacological treatment [2].

The second challenge, which is addressed in this chapter, is the promotion of adherence to treatment in people living with HIV. This challenge is linked to the facilitation of psychosocial processes that allow long-term adherence, while the previous challenge focuses mainly on the structural conditions associated with adherence. Unlike pharmacological treatment for other medical conditions, HAART requires an efficacy greater than 95% to control the number of copies of the virus in the body. The suboptimal medication intake is associated with higher levels of morbidity and mortality as well as the emergence of drug-resistant viral strains. This reduces the effectiveness of subsequent treatment schemes [3].

The lack of adherence to treatment has multiple consequences for the state: increased expenses for hospitalization, care for opportunistic infections, and changes in treatment schemes and laboratory studies. In turn, lack of adherence increases the risk of HIV transmission in populations and the development of new strains resistant to treatment [4].

The study of adherence to treatment in people living with HIV has focused mainly on pharmacological adherence. It is necessary to develop a comprehensive perspective on adherence, which not only includes medication intake but also the adoption of a healthy lifestyle in multiple areas. The following section analyzes the concept of adherence and its influence on the patient's relationship with health services.

2. Perspectives on adherence

The social construction of adherence influences the way in which patients are constituted as subjects, the type of relationships they establish with health personnel, and the policies of health services for patient care. Previously the term "compliance" was used to refer to the degree to which the patient followed medical recommendations for taking the medication or making lifestyle changes. The concept was criticized because it assumed a hierarchical relationship between the doctor and the patient, considered that the medical recommendations were correct and that the failure in the treatment was mainly the responsibility of the patient for not complying with the recommendations [5].

In contrast, the concept of adherence emerged in a historical moment where patients had greater access to information technologies, which expanded the possibilities of having information about their diagnosis and treatment. This allowed patients to develop a sense of agency, establish a dialog with health personnel and adopt a critical stance during the treatment process. Likewise, the emergence of chronic conditions sets limits to the power of health personnel and forced the incorporation of the patient in the planning and maintenance of long-term care.

Adherence means a different type of relationship to "compliance": a horizontal, democratic, and collaborative relationship for the maintenance of care over time. The concept not only implies a change in the relationship with health personnel; it also represents a change in the subject: the patient becomes an active agent in the treatment process. Health services not only attribute responsibility to the patient for taking the medication or following the health recommendations; they also encourage the patient to request information about their health status and to participate in decision-making during treatment. It should be noted that this notion of the patient is based on two assumptions: care depends on the patient's will, and the patient is interested in maintaining or improving their health status.

From biomedical discourse, it is assumed that subjects are able to choose; act rationally, intentionally, and responsibly; and make decisions in terms of costs and benefits. However, the possibility of deciding is determined structurally. This means that the subjects are not completely free to decide; they can select the possibilities available for their local context, according to their socioeconomic position and the dominant cultural values [6]. As previously mentioned, social inequality not only affects access to treatment; it also limits access to services that favor the maintenance of care and the patient's ability to become adherent.

In the particular case of HIV infection, there are two additional elements that affect the development of adherence. The social processes of stigma and discrimination [7] contribute to the exclusion of patients from health services, the delay in diagnosis, the rejection of the medical condition and treatment, the concealment of the diagnosis, and the reduction of social support. Close connection with these processes is the emotional discomfort, because the suffering caused by knowing the serological status can manifest itself in rejection toward diagnosis and health services; the development of risk practices or the appearance of a psychological disorder that limits the capacity for health care [8].

While it is important to consider that adherence requires an active agent in their self-care that maintains a collaborative relationship with health services, it is also assumed that the patient's agency is limited. There are different possibilities for patients to become adherents, due to structural inequalities, the processes of stigma and discrimination, and the emotional distress generated by the HIV diagnosis. Therefore, adherence is not a state that is achieved by all patients at the same time.

It is more appropriate to consider adherence as a dynamic process that develops over time [9], influenced by the social, economic, and cultural context surrounding the patient. Adherence is also affected by the learning process that arises from the patient's personal experience with diagnosis and treatment. This means that people living with HIV have different temporalities and rhythms to become adherent patients. Adherence is not a state that is reached once and for all, but a process that must be continually updated. At any point in treatment, the patient can become nonadherent, either intentionally or involuntarily [10].

From an integral perspective of patient care, it is assumed that there are two complementary dimensions of adherence. The first dimension is pharmacological adherence, which involves taking the medication and following the instructions in terms of the schedule and the food that accompanies the intake [3]. Previous studies have reported adherence rates ranging from

26–89% [11–14]. The variability in reported adherence rates depends on the operational definition of adherence and the instrument used for its measurement [15]. The pharmacological adherence is overestimated when it is calculated based on the ratio of pills forgotten and prescribed in the last days. A more precise evaluation requires the inclusion of aspects such as the follow-up of the schedule and special instructions or the last missed dose [16]. It is worth mentioning that several patterns of pharmacological nonadherence have been identified: difficulties to initiate treatment, temporary suspension (whose duration is variable), or definitive abandonment, which represents a long-term pattern [17]. Nonadherence may be due to error or forgetfulness of the medication intake, as well as the conscious decision to abandon the treatment or not follow it properly [10].

The patient not only decides whether or not to initiate HAART but also decides whether to adopt a new lifestyle. The second dimension is associated with nonpharmacological adherence, which encompasses a set of practices that promote the patient's health care. It includes practices in the areas of diet, physical activity, rest, sexual health, mental health, attendance at medical appointments and attendance to laboratory studies, and avoidance of alcohol, tobacco, or other substances. Medication intake needs to be complemented by a series of healthy practices to promote the care of the patient and the improvement of their quality of life.

Adherence can be conceived as a process that develops over time. This process is affected by the socioeconomic position of the patient in a certain context, the dominant cultural values, and his personal experience with illness. At any point of time, the patient may be adherent or nonadherent. To be adherent, the patient needs to follow both pharmacological and nonpharmacological treatment. However, there is a risk that the patient develops patterns of nonadherence (pharmacological or nonpharmacological), which occur in the short term (at a point in time) or in the medium and long terms (at multiple time points) (**Figure 1**).

Four possible scenarios can be contemplated in a single moment of the treatment: (1) The patient is adherent at the pharmacological and nonpharmacological level (ideal scenario);

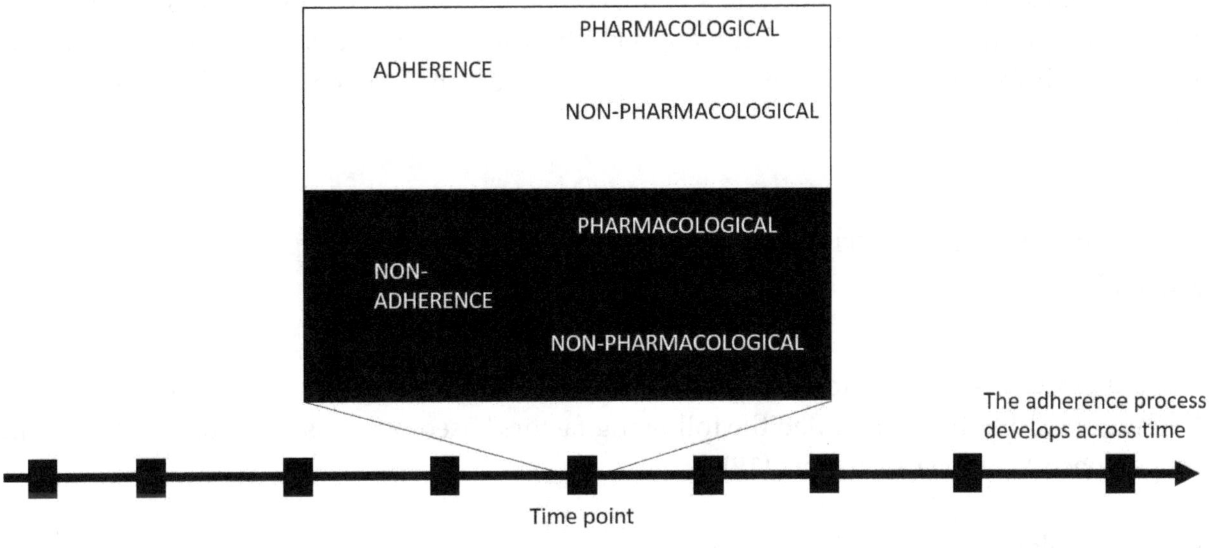

Figure 1. Adherence and nonadherence to treatment at a time point.

(2) the patient is adherent at the pharmacological level, but not at the nonpharmacological level (scenario where the patient takes the medication, but does not perform the other types of care); (3) the patient is adherent at the nonpharmacological level, but not at the pharmacological level (scenario where the patient performs healthcare practices, but does not take the medication according to the indications); and (4) the patient is not adherent in both dimensions (the worst-case scenario).

It should be mentioned that the identification of a patient as adherent will depend on the way in which the health personnel evaluate the taking of the medication and the recommendations of food and schedule (pharmacological adherence), as well as the evaluation of the degree of accomplishment of the practices in different areas of care (nonpharmacological adherence). Adherence can be considered in terms of degrees of a continuum; however, it is also necessary to establish what is the sufficient level of pharmacological and nonpharmacological adherence. This implies the need for a continuous dialog between the patient and the health personnel, in order to determine the levels of pharmacological and nonpharmacological adherence required, collaborate in the monitoring of the types of adherence, and receive feedback on the actions performed by both actors to maintain adherence.

Before reaching an optimal level of adherence, patients can alternate between periods of adherence and nonadherence until achieving an adequate and stable adherence. Traditionally it has been considered that patients are rational subjects who make a balance between the benefits and the costs of treatment to decide if they will remain adherent. However, it is necessary to consider the affective dimension, since patients not only accept treatment, they can also experience ambivalence or rejection toward treatment. It is necessary to remember that illness generates discomfort in function of the rupture it causes in the life of patients, since it affects their biography, identity, daily world, and social relations. Patients not only have the task of taking care of their health and adhering to treatment, simultaneously they embark on the tasks of giving meaning to life with the HIV infection and the reconstruction of their social world to incorporate illness in everyday life [18].

Adherence can be seen as a dialectical process where facilitators and barriers coexist during treatment. In the next section, the main facilitators and barriers to adherence reported in the literature, whether at the individual, interpersonal, or contextual levels will be reviewed.

3. Facilitators and barriers to adherence to treatment in people living with HIV

In the literature, several factors associated with adherence to treatment have been reported. A series of studies have identified the following factors based on cross-sectional studies, from the perspective of the researchers [19]:

- Factors related to personal attributes. They include the patient's clinical status, educational level, income, access to housing, and stability of the home.

- Factors related to the treatment regimen. It has been found that adherence is affected by the complexity of the regimen (depending on the number of pills or the type of indications for taking the medication), the ease of adapting the treatment to daily life, the use of devices for adherence (such as pillboxes or alarms), or side effects of treatment.

- Psychological factors. This level includes cognitive aspects such as concentration difficulties or forgetting, understanding of the role of antiretroviral treatment, or knowledge about the medical condition. Attitudes toward illness, treatment, and medications are also considered. Negative mental health factors include depression, hopelessness, anxiety or other types of psychiatric morbidity, alcohol or drug use, and coping through avoidance strategies. Positive factors include a positive attitude toward the future, long-term plans and goals, active coping, and stable mental health.

- Social factors. The relationship with the health service provider, the social support available, and the fear of revealing the diagnosis (linked to social processes of stigma and discrimination) have been identified.

- Structural factors. It includes access to treatment and health services, also economic resources to stay in treatment.

In another series of studies based on qualitative methods, facilitators and barriers to adherence have been identified from the perspective of people living with HIV. A facilitator is any individual attribute (physical, cognitive, emotional, or behavioral), characteristic of treatment, interpersonal process, or contextual aspect that favors the adherence process. In opposition, a barrier is the individual attribute, characteristic of treatment, interpersonal process, or contextual aspect that limits the adherence process.

At the individual level, beliefs that facilitate adherence have been found, such as the recognition of the drug's role in the prevention of death and illness, the perception of medicine as responsible for the improvement of health and well-being, the establishment of the maintenance of health as a priority, and religious beliefs. At an affective and motivational level, adherence is facilitated by the fear of experiencing opportunistic infections or hospitalizations, getting used to the presence of side effects, the emotional work of appropriating the suffering and feeling pride in their coping, having incentives as significant persons or future plans, adopting an optimistic perspective toward the future, or the will to live [20–25].

Other aspects that influence adherence are related to the impact of treatment, such as the absence of side effects or the clinical results of treatment. Among the practices that promote adherence are the use of external reminders, taking the medicine when the patient needs to leave the home, dealing with side effects, self-monitoring of symptoms and energy level, and conducting laboratory studies. Over time, taking the medication becomes a habit that is performed automatically [20–25].

Among the contextual aspects that facilitate adherence are having a stable lifestyle, the inclusion of treatment in the lifestyle, and the association of medication intake with daily routines. At the interpersonal level, there are facilitators such as access to positive sources of social support and the maintenance of a collaborative relationship with health personnel [20–26].

As has happened with the facilitators, the main barriers have been identified at the individual level. Adherence is affected by beliefs about antiretroviral treatment, lack of information about treatment, beliefs about illness, as well as minimizing the risks of living with HIV. It is also affected by aspects associated with the patient's physical condition, such as forgetfulness, fatigue, or feeling sick. Even self-care can be neglected when the patient perceives a good health status. At the affective level, adherence is limited by the emotional impact of diagnosis, lack of acceptance, or rejection of treatment because it remembers the presence of HIV. Other aspects that hinder adherence are the fatigue of medication, anger, depression, despair, or other vital concerns beyond health [23–27].

The barriers to adherence associated with the patient's context are the interference of treatment with the daily routine, the changes in the routine, and the workload or being out of home during the moment of medicine intake. At the interpersonal level, adherence is limited by the lack of social support and conflicts in the relationship with health personnel [20, 22, 25]. There are also barriers linked to social inequality. Some are of an economic nature, such as the difficulty to cover the expenses required for transportation to medical appointments or to maintain an appropriate diet [23, 24]. Other barriers are related to the internalization of stigma and the fear of discrimination. There are also barriers associated with gender inequality, such as differences in access to medical services and treatment or in the negotiation of condom use, especially when the couple denies the diagnosis of HIV [28]. Men may reject adherence as a form of resistance to "body discipline" [26].

In the previous section, it was mentioned that at any time during the treatment process, the patient faces the dilemma of adhering or not adhering. Adherence involves both taking the medication according to the specified conditions and adopting a healthy lifestyle in multiple areas. It should be added that at each moment of the treatment process, the patient encounters multiple facilitators and barriers to adherence (**Figure 2**).

At the individual level, there are facilitators and barriers of different types: physical, cognitive, affective, motivational, and practical. Traditionally, health psychology has focused on modifying these elements to promote adherence. However, there are also facilitators and barriers at the interpersonal level, specifically linked to social relationships established in areas such as family, friends, health services, or the community. At this level, different types of interventions are required: family interventions, interventions focused on providing social support or expanding the patient's network, interventions focused on improving interaction with health personnel, and interventions to modify the organization of health services.

Finally, there are facilitators and barriers that are part of the patient's life context: daily routines, work and home conditions, and economic conditions. There are also conditions that can limit access and permanence in health services, such as gender inequality and social processes of stigma and discrimination. This level needs to be considered not only to adjust the treatment

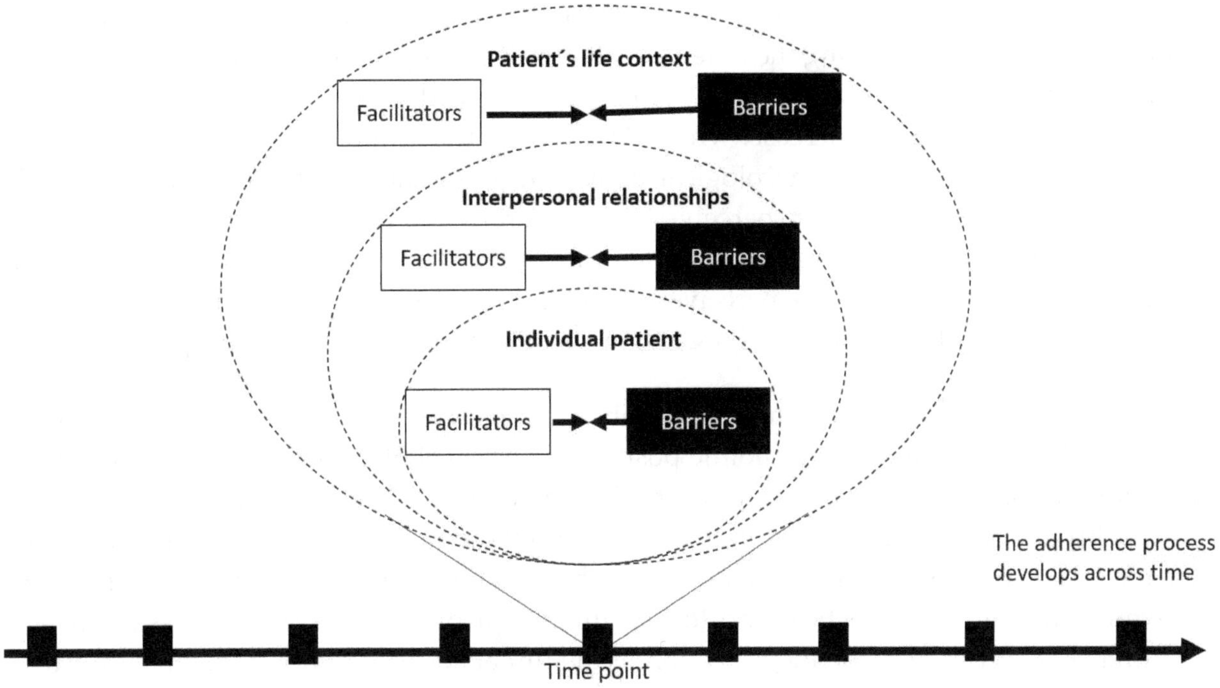

Figure 2. Facilitators and barriers to adherence to treatment, at different levels.

to the context of the patient's life but also to develop social interventions and public policies that benefit the adherence of patients in conditions of greater social vulnerability.

The identification of facilitators allows health personnel to understand the elements that contribute to the maintenance of good adherence by the patient, whether in the pharmacological or nonpharmacological dimension. The identification of barriers allows health personnel to provide feedback to the patient on those individual, interpersonal, or contextual aspects that limit the treatment and to plan the interventions required to improve the level of adherence (at the individual or collective level). It can even help in the anticipation of relapses, since both the patient and the health personnel can work collaboratively to design and implement strategies that reduce the impact of the barriers.

The following section shows how the facilitators interact to promote adherence, from the perspective of highly adherent patients. Likewise, barriers reported by these patients are identified, both for pharmacological and nonpharmacological adherence. This last type of adherence is not usually represented in adherence studies of people living with HIV.

4. Maintain adherence to antiretroviral treatment: perspective of highly adherent patients

From an individual level, the adherence process requires the interaction of different dimensions. The first dimension covers the beliefs that patients construct about illness and treatment.

Patients with high levels of adherence believe that HIV infection acts by replicating the virus within the body and decreasing the defenses, allowing the appearance of symptoms and diseases. In opposition to the beliefs about illness, they consider that HAART stops the virus and allows the defenses to increase, which strengthens the immune system. Although they recognize the benefits of pharmacological treatment, the main cost is the presence of side effects. The short-term effects are perceived as temporary and as indicators of an adaptation of the body. They mainly recognize gastrointestinal symptoms and alterations in mood or perception. Long-term effects are perceived as more damaging, due to their impact on physical appearance, metabolism, internal organs, or sensory and motor alterations [29].

Although the knowledge of common sense about illness can vary according to the cultural context of the patient, its socioeconomic position, or its level of education, it is important to point out that patients need to elaborate a basic explanatory model based on the relationship with health personnel and the education they get about their medical condition. This explanatory model establishes a common basis for collaboration with health services, since it allows to give meaning to care practices and to recognize their own vulnerability. Possibly beliefs about illness contribute to the identification of the threat and susceptibility to HIV infection, while beliefs about treatment favor the identification of the benefits in the care process. A crucial aspect is that the patient evaluates the benefits of the treatment more favorably than the costs of the side effects.

Patients also elaborate beliefs about adherence to treatment. This process is mainly associated with taking the medication, which may imply that greater importance is attached to the pharmacological adherence. This not only reflects the interests of the patient, since in the health services, there is also a greater concern for monitoring medication intake. In addition to taking the medication, patients consider that maintaining adherence requires two fundamental conditions. One of them is responsibility, because becoming a patient involves adopting the discipline of treatment.

The second condition is that patients maintain the desire to live, instead of "falling emotionally." This refers to the situation in which patients deny or reject the diagnosis, or they are depressed and put their health at risk. Therefore, in order to maintain the medication intake over time, patients need to accept the diagnosis and keep the will to live. Only in this way can patients take responsibility for their own care and incorporate the treatment discipline into their daily life, for a long period of time [29].

To stay under treatment, it is essential that patients anticipate the consequences if they do not adhere. These are the main consequences associated with nonadherence: (1) the treatment will stop working; (2) the virus is going to replicate; (3) the virus is going to become resistant; and (4) the problems will begin, such as the decrease of defenses and the emergence of diseases. It should be noted that the anticipated consequences are consistent with beliefs about illness and treatment. Another aspect that needs to be highlighted is the ability of the adherent patients to take care of themselves, even though the consequences of nonadherence are not visible (such as the replication of the virus or its mutation in resistant strains) or do not occur immediately.

The second dimension of the individual adherence process is affective. It is associated with the meaning they construct about illness, because this is an indicator of the relationship they establish with HIV infection and, in turn, the degree of acceptance of the diagnosis. From the perspective of patients, acceptance of HIV is one of the central conditions for maintaining adherence. There are different types of relationships established by highly adherent patients with their illness. Some consider that HIV infection is a motivation or challenge that drives them to get ahead, that is, a medical condition that acquires a positive meaning because it forces them to fight in life.

From a more pragmatic stance, there are patients who perceive illness as a "normal" and manageable health condition. In this case, patients normalize HIV infection in their daily lives, but they do not grant it a more transcendental meaning or consider it as a point of transformation of the self. However, they consider that they have some control over the medical condition. Finally, there are patients who conceive HIV infection as an opportunity to change toward a more moderate life. This position seems to make it easier for patients to adopt a healthier lifestyle, but at the same time, it may be linked to a desire to rebuild their social identity [29]. It seems that attributing a positive sense to illness contributes to adherence, regardless of the degree of transcendence granted in the patient's life or the impact on their identity.

In a third dimension, there are the motivational aspects that favor the adherence process. Highly adherent patients indicated three main aspects: (1) loving and taking care of themselves, (2) the family, and (3) the desire to live and "move forward" [29]. These motivational elements are not important only for the beginning of treatment but especially for its long-term maintenance. Adherence can be promoted when patients take care of themselves for the sake of their own well-being or because they want to be well for others. Possibly good adherence is an indicator of psychological well-being and positive relationships in the patient's social environment.

The fourth dimension of adherence is of a practical nature and includes the various actions or strategies that patients carry out to maintain adherence over time. For pharmacological adherence, short-term strategies were identified, such as, the use of external reminders (alarms, notes, diaries, or pillboxes), organizing the medication intake at specific moments of the daily routine, leaving the medication in special places to remember the intake, taking the medication in case of leaving home, reminder of medication intake by relatives, and not stop taking the medication if the schedule was not followed. The short-term strategies are focused on avoiding forgetfulness, which is the main barrier to pharmacological adherence even in highly adherent patients. In the long term, taking the medication is easier because it becomes a habit and is remembered mentally. There are also other strategies such as adapting to side effects and having willpower, which, unlike the previous strategies, seem to be more idiosyncratic and linked to stoicism [29, 30].

Regarding nonpharmacological adherence, patients indicated strategies according to each area of health care [29, 30]:

- Diet. Their strategies are to avoid harmful foods and try to eat healthy foods (low in fat and carbohydrates, high in vitamins and minerals).

- Physical activity. Patients establish an exercise routine or incorporate the activities of their daily routine as exercise.
- Rest. The strategies consist of sleeping 7 to 8 hours, not staying up late, and taking naps.
- Substance use. Some patients report having quit smoking or drinking (by willpower and not by specialized treatment, especially when there are low levels of previous consumption). In the case of patients who have not stopped drinking, they point out that consumption becomes occasional, only at parties or celebrations.
- Sexual health. Patients use strategies such as refusing to have sex without a condom, having condoms available, or creating justifications for condom use (such as avoiding pregnancy), especially when there is a difference in power in the couple or they are afraid of being discriminated against because of their medical condition. One facilitator of these practices is the fear of reinfection or contracting another sexually transmitted disease.
- Mental health. Patients resort to strategies such as attending psychological care (individual therapy or self-groups), obtaining social support in the family or in religious groups, and thinking positively.
- Attendance at medical appointments. Strategies were mentioned such as the use of external reminders, saving money to attend the appointment (due to transportation expenses), "keeping an eye on the appointment," or remembering it internally.
- Attendance to laboratory tests. The use of external reminders was pointed out as the only strategy. One aspect that facilitates attendance at appointments is the desire to know the health status, specifically the viral load and the level of CD4 cells.

The adherence process from the perspective of the individual patient involves the interaction between four dimensions. The first dimension comprised beliefs about illness, treatment and adherence. These beliefs require coherence with each other and with the explanatory model of health personnel. To promote adherence at this level, health education is required to provide knowledge on critical aspects of HIV infection. At the same time, it is important that a relationship be established between the patient and the health personnel where the agreement between explanatory models is verified and the dialog is facilitated for the modification of beliefs that affect the adherence process.

The second dimension is affective and focuses on the relationship that patients establish with their illness. This is an indicator of the degree of acceptance of HIV infection. Patients will not elaborate the same meaning about illness, as this depends on the psychosocial impact that HIV infection has on their lives. The impact can be diminished by coping strategies and the sources of social support they have to manage the consequences of the medical condition in daily life. It is important not to force the patient to perceive the HIV infection in a certain way; it is necessary to respect his time for acceptance. It is not necessary for the patient to perceive the diagnosis as a transcendental event that has transformed their existence or their identity, but it is a good indicator for adherence when the patient constructs a positive meaning of illness and considers it a manageable condition. Although the meaning of illness is elaborated over time, its acceptance can be promoted through individual therapy. Especially useful are the support groups, because the construction of new discourses about living with HIV is promoted within the framework of these social relations.

The third dimension is motivational and consists of identifying those elements that encourage the patient to start treatment but, above all, maintain adherence in the long term. The main sources of motivation are individual (like the desire to continue living and taking care of oneself) and interpersonal (taking care of oneself to be well for others). Both sources are important and complement each other, but individual motivations should be emphasized, especially when patients have scarce social networks or persistent conflicts exist in their social network. Individual or group psychotherapy can strengthen individual motivation, but it is also necessary to take into account the role of social support from family members, friends, or the couple in patient care to promote interpersonal motivation. It is worth mentioning that other possible motivations that can be explored with patients are future goals or plans, since self-care is strengthened when there is a specific purpose that is to be achieved in the short, medium, or long terms.

The fourth dimension is practical and includes strategies for the two types of adherence. The strategies for pharmacological adherence are mainly focused on remembering the medication, so they can be promoted from health education, by behavioral modeling of strategies by health personnel, or through social learning in support groups. Another aspect that needs to be addressed is the management of side effects of treatment, which implies a close dialog with the health personnel for the monitoring of side effects, to assess whether the patient can benefit from medications to reduce side effects or if a change in the treatment scheme is required.

Strategies for nonpharmacological adherence can also be promoted from health education, individual counseling, or support groups. In each area of health care, it is necessary to monitor the patient's behavior to establish minimum goals and to evaluate the follow-up of health recommendations. In areas where difficulties are detected, problem-solving therapy can be used to address the barriers that limit health care and prevent relapse. In case the difficulties are maintained, it is necessary to channel the patient with specialized personnel in each area, such as nutritionists, psychotherapists specialized in addictions, or self-support groups (**Figure 3**).

Different barriers may appear through the adherence process, either individual or contextual. For pharmacological adherence, the following individual barriers have been identified: forgetfulness of medicine intake, physical discomfort, side effects, and emotional distress. It should be noted that patients' emotional distress is not only linked to their biography and personality; it is a suffering with a social origin, because it is linked to stigma and discrimination processes. As contextual barriers were mentioned, the pending tasks in the domestic or work environment that interfere with medication intake. The barriers to nonpharmacological adherence for each area of health care are the following [29, 30]:

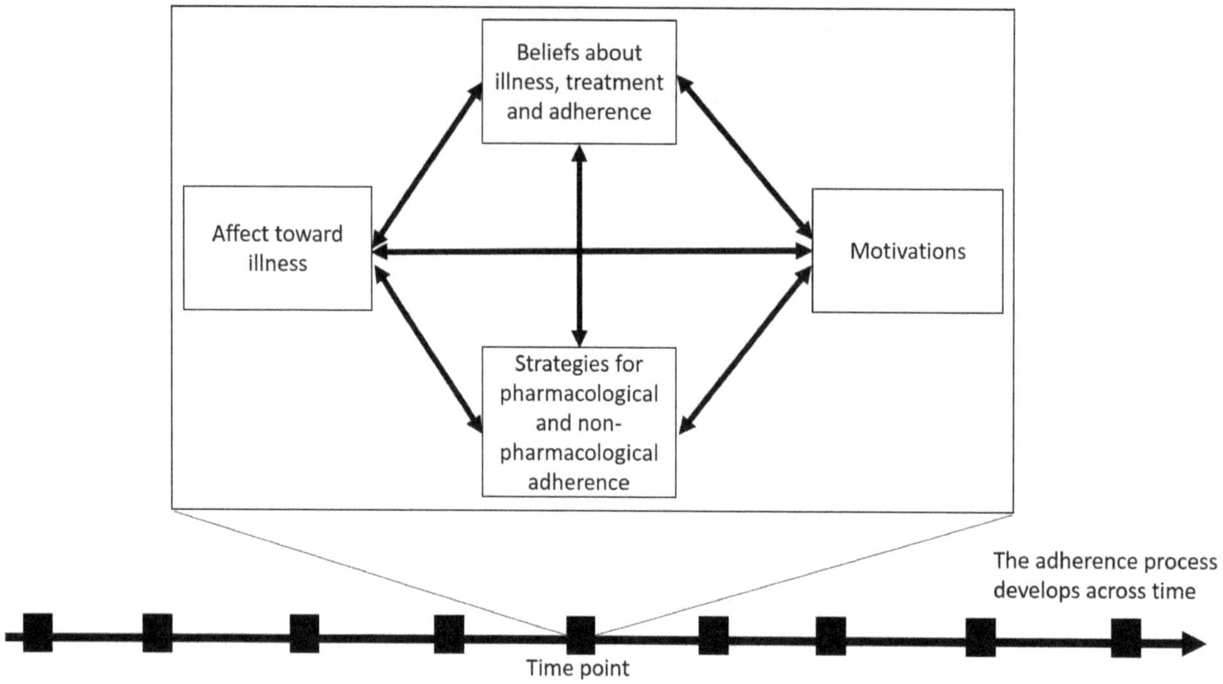

Figure 3. Dimensions of the adherence process at the individual level.

- Diet. The individual barrier is the difficulty in leaving junk food. The contextual barrier is the economic difficulty to buy healthy foods.
- Physical activity. The main individual barrier is feeling weak or tired. The contextual barrier is the lack of time to exercise.
- Rest. The most frequently mentioned individual barrier was physical discomfort. The main contextual barrier was the work schedule.
- Substance use. The individual barriers identified were tobacco addiction and not attending specialized help to quit smoking. The contextual barriers identified were friendships that consume substances.
- Sexual health. The barriers were identified in the context of the couple relationship. Some mentioned that at certain times they did not use the condom because they did not care about risk. Also mentioned was the avoidance of sexual relations with a stable partner due to the fear of transmitting HIV.
- Mental health. Depression and stigma were the main barriers to mental health. A situation mentioned by some patients was the rejection of psychological services or the desire to get ahead by themselves.
- Attendance at medical appointments. The individual barriers were forgetfulness and physical discomfort. The main contextual barriers were work and not having money for transportation.

- Attendance to laboratory tests. The barrier identified was forgetfulness. It should be mentioned that laboratory studies are performed less frequently than medical appointments.

Diet is affected not only by the habits developed in the past by the patient but also by the influence of culture on food preferences, the supply of healthy food in its sociocultural context, and feeding practices in the family. It is therefore essential that overweight and obese patients can attend a nutritional consultation to continuously monitor their weight and develop a meal plan that fits their daily routine and economic capacity.

Physical activity and rest are two areas of health care closely linked to the work context and the demands of home. The overload of daily tasks can reduce the time available for rest and exercise. If the patient cannot access a job with better conditions for their health, it is important to focus on the organization of time to get more rest hours and design a physical activity plan that adapts to the patient's daily routine and can be performed in a short time.

Substance use is an area that requires greater attention in health services. Tobacco addiction is usually minimized, and specialized care services are not frequently visited for treatment. The consumption of alcohol can be difficult to avoid in a sociocultural context where it is promoted as a ritual of socialization, which is why in health services a compromise solution is usually established: allow the patient to consume alcohol occasionally during special situations. However, health services need to send a clear message to patients regarding substance use during treatment. It is necessary for health personnel to identify the level of substance use in the patient, clearly communicate the consequences of consumption for their health and the treatment process, and conduct referral to specialized services in addiction care when required.

In the area of sexual health, adherent patients usually adopt condom use in a systematic way. However, the problems can be due to a tiredness of the use of the condom, because they perceive it as a routine act, which affects spontaneity and eroticism. These situations are not usually reported to health personnel, so it is necessary to establish a trust relationship with the patient so that they can talk about these issues and request help when necessary. In the care services, interventions that address the eroticization of condom use can be implemented.

Especially, it is necessary to be alert when patients are immersed in power relations where the negotiation of condom use is limited. On the other hand, some patients report that they have stopped having sex for fear of transmitting HIV. In these cases, it may be necessary to provide relevant information about transmission risks and protected sex practices. Counseling sessions for the couple can also be developed to clarify doubts about the transmission of HIV and provide alternatives for safe sex and protected sex.

The mental health of patients can be compromised from the moment of diagnosis, because it generates emotional distress and limits the acceptance of HIV. This is due not only to a patient's vulnerability in psychological terms but also because of the social vulnerability associated with their socioeconomic position and the processes of stigma and discrimination. Psychological care (at the individual or group level) is essential before starting treatment so that the patient can accept the illness and emotionally prepare to maintain adherence. A problem is that in health services, care is not usually promoted in an integral way, but mainly physical health care is considered and mental health is not sufficiently attended. Another difficulty lies in the rejection of patients to psychological care, either because of the stigma toward mental illness or the desire to solve their psychosocial problems individually.

Finally, attendance at medical appointments or laboratory tests is often affected by forgetfulness. Reminders via telephone, text message, or social networks can be useful to promote adherence in this area. Some patients pointed to work as a barrier, which can be reduced if health centers establish a policy for extending the schedules of service. Physical discomfort can be a barrier when a health problem makes it difficult to attend the health center, so they can benefit from special procedures for changing appointments in such circumstances. Certain patients' report has economic difficulties for transport payment. In certain vulnerable groups, financial support may be granted for attendance at medical appointments (**Figure 4**).

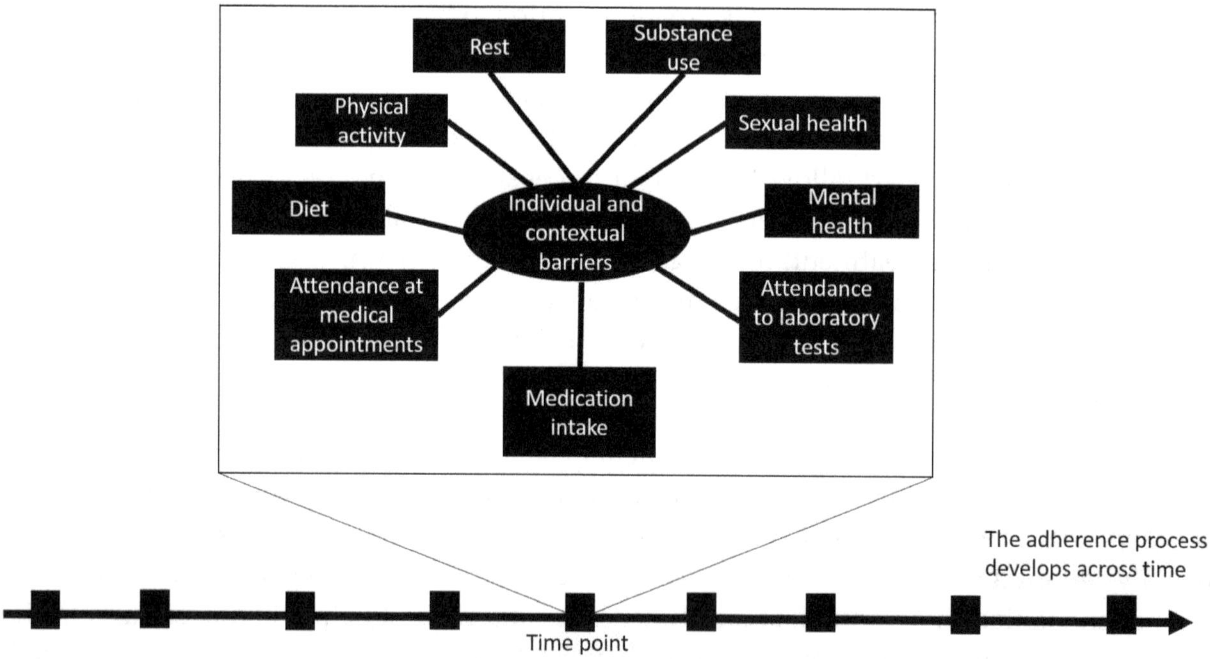

Figure 4. Individual and contextual barriers during the adherence process.

5. Conclusions

Adherence is a process that develops over time, where people living with HIV need to identify as patients, take an active role in their health care, and establish a collaborative relationship with health personnel. The agency capacity is not the same for all patients; it depends on their level of social vulnerability. This means that there are structural conditions that reduce the capacity of agency and the options of patients in their daily lives. Patients are not only rational subjects who make decisions regarding treatment based on a cost–benefit analysis;

they are at the same time affective subjects who need to deal with the rupture of their social world caused by a medical condition that is stigmatized in his cultural context.

Adherence has two dimensions: pharmacological and nonpharmacological. At any time in the adherence process, patients may become nonadherent, in one or both dimensions. The patterns of nonadherence can be generated in the short, medium, and long terms; persistent patterns that extend over time are more problematic. From the perspective of the individual patient, adherence is maintained at any point of time due to the interaction of the following elements: beliefs about illness, treatment and adherence, affection toward HIV infection, motivations, and strategies for taking medication and health care. However, the patient may encounter individual and contextual barriers in multiple areas: medication intake, diet, rest, physical activity, substance use, sexual health, mental health, attendance at medical appointments, and attendance to laboratory tests. Health services require a comprehensive evaluation of the patient in each of the areas indicated, in order to understand the resources available to the patient for adherence and the barriers that require specific interventions.

Author details

Ariagor Manuel Almanza Avendaño[1]*, Martha Patricia Romero Mendoza[2] and Anel Hortensia Gómez San Luis[1]

*Address all correspondence to: manuelalmanzaavendano@gmail.com

1 Universidad Autónoma de Baja California, Mexicali, Baja California, Mexico

2 Instituto Nacional de Psiquiatría "Ramón de la Fuente Muñiz", Ciudad de México, Mexico

References

[1] Magis C, Hernández M. Epidemiología del SIDA en México. In: Córdova J, Ponce de León S, Valdespino J, editors. 25 años de SIDA en México: logros, desaciertos y retos. México: Instituto Nacional de Salud Pública; 2008

[2] Biehl J. Will to Live. Aids Therapies and the Politics of Survival. New Jersey: Princeton University Press; 2007

[3] Centro Nacional para la Prevención y el Control del VIH y el SIDA. Guía de manejo antirretroviral de las personas con VIH [Internet]. México: CENSIDA; 2014. Available from: http://www.censida.salud.gob.mx/descargas/biblioteca/Guia_ARV_ISBN.pdf [Accesed: March 15, 2017]

[4] Scalera A, Bayoumi A, Oh P, Risebrough N, Shear N, Lin-In A. Clinical and economic implications of non-adherence to HAART in HIV infection. Disease Management & Health Outcomes. 2002;**10**(2):85-91

[5] Chesney M, Morin M, Sherr L. Adherence to HIV combination therapy. Social Science & Medicine. 2000;**50**(11):1599-1605

[6] Menéndez EL. De sujetos, saberes y estructuras. Lugar Editorial: Buenos Aires, Argentina; 2009

[7] Aggleton P, Parker R. Documento de trabajo no. 9. Estigma y discriminación relacionados con el VIH/SIDA: un marco conceptual e implicaciones para la acción. México: El Colegio de México; 2002

[8] Almanza A. Narrativas acerca del VIH: la mirada del paciente y de su red social. Saarbrücken: Publicia; 2015

[9] Spire B, Duran S, Souville M, Leport C, Raffi F, Moatti JP. The APROCO cohort study group. Adherence to highly active antiretroviral therapies (HAART) in HIV-infected patients: from a predictive to a dynamic approach. Social Science & Medicine. 2002; **54**(10):1481-1496

[10] Norton W, Rivet K, Fisher W, Shuper P, Ferrer R, Cornman D, Trayling C, Reeding C, Fisher J. Information-motivation-behavioral skills barriers associated with intentional versus unintentional ARV non-adherence behavior among HIV+ patients in clinical care. AIDS Care. 2010;**22**(8):979-987

[11] Applebaum A, Richardson M, Brady S, Brief D, Keane T. Gender and other psychosocial factors as predictors of adherence to highly active antiretroviral therapy (HAART) in adults with comorbid HIV/AIDS, psychiatric and substance-related disorder. AIDS and Behavior. 2008;**13**:60-65

[12] Mo P, Mak W. Intentionality of medication non-adherence among individuals living with HIV/AIDS in Hong Kong. AIDS Care. 2009;**21**(6):785-795

[13] Puskas C, Forrest J, Parashar S, Salters K, Cescon A, Kaida A, Miller C, Bangsberg D, Hogg R. Women and vulnerability to HAART non-adherence: A literature review of treatment adherence by gender from 2000 to 2011. Current HIV/AIDS Reports. 2011;**8**:277-287

[14] Ubbiali A, Donati D, Chiorri C, Bregani V, Cattaneo E, Maffei C, Visintini R. Prediction of adherence to antiretroviral therapy: Can patients´ gender play some role? An italian pilot study. AIDS Care. 2008;**20**(5):571-575

[15] Gagné C, Godin G. Improving self-report measures of non-adherence to HIV medications. Psychology and Health. 2005;**20**(6):803-816

[16] Balandrán D, Gutiérrez J, Romero M. Evaluación de la adherencia antirretroviral en México: adherencia de cuatro días vs índice de adherencia. Revista de Investigación Clínica. 2013;**65**(5):384-391

[17] Murphy D, Johnston K, Martin D, Marelich W, Hoffman D. Barriers to antiretroviral adherence among HIV-infected adults. In: Laurence J, editor. Medication adherence in HIV/AIDS. Nueva York: Mary Ann Liebert Publishers; 2004

[18] Good B. Medicina, racionalidad y experiencia. Una perspectiva antropológica. Barcelona: Bellaterra; 2003

[19] Fogarty L, Roter D, Larson S, Burke J, Gillespie J, Levy R. Patient adherence to HIV medication regimens: A review of published and abstract reports. Patient Education and Counseling. 2002;**46**:93-108

[20] Brion J, Menke E. Perspectives regarding adherence to prescribed treatment in highly adherent HIV-infected gay men. Journal of the Association of Nurses in AIDS Care. 2008;**19**(3):181-191. DOI: 10.1016/j.jana.2007.11.006

[21] Lewis M, Colbert A, Erlen J, Meyers M. A qualitative therapy of persons who are 100% adherent to antiretroviral therapy. AIDS Care. 2006;**18**(2):140-148. DOI: 10.1080/09540120500161835

[22] Sidat M, Fairley C, Grierson J. Experiences and perceptions of patients with 100% adherence to highly active antiretroviral therapy: A qualitative study. AIDS Patient Care and STDs. 2007;**21**(7):509-520. DOI: 10.1089/apc.2006.0201

[23] dos Santos W, Freitas E, da Silva A, Marinho C, Freitas MI. Barreiras e aspectos facilitadores da adesão á terapia antirretroviral em Belo-Horizonte-MG. Revista Brasileira de Enfermagem. 2011;**64**(6):1028-1037

[24] Krummenacher I, Spencer B, Du Pasquier S, Bugnon O, Cavassini M, Schneider M. Qualitative analysis of barriers and facilitators encountered by HIV patients in an ART adherence programme. International Journal of Clinical Pharmacy. 2014;**36**(4):716-724. DOI: 10.1007/s11096-014-9930-0

[25] Remien R, Hirky E, Johnson M, Weinhardt L, Whittier D, Minh Le G. Adherence to medication treatment: A qualitative study of facilitators and barriers among a diverse sample of HIV+ men and women in four U.S. cities. AIDS and Behavior. 2003;**7**(1):61-73. DOI: 1090-7165/03/0300-0061/10

[26] Herrera C, Kendall T, Campero L. Vivir con VIH en México: experiencias de mujeres y hombres desde un enfoque de género. México: El Colegio de México; 2014

[27] Sabin L, Bachman M, Hamer D, Keyi X, Yue Y, Wen F, Tao L, Heggenhougen H, Seton L, Wilson I, Gill C. Barriers to adherence to antiretroviral medications among patients living with HIV in southern China: A qualitative study. AIDS Care. 2008;**20**(10):1242-1250. DOI: 10.1080/09540120801918651

[28] Skovdal M, Campbell C, Nyamukapa C, Gregson S. When masculinity interferes with women's treatment of HIV infection: A qualitative study about adherence to antiretroviral therapy in Zimbabwe. Journal of the International AIDS Society. 2011;**14**(29):1-7. DOI: 10.1186/1758-2652-14-29

[29] Almanza AM. Estrategias y barreras para la adherencia terapéutica en pacientes con VIH del estado de Tamaulipas. In: Etienne C, editor. Nuevos profesores de tiempo completo. Nueva generación de investigadores. México: Colofón; 2017

[30] Almanza AM, Gómez AH. Barreras para la adherencia al tratamiento farmacológico y no farmacológico en mujeres con VIH. Psicología y Salud. 2017;**27**(1):29-39

6

Brain Aging in HIV-1 Infection

Maryline Santerre and Bassel Sawaya

Abstract

It has been shown that patients carrying HIV-1 accumulate damage to cells and tissues that are not directly infected by the virus itself (e.g., neurons). Importantly, these include changes known as HIV-Associated Neurodegenerative Disorder (HAND) leading to the loss of neuronal functions. HAND is an outstanding problem in the clinical management of HIV-1 patients because suppression of infectious virus by c-ART does not completely block neurodegenerative changes. Neuropsychological studies disclose cognitive alteration (such as loss of Spatial and Declarative Memory) in a substantial proportion of HIV-1 infected patients, and analysis of post-mortem brain tissues isolated from HIV-1 patients treated with c-ART show signs of neurodegeneration. In the absence of HIV-1 infection of neurons, several mechanisms have been proposed for HAND, including indirect inflammatory effects in the CNS and direct effects of viral proteins (e.g., gp120) shed from activated HIV-1-infected cells. The fact that these viral proteins enter the neurons through several pathways suggests the presence of many competing mechanisms that can contribute to HAND, each of which has its advocates. Their relative contributions to clinical disease in vivo remain to be sorted out, and this is an outstanding problem in HIV research. This chapter will shed some light on the mechanisms used by HIV-1 leading to memory impairments and premature brain aging.

Keywords: HIV, brain, aging, mitochondria

1. HIV-1 and structural changes

1.1. Thinning of the cortex: white/gray matter (methods and results)

Physiological brain aging is associated with a decrease in gray matter (GM) volume between adulthood and old age, while the volume of white matter (WM) increase from age 19 to 40 and will regress after that [1]. *The reduction of gray matter is probably the result of neuronal shrinkage and the reduction of synaptic spines* [2]. Ventricular enlargement associated with normal aging and the Evans' index is used to distinguish normal and pathological enlargement [3].

Different techniques are used to evaluate different categories of brain changes: neurophysiology, neurochemistry, brain structure, and brain activation networks. Structural magnetic resonance imaging (MRI), diffusion MRI, and X-ray computed tomography (CT) are the tools for structural neuroimaging. Neurometabolites or neurochemicals can be tracked with positron emission tomography (PET) using radiotracers and by magnetic resonance spectroscopy (MRS). Brain activation networks can be studied by functional magnetic resonance imaging (fMRI) methods based on blood oxygenation level-dependent (BOLD) contrast, and arterial spin labeling (ASL) perfusion contrast shows changes in cerebral blood flow (CBF) and blood oxygenation.

Using imaging techniques, scientists and clinicians determined that the global cerebral volume is smaller in HIV-1 patients than in the seronegative population [4]. The HIV+ subjects also present a higher neuronal loss [5] and the patients with detectable viral loads had the highest rates of gray (GM) and white (WM) matter loss [6].

MRI technique also revealed that the gray matter of HIV+ subjects may present cortical atrophy [7, 8] and volumetric loss in the caudate, amygdala, and hippocampus [4, 7, 9–12]. Moreover, the medial and superior frontal gyri can show an atrophy [13], as well as the posterior and inferior temporal lobe, parietal lobe, and cerebellum [14].

If changes of white matter integrity are common with age, the abnormalities are more pronounced in aged HIV+ subjects [15]. The white matter of HIV+ subjects displayed some changes, like a tissue loss in the corpus callosum [9], as well as corpus callosum thinning and ventricular expansion [16]. HIV+ subjects showed increased mean diffusivity in frontal and parietal white matter, putamen, and genu [17]. Lower fractional anisotropy is also found at an older age in HIV+ subjects in white matter of frontal, temporal, and parietal lobes but a higher mean diffusion only in the occipital white matter [18]. Small white matter hyperintensities (WMH) are associated with age in seronegative adults [19, 20] and are attributed to inflammatory, vascular, or blood–brain barrier changes [21, 22]. However, these WMHs can be connected to dementia, multiple sclerosis, and cerebrovascular diseases [23, 24]. The increase of WMH volume is linked to lesser brain integrity in the sagittal stratum and the corpus callosum. HIV+ adults over age 60 showed a higher ratio from abnormal to normal WMH, with a subset of individuals in this age group with a significantly high WMH. This high ratio is associated with cardiovascular and is inversely correlated with global psychomotor and cognitive performance. The examination of the microstructure of the white matter by diffusion tensor imaging (DTI) brings a promising disease-activity marker [25]. A disease more advanced associated with a higher rate of decline of the CD4 count is linked to a greater atrophy of the gray and white matter in the brain [26].

Away from human, this degeneration in gray and white matter was also observed in HIV-1 Tat transgenic mice model. The expression of Tat protein diminishes cortical gray matter density in young Tat transgenic mice [27] and alters the structure of myelin examined by either DTI imaging [28] or electron microscopy [29], with declines of fractional anisotropy and behavioral changes.

Finally, more developed tools and methods (e.g., brain PAD) were also used to measure the influence of HIV-1 on aging. This integrative tool measures brain-predicted age difference (brain-PAD) scores. It associates structural neuroimaging data with neuropsychological test scores, trying to predict brain age and to assess the correlation of brain age to chronological age [30].

1.2. Loss of neural circuits and brain plasticity: implication of long-term potentiation in learning and memory

Long-term potentiation (LTP) is a persistent increase in the synaptic activity leading to the signal transmission between two neurons. The canonical mode of LTP induction at CA1 hippocampal synapses relies on the glutamate receptor NMDAR and the following biochemical cascade triggered and maintained by the synaptic protein calcium/calmodulin-dependent protein kinase II (CaMKII). The impairment of this cascade would lead to an acute deficit in learning and memory storage. LTP is involved in learning and memory functions in structures like the hippocampus or the amygdala. It is generated by short repetitive high-frequency stimulation (HFS) and may persist for hours or days.

An early study in 1999 demonstrated that some factors secreted by HIV-1-infected monocytes-derived macrophages (MDMs) inhibit the induction of LTP in the CA1 region of the rat hippocampus [31]. Later, a study shows that mice with severe combined immunodeficiency (SCIDs) injected by HIV-1-infected human monocyte-derived macrophages (MDMs) into the basal ganglia present a gradual decrease in synaptic function, followed by decreased cognition and later by an impairment of multiple phases of synaptic potentiation [32]. Impairment of synaptic functions, as well as the induction and maintenance of LTP, is described in mice with HIVE [33]. HIV-infected brain mononuclear phagocytes (MP) (macrophages and microglia) are the reservoirs for persistent viral infection. They secrete soluble factors like chemokines, free radicals, proinflammatory cytokines, nitric oxide, and eicosanoids. HIV-infected MDM culture supernatants containing same soluble factors have the capability to inhibit synaptic transmission and block LTP from the CA1 part of the hippocampus of rats. A deeper investigation of the mechanism involved shows that IL-8 severely reduces Ca^{2+} currents in the septal neurons, triggering the closure of L- and N-type Ca^{2+} channels [34]. Without an increase of the intracellular Ca^{2+} flux, the LTP in the CA1 region of the hippocampus is impaired [35].

The study of isolated HIV-1 proteins on CA1 long-term potentiation (LTP) gave us more information about the mechanisms involved in the impairment of learning and memory by HIV-1. Mice-expressing HIV-1 gp120 are showing a significant decrease in CA1 hippocampal LTP. Gp120-induced impairment is prevented by a pre-treatment with the NMDA receptor antagonist, suggesting that excessive activation of the NMDA receptor, that can lead to excitotoxic cell death, is responsible for the degenerative process triggered by gp120 [36]. HIV-1 gp120 protein inhibits LTP via the chemokine receptor CXCR4 and binds to it through the V3 loop epitope KRIHI [37]. Gp120-associated reduction of LTP is alleviated by a systemic administration of 4-AP, a Kv, channel antagonist. This result supports the evidence that the neuronal voltage-gated potassium (K^+) channels (Kv) are targeted by gp120 during the inhibition of LTP and that Kv channels are linked learning and memory deficiencies in HAND [38]. With normal, non-pathological aging, dendritic trees experience gradual regression in dendritic arbors of pyramidal neurons situated in the superior temporal, precentral, and prefrontal cortices in humans [8]. HIV-1 Tat expression in pyramidal CA1 neurons decrease the number of apical dendritic spines, without the evidence of pyramidal death but with the disruption of the distribution of the synaptic proteins gephyrin and synaptogtagmin2 [39]. The Tat expression induces synapto-dendritic modifications in the hippocampus that will disrupt the LTP in CA1 pyramidal neurons and subsequently bring deficits in learning and memory.

HIV-1 Tat protein injection into the hippocampus showed that Tat plays on extra-synaptic NMDA receptors but not on synaptic. Additionally, it suppresses long-term potentiation (LTP) followed by a diminution of spatial learning. Tat protein induces the phosphorylation of NMDA receptor subunits NR2A and NR2B in a tyrosine kinase-dependent manner, which triggers Ca^{2+} flux. Ca^{2+} entry through synaptic NMDA receptors activates cAMP response element binding protein (CREB) activity, and confers antiapoptotic ability, while Ca^{2+} entry through extrasynaptic NMDA receptors shuts off CREB pathway [40]. Some recent work shows that CREB protein holds an essential role in memory formation. CREB protein brings changes in global neuronal excitability. CREB overexpression results in more action potential for each pulse and a smaller after-hyperpolarization (AHP) after a chain of action potentials. AHP is usually engendered by K^+ channels, and CREB might be involved in variations in K^+ conductance. By enhancing neuronal excitability, CREB might increase the inclusion of neurons into the memory trace [41].

2. Neuropsychological changes

2.1. Depression: serotonin loss

With normal aging, the brain suffers from serotonin (5-HT) neuron and neurotransmitter loss. This deficit in serotonergic neurotransmission might promote the occurrence of depression in the elderly population [42]. The incidence of major depression is estimated from 1 to 10% in a population older than 60 years of age, while depressive symptoms may affect up to 20% [43, 44]. Even if it is not considered as a normal aging event, the loss of serotonin and subsequent depression is a common even among the elderly.

Depression is significant comorbidity with a prevalence superior to 30% in some studies in HIV-infected patients [45, 46]. Among a cohort of 13,874 HIV-infected patients, 44% percent of the study population had depression, and 15% of the whole cohort was prescribed SSRIs [47].

The essential amino acid l-tryptophan (Trp) is the precursor of some essential metabolites produced during the course of its degradation, along with different pathways, like the kynurenine (KYN) pathway and the serotonin, 5-hydroxytryptamine or 5-HT pathway. During the kynurenine pathway, the tryptophan is converted by the enzymes Tryptophan 2,3-dioxygenase (TDO) or indoleamine 2,3-dioxygenase 1 (IDO1), IDO2. The resulting product is further degraded to kynurenine (KYN), which is a precursor of bioactive compounds, including quinolinic acid (QUIN), that subsequently activate or inhibit NMDA neurotransmission. Pro-inflammatory cytokines, including interferon-γ (IFN-γ), interleukin-1 β (IL-1β), and IL-6, can further induce IDO-1 and TDO and thus activate this pathway, reducing the availability of TRP for the serotonin synthesis pathway [48–51].

HIV-1 clade B Tat is responsible for the up-regulation of IDO and the down-regulation of 5-HT gene and protein expressions. Also, HIV-1 clade B Tat reduces 5-HT with a concomitant increase in KYN levels as compared to HIV-1 clade C Tat [52].

HIV+ subjects present a reduced breakdown of Phe to tyrosine (Tyr) [53, 54] and a faster conversion of trp to kynurenine (Kyn) [55], which is correlated with higher levels of immune activation markers like interferon-γ (IFN-γ) or neopterin in HIV-1 individuals [56]. Accelerated trp breakdown was correlated with neuropsychiatric symptoms in HIV patients [55, 57].

It is interesting to note that serotonin treatment decreases the HIV-I replication in human macrophages. Indeed 5-HT decreases the β-chemokine receptor, CCR5, and increases the CCL5 chemokine, MIP-1α, implying an effect of 5-HT on 5-HT1A receptors on macrophages [58]. Further, some studies show that in HIV+ individuals the blocking of the re-uptake of serotonin (SSRIs) is associated with the up-regulation of NK cells [59, 60]. Serotonergic pathways are important in the function of natural killer (NK) cells and CD8 + T cells [61].

2.2. HIV-1 and risks of Alzheimer's disease (AD) pathogenesis

Apolipoprotein (apo) E isoforms (apoE2, apoE3, and apoE4) play a role in cardiovascular disease and lipoprotein metabolism but are mainly studied for their contribution in neurodegeneration in Alzheimer's disease [62–64]. HIV-associated dementia (HAD) is a neurological condition with clinicopathological features similar to Alzheimer's disease [65].

Early research presented in Nature Medicine in 1998 measures the risk of dementia in patients who presented E4 isoform for apolipoprotein E (APOE). Compared to the normal subjects, they presented twice more dementia and peripheral neuropathy, concluding that a long-term infection brings an increased risk of dementia for E4(+) subjects [66], with an even bigger risk with low CD4+ cell count and length of infection. It is today widely accepted that the *APOE* ε4/ε4 genotype is associated with a faster disease course and progression to death compared with the *APOE* ε3/ε3 genotype. However, an association between the ε4/ε4 genotype and HIV-associated dementia (HAD) was not identified [67].

APOEε4 allele(s) may lead to premature aging with neurodegeneration in younger HIV patients preceding the development of HAND, potentially because of greater neuroinflammation or more abundant amyloid deposition in younger HIV subjects with APOEε4 allele(s) [4, 68]. Recent neuroimaging studies present conflicting results. One study on 237 patients shows that the ApoEε4 allele does not affect brain integrity, gray, or white matter, in their cohort of HIV+ individuals [69]. Another study on 76 patients shows brain atrophy, especially in the posterior corpus callosum, thalamus, and brainstem [70]. These individuals were older than 60, which could explain the discrepancy between the studies; the deleterious effects could be age dependent [71].

The APOEε4 genotype is a risk factor for elevated cholesterol in ART-adherent HIV(+) men aged >50 years [72] with a risk for a higher cognitive decline associated and cardiovascular problems.

All these studies taken together, it is now clear that individuals with HIV and the ApoE gene exhibited greater cognitive deficits when tested for attention, executive function, and working memory than HIV-infected individuals with ApoE4 genotype carriers.

3. Gait/balance

Aging is associated with a cascade of events affecting the function of the Substantia Nigra (SN) neurons, from the dopamine metabolism to the mitochondrial dysfunction and the alteration in protein degradation. The addition of cellular defects linked to aging increases the risks of developing Parkinson's disease [73, 74].

With aging, the density of dopamine transporters and dopaminergic neurons decreases, and there is a correlation between the decline of the dopamine system function and the executive function [75]. Several studies show evidence of a link between aging, memory, learning, and dopaminergic change [76–79]. HIV-1 penetrates the brain immediately after the initial infection and is disseminated in various concentrations in different parts of the brain, with a particular affinity for the subcortical regions like the basal ganglia, including the putamen, caudate nucleus, globus pallidus, and Substantia Nigra [80]. HIV-1 RNA is also identified in different regions of the postmortem brain, especially in different nuclei of the basal ganglia [81–83]. Since basal ganglia is the main target of HIV infection in the brain, it is not surprising that the dopaminergic function located in the Substantia Nigra will be altered. Neuropathological assessments of HIV+ patients show that the degeneration of Substantia Nigra is common. Moreover, it could explain the sensitivity of some patients to drug-induced Parkinsonism [84].

HIV-1 and Parkinson's disease both affect nigrostriatal structures with subsequent dopaminergic dysfunction. HIV-1 patients display signs of hypomimia, bradykinesia, poor hand agility, and action or postural tremor exacerbated by age [85]. The aging HIV+ population treated with HAART shows more frequent presentation of HIV-1 Parkinsonism. A significant decrease of dopamine in the Substantia Nigra was subsequently found in the postmortem examination of the HIV+ brains [86]. Alpha-synuclein is one of the major factors in Parkinson's disease pathology, and its expression was found to have increased in the Substantia Nigra of HIV+ postmortem brain [87]. Alpha-synuclein plays a role in the apoptosis of dopamine cells and reinforces the idea that the aging brain of HIV+ individuals may develop PD. Different studies report that the dopamine concentration in the HIV-infected brain can decrease by 50% [80, 86, 88]. The decrease in DA levels in SN was significantly correlated with the decrease in performance in learning, memory, speed of processing information, and verbal fluency.

The presynaptic dopamine transporter (DAT)-mediated dopamine reuptake is crucial for regular dopamine homeostasis and subsequent brain functions like memory, learning, and attention. However, it has been reported that HIV patients with dementia had substantially lower DAT availability in ventral striatum and putamen [89]. The DAT expression and function is also altered by HIV proteins in animals. HIV-1 Tat induces inhibition of the transporter by an allosteric binding to DAT [90]. DAT function and expression is modified in the HIV-1-tg rats [91]. HIV-1 gp120 was similarly described to cause a loss of dopamine-secreting neurons in rats [92–94]. HIV-1 Nef is another viral protein disturbing the dopamine functions, reducing striatal dopamine levels in HIV-1 mice. The animal will consequently develop mania-like behaviors and present a reduced content of dopamine and DAT [95].

HIV+ subjects present a diminished motor performance at multitasking and a decreased velocity compared to the control group. This may affect the daily life and require more attention to every motor task [96]. A psychomotor slowing of HIV patients was already described in early neuropsychological studies [97], which was presumed to be from the frontostriatal origin. The first hypothesis for the gait and balance problems was a neuropathy of the peripheral nervous system [98, 99]. However, the cerebellum, and the pons more exactly, is also implicated in HIV infection [100–105].

There is evidence of cerebellar damage [105–107] and an important degeneration of the cerebellar granular cell layer and axonal swelling. CT and MRI show pontocerebellar damage in HIV infection [108] and 3–6% of an HIV-infected group [109]. Men and women show tissue volume deficits in combined pons, vermis tissue, and cerebellar hemispheres. This will result in a deficit in motor performance like static postural stability, and tandem walking, particularly when the patients have their eyes closed during the test. The psychomotor speed and the finger dexterity were also impaired.

The pediatric HIV-1 infection will present different complications, involving deep abnormalities in the striatal dopamine system including the basal ganglia. The HIV-infected children present a slower-than-normal information processing and poor attentional abilities [110–112].

4. Epigenetic changes

4.1. Methylation levels

Epigenetic alterations are one of the hallmarks of aging. As epigenetic changes accumulate upon aging, DNA methylation can be a precise predictor of chronological age [113, 114], since certain CpG sites are highly associated with age [115].

A first large-scale epigenome-wide association study in 2016 analyzed DNA methylation during HIV infection [116] and found a differential DNA methylation associated with the infection. HIV-1, as other viruses, can alter the expression of DNA methyltransferases (DNMTs), like DNMT1 [117, 118] and DNMT3b [119], affecting maintenance and de novo DNA methylation maintenance. The alteration of methylation could be an epigenetic outcome of the integration of HIV-1 DNA into the host genome and could decrease genome stability. These studies were made in blood, and because of the presence of the blood-brain barrier, it was necessary to analyze methylation directly in the brain tissue.

A 2015 study uses blood and brain tissue to find a relationship between HIV status and epigenetic age acceleration [120]. It eliminates different hypothesis explaining age acceleration effects in the brain tissue. It concluded that the telomere length is not involved and finds difficult to explain the age acceleration in the brain by the increase in the amount of senescent or exhausted T-cells like it is working in the blood, because of the blood-brain barrier. The retained hypothesis is an effect of the age acceleration, and independently the T-cells exhaust, confounding the relationship between these two events. In 2016, a comparative DNA methylation profiling on monocytes derived from HIV-infected individuals, with or without impairment, identifies a specific immunoepigenetic signature of cognitive impairment [121]. A total of 1032 loci differentially methylated are associated with cognitive impairment, with loci connected to gene networks in the central nervous system and preferentially located in intergenic regions of the gene and over gene bodies. A more recent analysis was made on DNA from the occipital cortex of 58 HIV+ subjects that were followed for neurocognitive evaluation within 1 year of death [122]. It is the first study to associate HAND status with the epigenetic age of frontal cortex tissue, with an average relative acceleration of 3.5 years. This accelerated epigenetic aging was not the consequence of CD4+ cell count or viral load, the activity of HAART on the CNS, or comorbidities. Interestingly, the entire HAND group presented accelerated aging in the brain tissue, but that was not correlated with HAND gravity or neurocognitive performance. This accelerated aging seems linked to the duration of the infection and suggests that a low level but chronic HIV replication in brain reservoirs maintains pathological processes.

4.2. microRNA

The genome-wide expression analysis of miRNA in aging brains showed a unique expression profile which emphasizes how crucial their role is in the neurodegeneration and the aging process [123].

MiR-34a has been linked to the regulation of several proteins including sirtuin 1 (SIRT1) [124]. SIRT1 is an enzyme implicated in the deacetylation of proteins involved in cell stress, longevity, and glucose metabolism [125]. Mir-34a up-regulation, the reciprocal decline of its target SIRT1, is the biomarker for aging in the brain and a good predictor of deterioration of the brain function. The miR-34a expression is significantly increased in HIV-infected vascular endothelial cells (ECs) [126] as well as in primary neuronal cultures and neuronal cell lines [127]. MiR-146a was also up-regulated in these cells. HIV-1 vpr has the same ability to strongly overexpress miR-34a and miR-146a in neuronal cells and to down-regulate miR-106a [128]. The up-regulation of miR-34a and miR146a [129] and the down-regulation of miR-106a [130] are described to be associated with aging. The increase of miR-34a can cause abnormal mitochondrial dynamics and dysfunctional autophagy [131].

4.3. HIV-1 disrupts the calcium signaling in the brain

Changes in calcium signaling are major factors leading to aging, as many vital functions of the brain depend on precise calcium homeostasis [132]. Khachaturian presented in 1994 his hypothesis of aging [133] to try to elucidate the neurophysiological mechanisms of Ca^{2+} signaling that they are associated with aging and neurodegeneration.

HIV-1 disturbs the functional expression and activity of voltage-gated calcium channel (VGCCs) (changes in evoked Ca^{2+} spikes and L-channel expression) in the mPFC in an age-dependent way and implies that ion-channel dysfunction associated with HIV-induced medial PreFrontal Cortex (mPFC) hyper-excitability progresses with age/HIV duration [134].

HIV-infected individuals, especially as they age, are subject to neuronal Ca^{2+} dysregulation and neurotoxicity elicited by the HIV-1 proteins gp120, Tat, and Vpr [135–137]. Tat protein increases neuronal Ca^{2+} levels via IP3R and NMDAR and L-type Ca^{2+} channels, followed by mitochondrial Ca^{2+} uptake and ROS production, leading to caspase activation and neuronal apoptosis [137–139]. In microglia and astrocytes, Tat and gp120 can interact and trigger the production of cytokines, nitric oxide, and excitotoxins which can intensify the neurotoxic effects of Tat and gp120 [137]. HIV-1 Vpr is also able to activate the expression of cytokines, ROS, and inflammatory proteins in uninfected and infected cells. Vpr will elicit a slow but persistent elevation of Ca^{2+} leading to glutamate signaling impairment in neuronal cells. Moreover, the calcium homeostasis is disturbed by Vpr via down-regulation of endogenous PMCA [136].

4.4. Inflammation links aging to the brain

The neuroinflammation is present even in the absence of productive infection and may have a different cause, like an undetectable level of virus production, the effects of combination antiretroviral therapy (cART) itself, and/or a chronic and systemic immune action. Together, these factors contribute to HIV-1 neurodegeneration. The stimulated microglia will synthesize neurotoxic molecules, inflammatory mediators like cytokines/chemokines, and provoke glutamate receptor-mediated excitotoxicity, disrupt intracellular calcium concentration and ion channel expression, and mechanisms controlling cAMP levels. Viral latency and residual inflammation are codependent mechanisms promoting each other [140]. The peripheral immune activation and production of peripheral cytokines increase inflammation within the CNS and have been associated with lower cognitive performance [141–148].

In the HIV-infected brain, the microglia will produce NF-kappa B, triggering the secretion of the pro-inflammatory cytokine TNFα which stimulates NF-kappa B signaling in neurons of the medial basal hypothalamus in a feed-forward loop. IKKβ/NF-κB inhibits GnRH and activates aging-related hypothalamic GnRH degeneration. The inhibition of IKKβ/NF-κB activation or GnRH treatment can reverse the aging effects of HIV-1 and increase the lifespan [149]. This feedback loop has been linked to the hypothalamic programming of systemic aging [149]. In primary astrocytes, HIV stimulates C3 expression indirectly, via NF-κB-dependent induction of IL-6, which will activate the C3 promoter [150].

A senescence-associated secretory phenotype (SASP), a central aspect of cellular senescence, is activated when the certain chemokines/cytokines, especially IL-6, IL-8, and IL-1 α, are secreted. These interleukins play a major role in brain aging [151–153]. HIV-1 infection is quickly followed by the inflammasome activation, allowing the release of IL-6, IL-8, IL-18, IFN-γ, IL-1β, IL-2Rα, IL-3, IL-6, TNFα, IL-1Rα, IL-10, IL-1α, and TNFβ [154, 155].

4.5. Influence of cART on neurotoxicity

The development of highly active antiretroviral therapy (HAART) has changed the neurodegeneration pattern and prevented the major cognitive impairments of AIDS, increasing survival times.

To be effective in the brain, combination antiretroviral therapy (cART) has to cross the blood–brain barrier and be metabolized. However, if these drugs made it possible to alleviate cognitive impairment, they can contribute to it and damage nerve cells. Indeed, long-term cART can generate toxic effects and contribute to HAND. The efavirenz (EFV) metabolites 7-hydroxyefavirenz (7-OH-EFV) and especially 8-hydroxyefavirenz (8-OH-EFV) can provoke damage to dendritic spines. Furthermore, the 8-OH-EFV metabolite can trigger calcium flux in neurons, mainly mediated by L-type voltage-operated calcium channels (VOCCs), and acts as a potent neurotoxin [156]. The mitochondrial respiratory capacity (SRC) is reduced by maraviroc, raltegravir, lopinavir, darunavir, zidovudine, emtricitabine, abacavir, nevirapine, and efavirenz but not by indinavir. Efavirenz and maraviroc provoke a reduction of ATP at the synapse that may contribute to its dysfunction [157, 158]. Additionally, the non-nucleoside reverse transcriptase inhibitor efavirenz can decrease neural stem cell proliferation [159]. Non-nucleoside reverse transcriptase inhibitors (NRTIs) are key players in HAART-induced mitochondrial toxicity due to their capacity to inhibit the DNA polymerase in charge of the synthesis of mitochondrial DNA, Pol-γ [160–162]. Some brains under HAART present neuroinflammation combined with mononuclear phagocyte activation, notably in the hippocampus, and can reach the level seen in AIDS and HIVE pre-HAART [163].

4.6. Anti-oxidant defense

Oxidative phosphorylation is a highly efficient way of generating energy to produce adenosine triphosphate (ATP). Oxygen is a key player in this metabolic pathway in mitochondria to break down the glucose. Reactive oxygen species (ROS), hydroxyl radical (OH^-), hydrogen peroxide (H_2O_2), and superoxide (O_2^-) are usually produced at low levels. If the balance between antioxidants and pro-oxidant is disturbed, oxidative damage can occur, followed by mitochondrial dysfunction and accumulation of cytotoxins leading to cell death. The brain is rich in fatty acids, which make neurons highly sensitive to oxidative alteration and peroxidation [164], in particular because it has fewer antioxidants than other tissue and higher iron levels. Under oxidation, the membrane lipids can undergo lipid peroxidation producing malondialdehyde (MDA) and 4-hydroxynonenal (4-HNE). The endogenous brain defense against oxidative stress is composed of glutathione peroxidase (GPx1), superoxide dismutases (SOD), catalase, and glutathione (γ-l-glutamyl-l-cysteinylglycine, GSH) [165].

In HAND, oxidative stress increased levels of oxidized proteins and lipid peroxidation products, at the same time than a deficit in GSH and GPx1 [166–169]. The lipid peroxidation induced by HIV-1 affects the specific region of the brain [170] and is correlated with the gravity of HAND [171]. Several viral proteins are involved in this mechanism. Tat is inducing the reactive oxygen species (ROS) superoxide (O_2^-) and hydrogen peroxide (H_2O_2), increasing at the same time the levels of lipid peroxidation. It is able also to induce nitric oxide synthase (iNOS) to generate nitric oxide (NO), which when combined with superoxide (O_2^-) will form the peroxynitrite (ONOO) [172]. Gp120 triggers the release of arachidonic acid in glial cells [173], from the lipoxygenase and cyclooxygenase pathways [173]. Gp41 can provoke neuronal cell death by a mechanism involving NO formation, iNOS, and a deficit in glutathione, which will subsequently disrupt the mitochondrial function [174, 175]. Vpr induces the production of ROS after a reduction in the total GSH/GSSG ratio and an increase in the level of oxidized glutathione (GSSG) [176].

4.7. Mitochondria

In the mitochondrial theory of aging (or free-radical theory of aging), the reactive oxygen species, which are the products of respiration, damage the membranes, mitochondrial DNA (mtDNA), and proteins, causing an accumulation of cellular and molecular injuries subsequently responsible for aging. It creates a "vicious cycle" when the mtDNA damage increases ROS production, which will damage even more the mtDNA [177].

The HIV-1 infection initiates changes in mitochondrial electron transport chain (ETC), mitochondrial trafficking proteins, glycolytic pathways, and proteins implicated in several energy pathways. In the presence of HIV-1 proteins, the mitochondria face a higher energy demand, will consume more oxygen, and show a higher capacity to produce ATP. These mechanisms are usually observed when there is cellular damage leading to ROS production [178].

During HAND, mitochondrial fission/fusion mechanism is dysregulated. The mitochondrial fission protein (dynamin 1-like, DNM1L) is decreased in frontal cortex tissues of HAND patients, and the soma of damaged neurons presents elongated and enlarged mitochondria. The GFAP-gp120 mice present the same phenotype, and gp120 also decreases the DNML1 levels. The mitochondrial fusion seems to be the predominant mitochondrial dynamic in the brains of HAND patients [179]. HIV-1 Tat provokes a massive diminution in the mitochondrial membrane potential, a mechanism closely linked to fusion and fission. It is probably the consequence of the quick increase Tat caused on the intracellular Ca^{2+}, whether via the NMDA receptor or L-type calcium channels. The levels of mitochondrial fission protein Drp1 are consequently increased and the mitochondrial morphology is altered by Tat. Unbalanced mitochondrial fission and fusion are responsible for several neurodegenerative disorders [180]. HIV-1 Vpr promotes the formation of permeability transition pores in mitochondria, which disturbs the transmembrane potential and the ATP synthesis. This process permeabilizes the mitochondria and allows the release of cytochrome *c* via a cascade of caspase and leads to apoptosis [181]. Moreover, Vpr decreases rapidly the mitochondrial membrane potential [182], which provokes the formation of the permeability transition pore complex (PTPC) [183], composed by the adenine nucleotide translocator (ANT) on the inner mitochondrial membrane and the voltage-dependent anion channel (VDAC) on the outer mitochondrial membrane. This creation of mitochondrial conductance channels will allow the release of apoptosis-inducing factor cytochrome *c* into the cytoplasm, as described in striatal and cortical neurons of rats [184]. Following HIV-1 Vpr treatment, the intracellular glutathione is reduced, maybe the result of decreased ATP availability when Vpr binds to the ANT on the inner mitochondrial membrane [185]. HIV-1 Vpr is also described to impair the mitochondria axonal transport [186].

4.8. Autophagy

Defects in autophagy can lead to several neurodegenerative diseases like Parkinson's disease, Alzheimer's disease, and amyotrophic lateral sclerosis (ALS) for the most common [187]. Without autophagic cleaning, protein aggregates will accumulate and become toxic to the cells. Aging is slowing down the efficiency of cell autophagy (macroautophagy and chaperone-mediated autophagy) either by diminishing the autophagic flux or by too much cargo accumulation from chronic cell injury [187]. Some interventions intend to increase the autophagy levels like caloric restriction or autophagy-inducing drugs can attenuate age-linked pathologies and lengthen the lifespan [188–190].

The activation of autophagy is beneficial for the virus during the initial phase of HIV-1 infection in many cell types [191]. However, the autophagy inhibition is necessary for virus replication in later phases of infection, stimulating the biogenesis of exosomes enclosing viral products [192]. In HIV-1 dementia, the neurodegeneration seems to be associated with the inhibition of neuronal autophagy, a decrease in autophagy-inducing protein, and an increase in sequestosome-1/p62 [193]. Autophagy genes like *SQSTM1*, *ATG5*, and *LAMP1* appear to be differentially regulated at the transcriptional, translational, and post-translational levels by HIV-1 in the brain at a different stage of the disease [194]. Basal autophagy is inhibited by the HIV-1 infection in CD4+, monocyte/macrophage lineage [195], as well as in neurons and astrocytes and leads to neuro-glial toxicity [196].

Nef binds BECN1 and inhibits the proteolytic stages of autophagy in HIV-infected macrophages [197, 198]. In astrocytes, Nef is also blocking the fusion of autophagosome to lysosome to escape the viral degradation, increasing LC3II and p62/SQSTM1 levels. It is interesting to note that LC3 and Gag interact and that basal autophagy promotes optimal Gag processing and yields of HIV in macrophages [195]. Gag processing is increased when autophagy is induced, manipulating the autophagy process to maximize the viral replication in infected macrophages. The Gag protein is the main target of autophagy, but HIV-1 has taken advantage of Gag targeting for its replication, especially in macrophages. HIV-1 Tat is targeted for degradation via an ubiquitin-independent pathway, as an anti-HIV effect, interacting with p62/SQSTM1 in CD4+ T lymphocytes. However, Tat can counteract this degradation by decreasing the quantity of the autophagy markers LC3II andp62/SQSTM1 coupled with the membrane in neurons [199]. Moreover, Tat can bind to the lysosomal-associated membrane protein 2A (LAMP2A) to regulate the fusion of autophagosomes with lysosomes. Through this interaction with LAMP2, Tat may allow abnormal autophagolysosome formation, leading to neurodegeneration [199]. Gp120 on the opposite is inducing autophagy in neuronal cells [200], probably as a protective mechanism from the toxic effects of gp120 [201].

5. Conclusion

The aging mechanism linked to aging is the consequence of multiple heterogeneous processes and is the interplay of several areas including physiological changes, metabolical aging, or cognitive impairment. The HIV-associated aging is distinct from chronological aging and should be treated as well. It will be influenced by the cognitive reserve of the patient, modeled by its social, cultural, physical, and economic environment.

Author details

Maryline Santerre[1] and Bassel Sawaya[1,2*]

*Address all correspondence to: sawaya@temple.edu

1 Molecular Studies of Neurodegenerative Diseases Lab, Fels Institute for Cancer Research and Molecular Biology, Lewis Katz School of Medicine, Temple University, Philadelphia, PA, USA

2 Department of Neurology, Lewis Katz School of Medicine, Temple University, Philadelphia, PA, USA

References

[1] Sowell ER et al. Mapping cortical change across the human life span. Nature Neuroscience. 2003;**6**:309-315

[2] Fjell AM, Walhovd KB. Structural brain changes in aging: Courses, causes and cognitive consequences. Reviews in the Neurosciences. 2010;**21**:187-221

[3] Missori P et al. In normal aging ventricular system never attains pathological values of Evans' index. Oncotarget. 2016;**7**:11860-11863

[4] Chang L et al. Impact of apolipoprotein E ε4 and HIV on cognition and brain atrophy: Antagonistic pleiotropy and premature brain aging. NeuroImage. 2011;**58**:1017-1027

[5] Bell JE. The neuropathology of adult HIV infection. Revue Neurologique (Paris). 1998;**154**:816-829

[6] Cardenas VA et al. Evidence for ongoing brain injury in human immunodeficiency virus-positive patients treated with antiretroviral therapy. Journal of Neurovirology. 2009;**15**:324-333

[7] Archibald SL et al. Correlation of in vivo neuroimaging abnormalities with postmortem human immunodeficiency virus encephalitis and dendritic loss. Archives of Neurology. 2004;**61**:369-376

[8] Ghafouri M, Amini S, Khalili K, Sawaya BE. HIV-1 associated dementia: Symptoms and causes. Retrovirology. 2006;**3**:28

[9] Chiang MC et al. 3D pattern of brain atrophy in HIV/AIDS visualized using tensor-based morphometry. NeuroImage. 2007;**34**:44-60

[10] Harezlak J et al. Persistence of HIV-associated cognitive impairment, inflammation, and neuronal injury in era of highly active antiretroviral treatment. AIDS. 2011;**25**:625-633

[11] Lepore N et al. Generalized tensor-based morphometry of HIV/AIDS using multivariate statistics on deformation tensors. IEEE Transactions on Medical Imaging. 2008;**27**:129-141

[12] Ances BM, Ortega M, Vaida F, Heaps J, Paul R. Independent effects of HIV, aging, and HAART on brain volumetric measures. Journal of Acquired Immune Deficiency Syndromes. 2012;**59**:469-477

[13] Towgood KJ et al. Mapping the brain in younger and older asymptomatic HIV-1 men: Frontal volume changes in the absence of other cortical or diffusion tensor abnormalities. Cortex. 2012;**48**:230-241

[14] Becker JT et al. Factors affecting brain structure in men with HIV disease in the post-HAART era. Neuroradiology. 2012;**54**:113-121

[15] Seider TR et al. Age exacerbates HIV-associated white matter abnormalities. Journal of Neurovirology. 2016;**22**:201-212

[16] Thompson PM et al. 3D mapping of ventricular and corpus callosum abnormalities in HIV/AIDS. NeuroImage. 2006;**31**:12-23

[17] Chang L, Yakupov R, Nakama H, Stokes B, Ernst T. Antiretroviral treatment is associated with increased attentional load-dependent brain activation in HIV patients. Journal of Neuroimmune Pharmacology. 2008;**3**:95-104

[18] Gongvatana A et al. Clinical contributors to cerebral white matter integrity in HIV-infected individuals. Journal of Neurovirology. 2011;**17**:477-486

[19] Boone KB et al. Neuropsychological correlates of white-matter lesions in healthy elderly subjects. A threshold effect. Archives of Neurology. 1992;**49**:549-554

[20] Ylikoski A et al. White matter hyperintensities on MRI in the neurologically nondiseased elderly. Analysis of cohorts of consecutive subjects aged 55 to 85 years living at home. Stroke. 1995;**26**:1171-1177

[21] Maniega SM et al. White matter hyperintensities and normal-appearing white matter integrity in the aging brain. Neurobiology of Aging. 2015;**36**:909-918

[22] Shoamanesh A et al. Inflammatory biomarkers, cerebral microbleeds, and small vessel disease: Framingham Heart Study. Neurology. 2015;**84**:825-832

[23] Debette S, Markus HS. The clinical importance of white matter hyperintensities on brain magnetic resonance imaging: Systematic review and meta-analysis. BMJ. 2010;**341**:c3666

[24] Fern RF, Matute C, Stys PK. White matter injury: Ischemic and nonischemic. Glia. 2014;**62**:1780-1789

[25] O'Connor EE, Jaillard A, Renard F, Zeffiro TA. Reliability of white matter microstructural changes in HIV infection: Meta-analysis and confirmation. AJNR. American Journal of Neuroradiology. 2017;**38**:1510-1519

[26] Stout JC et al. Progressive cerebral volume loss in human immunodeficiency virus infection: A longitudinal volumetric magnetic resonance imaging study. HIV Neurobehavioral Research Center Group. Archives of Neurology. 1998;**55**:161-168

[27] Carey AN et al. Conditional Tat protein expression in the GT-tg bigenic mouse brain induces gray matter density reductions. Progress in Neuro-Psychopharmacology & Biological Psychiatry. 2013;**43**:49-54

[28] Carey AN et al. Conditional Tat protein brain expression in the GT-tg bigenic mouse induces cerebral fractional anisotropy abnormalities. Current HIV Research. 2015;**13**:3-9

[29] Hahn YK et al. Effects of chronic HIV-1 Tat exposure in the CNS: Heightened vulnerability of males versus females to changes in cell numbers, synaptic integrity, and behavior. Brain Structure & Function. 2015;**220**:605-623

[30] Cole JH et al. Increased brain-predicted aging in treated HIV disease. Neurology. 2017;**88**:1349-1357

[31] Xiong H, Zeng YC, Zheng J, Thylin M, Gendelman HE. Soluble HIV-1 infected macrophage secretory products mediate blockade of long-term potentiation: A mechanism for cognitive dysfunction in HIV-1-associated dementia. Journal of Neurovirology. 1999;**5**:519-528

[32] Zink WE et al. Impaired spatial cognition and synaptic potentiation in a murine model of human immunodeficiency virus type 1 encephalitis. The Journal of Neuroscience. 2002;**22**:2096-2105

[33] Anderson ER et al. Hippocampal synaptic dysfunction in a murine model of human immunodeficiency virus type 1 encephalitis. Neuroscience. 2003;**118**:359-369

[34] Xiong H et al. Inhibition of long-term potentiation by interleukin-8: Implications for human immunodeficiency virus-1-associated dementia. Journal of Neuroscience Research. 2003;**71**:600-607

[35] Bliss TV, Collingridge GL. A synaptic model of memory: Long-term potentiation in the hippocampus. Nature. 1993;**361**:31-39

[36] D'hooge R, Franck F, Mucke L, De Deyn PP. Age-related behavioural deficits in transgenic mice expressing the HIV-1 coat protein gp120. The European Journal of Neuroscience. 1999;**11**:4398-4402

[37] Dong J, Xiong H. Human immunodeficiency virus type 1 gp120 inhibits long-term potentiation via chemokine receptor CXCR4 in rat hippocampal slices. Journal of Neuroscience Research. 2006;**83**:489-496

[38] Keblesh JP, Dou H, Gendelman HE, Xiong H. 4-Aminopyridine improves spatial memory in a murine model of HIV-1 encephalitis. Journal of Neuroimmune Pharmacology. 2009;**4**:317-327

[39] Fitting S et al. Synaptic dysfunction in the hippocampus accompanies learning and memory deficits in human immunodeficiency virus type-1 Tat transgenic mice. Biological Psychiatry. 2013;**73**:443-453

[40] Li ST et al. HIV-1 Tat inhibits long-term potentiation and attenuates spatial learning [corrected]. Annals of Neurology. 2004;**55**:362-371

[41] Lisman J, Cooper K, Sehgal M, Silva AJ. Memory formation depends on both synapse-specific modifications of synaptic strength and cell-specific increases in excitability. Nature Neuroscience. 2018;**21**:309-314

[42] Morgan DG, May PC, Finch CE. Dopamine and serotonin systems in human and rodent brain: Effects of age and neurodegenerative disease. Journal of the American Geriatrics Society. 1987;**35**:334-345

[43] Blazer D, Hughes DC, George LK. The epidemiology of depression in an elderly community population. Gerontologist. 1987;**27**:281-287

[44] Casey DA. Depression in the elderly. Southern Medical Journal. 1994;**87**:559-563

[45] Israelski DM et al. Psychiatric co-morbidity in vulnerable populations receiving primary care for HIV/AIDS. AIDS Care. 2007;**19**:220-225

[46] Bing EG et al. Psychiatric disorders and drug use among human immunodeficiency virus-infected adults in the United States. Archives of General Psychiatry. 2001;**58**:721-728

[47] Horberg MA et al. Effects of depression and selective serotonin reuptake inhibitor use on adherence to highly active antiretroviral therapy and on clinical outcomes in HIV-infected patients. Journal of Acquired Immune Deficiency Syndromes. 2008;**47**:384-390

[48] Maes M, Leonard BE, Myint AM, Kubera M, Verkerk R. The new '5-HT' hypothesis of depression: Cell-mediated immune activation induces indoleamine 2,3-dioxygenase, which leads to lower plasma tryptophan and an increased synthesis of detrimental tryptophan catabolites (TRYCATs), both of which contribute to the onset of depression. Progress in Neuro-Psychopharmacology & Biological Psychiatry. 2011;**35**:702-721

[49] Schröcksnadel K, Wirleitner B, Winkler C, Fuchs D. Monitoring tryptophan metabolism in chronic immune activation. Clinica Chimica Acta. 2006;**364**:82-90

[50] Widner B, Laich A, Sperner-Unterweger B, Ledochowski M, Fuchs D. Neopterin production, tryptophan degradation, and mental depression—What is the link? Brain, Behavior, and Immunity. 2002;**16**:590-595

[51] Schroecksnadel K et al. Quality of life and immune activation in patients with HIV-infection. Brain, Behavior, and Immunity. 2008;**22**:881-889

[52] Samikkannu T, Rao KV, Gandhi N, Saxena SK, Nair MP. Human immunodeficiency virus type 1 clade B and C Tat differentially induce indoleamine 2,3-dioxygenase and serotonin in immature dendritic cells: Implications for neuroAIDS. Journal of Neurovirology. 2010;**16**:255-263

[53] Zangerle R et al. Increased blood phenylalanine to tyrosine ratio in HIV-1 infection and correction following effective antiretroviral therapy. Brain, Behavior, and Immunity. 2010;**24**:403-408

[54] Neurauter G et al. Chronic immune stimulation correlates with reduced phenylalanine turnover. Current Drug Metabolism. 2008;**9**:622-627

[55] Fuchs D et al. Immune activation and decreased tryptophan in patients with HIV-1 infection. Journal of Interferon Research. 1990;**10**:599-603

[56] Fuchs D et al. Interferon-gamma concentrations are increased in sera from individuals infected with human immunodeficiency virus type 1. Journal of Acquired Immune Deficiency Syndromes. 1989;**2**:158-162

[57] Fuchs D et al. Decreased serum tryptophan in patients with HIV-1 infection correlates with increased serum neopterin and with neurologic/psychiatric symptoms. Journal of Acquired Immune Deficiency Syndromes. 1990;**3**:873-876

[58] Manéglier B et al. Serotonin decreases HIV-1 replication in primary cultures of human macrophages through 5-HT(1A) receptors. British Journal of Pharmacology. 2008;**154**:174-182

[59] Frank MG, Hendricks SE, Johnson DR, Wieseler JL, Burke WJ. Antidepressants augment natural killer cell activity: In vivo and in vitro. Neuropsychobiology. 1999;**39**:18-24

[60] Evans DL et al. Selective serotonin reuptake inhibitor and substance P antagonist enhancement of natural killer cell innate immunity in human immunodeficiency virus/acquired immunodeficiency syndrome. Biological Psychiatry. 2008;**63**:899-905

[61] Fauci AS, Mavilio D, Kottilil S. NK cells in HIV infection: Paradigm for protection or targets for ambush. Nature Reviews. Immunology. 2005;**5**:835-843

[62] Strittmatter WJ et al. Apolipoprotein E: High-avidity binding to beta-amyloid and increased frequency of type 4 allele in late-onset familial Alzheimer disease. Proceedings of the National Academy of Sciences of the United States of America. 1993;**90**:1977-1981

[63] Travis J. New piece in Alzheimer's puzzle. Science. 1993;**261**:828-829

[64] Corder EH et al. Gene dose of apolipoprotein E type 4 allele and the risk of Alzheimer's disease in late onset families. Science. 1993;**261**:921-923

[65] Grant I et al. Evidence for early central nervous system involvement in the acquired immunodeficiency syndrome (AIDS) and other human immunodeficiency virus (HIV) infections. Studies with neuropsychologic testing and magnetic resonance imaging. Annals of Internal Medicine. 1987;**107**:828-836

[66] Corder EH et al. HIV-infected subjects with the E4 allele for APOE have excess dementia and peripheral neuropathy. Nature Medicine. 1998;**4**:1182-1184

[67] Burt TD et al. Apolipoprotein (apo) E4 enhances HIV-1 cell entry in vitro, and the APOE epsilon4/epsilon4 genotype accelerates HIV disease progression. Proceedings of the National Academy of Sciences of the United States of America. 2008;**105**:8718-8723

[68] Soontornniyomkij V et al. Cerebral β-amyloid deposition predicts HIV-associated neurocognitive disorders in APOE ε4 carriers. AIDS. 2012;**26**:2327-2335

[69] Cooley SA et al. Apolipoprotein E ε4 genotype status is not associated with neuroimaging outcomes in a large cohort of HIV+ individuals. Journal of Neurovirology. 2016;**22**:607-614

[70] Wendelken LA et al. ApoE ε4 is associated with cognition, brain integrity, and atrophy in HIV over age 60. Journal of Acquired Immune Deficiency Syndromes. 2016;**73**:426-432

[71] Pomara N, Belzer K, Sidtis JJ. Deleterious CNS effects of the APOE epsilon4 allele in individuals with HIV-1 infection may be age-dependent. Proceedings of the National Academy of Sciences of the United States of America. 2008;**105**:E65; author reply E67-68

[72] Mukerji SS et al. Lipid profiles and APOE4 allele impact midlife cognitive decline in HIV-infected men on antiretroviral therapy. Clinical Infectious Diseases. 2016;**63**:1130-1139

[73] Reeve A, Simcox E, Turnbull D. Ageing and Parkinson's disease: Why is advancing age the biggest risk factor? Ageing Research Reviews. 2014;**14**:19-30

[74] Rodriguez M, Rodriguez-Sabate C, Morales I, Sanchez A, Sabate M. Parkinson's disease as a result of aging. Aging Cell. 2015;**14**:293-308

[75] Bäckman L, Lindenberger U, Li SC, Nyberg L. Linking cognitive aging to alterations in dopamine neurotransmitter functioning: Recent data and future avenues. Neuroscience and Biobehavioral Reviews. 2010;**34**:670-677

[76] Colzato LS, van den Wildenberg WP, Hommel B. The genetic impact (C957T-DRD2) on inhibitory control is magnified by aging. Neuropsychologia. 2013;**51**:1377-1381

[77] Li SC et al. Aging magnifies the effects of dopamine transporter and D2 receptor genes on backward serial memory. Neurobiology of Aging. 2013;**34**(358):e351-e310

[78] Nagel IE et al. Human aging magnifies genetic effects on executive functioning and working memory. Frontiers in Human Neuroscience. 2008;**2**:1

[79] Störmer VS, Passow S, Biesenack J, Li SC. Dopaminergic and cholinergic modulations of visual-spatial attention and working memory: Insights from molecular genetic research and implications for adult cognitive development. Developmental Psychology. 2012;**48**:875-889

[80] Kumar AM, Ownby RL, Waldrop-Valverde D, Fernandez B, Kumar M. Human immunodeficiency virus infection in the CNS and decreased dopamine availability: Relationship with neuropsychological performance. Journal of Neurovirology. 2011;**17**:26-40

[81] Kumar AM, Borodowsky I, Fernandez B, Gonzalez L, Kumar M. Human immunodeficiency virus type 1 RNA levels in different regions of human brain: Quantification using real-time reverse transcriptase-polymerase chain reaction. Journal of Neurovirology. 2007;**13**:210-224

[82] Reyes MG, Faraldi F, Senseng CS, Flowers C, Fariello R. Nigral degeneration in acquired immune deficiency syndrome (AIDS). Acta Neuropathologica. 1991;**82**:39-44

[83] Itoh K, Mehraein P, Weis S. Neuronal damage of the substantia nigra in HIV-1 infected brains. Acta Neuropathologica. 2000;**99**:376-384

[84] Hriso E, Kuhn T, Masdeu JC, Grundman M. Extrapyramidal symptoms due to dopamine-blocking agents in patients with AIDS encephalopathy. The American Journal of Psychiatry. 1991;**148**:1558-1561

[85] Valcour V et al. Aging exacerbates extrapyramidal motor signs in the era of highly active antiretroviral therapy. Journal of Neurovirology. 2008;**14**:362-367

[86] Kumar AM et al. Human immunodeficiency virus type 1 in the central nervous system leads to decreased dopamine in different regions of postmortem human brains. Journal of Neurovirology. 2009;**15**:257-274

[87] Khanlou N et al. Increased frequency of alpha-synuclein in the substantia nigra in human immunodeficiency virus infection. Journal of Neurovirology. 2009;**15**:131-138

[88] Silvers JM et al. Dopaminergic marker proteins in the substantia nigra of human immunodeficiency virus type 1-infected brains. Journal of Neurovirology. 2006;**12**:140-145

[89] Wang GJ et al. Decreased brain dopaminergic transporters in HIV-associated dementia patients. Brain. 2004;**127**:2452-2458

[90] Yuan Y et al. Molecular mechanism of HIV-1 Tat interacting with human dopamine transporter. ACS Chemical Neuroscience. 2015;**6**:658-665

[91] Zhu J et al. HIV-1 transgenic rats display an increase in [(3)H]dopamine uptake in the prefrontal cortex and striatum. Journal of Neurovirology. 2016;**22**:282-292

[92] Bennett BA, Rusyniak DE, Hollingsworth CK. HIV-1 gp120-induced neurotoxicity to midbrain dopamine cultures. Brain Research. 1995;**705**:168-176

[93] Mocchetti I, Nosheny RL, Tanda G, Ren K, Meyer EM. Brain-derived neurotrophic factor prevents human immunodeficiency virus type 1 protein gp120 neurotoxicity in the rat nigrostriatal system. Annals of the New York Academy of Sciences. 2007;**1122**:144-154

[94] Bachis A, Aden SA, Nosheny RL, Andrews PM, Mocchetti I. Axonal transport of human immunodeficiency virus type 1 envelope protein glycoprotein 120 is found in association with neuronal apoptosis. The Journal of Neuroscience. 2006;**26**:6771-6780

[95] Acharjee S et al. HIV-1 Nef expression in microglia disrupts dopaminergic and immune functions with associated mania-like behaviors. Brain, Behavior, and Immunity. 2014;**40**:74-84

[96] Kronemer SI, Mandel JA, Sacktor NC, Marvel CL. Impairments of motor function while multitasking in HIV. Frontiers in Human Neuroscience. 2017;**11**:212

[97] Butters N et al. Assessment of AIDS-related cognitive changes: Recommendations of the NIMH workshop on neuropsychological assessment approaches. Journal of Clinical and Experimental Neuropsychology. 1990;**12**:963-978

[98] Goodkin K et al. Aging and neuro-AIDS conditions and the changing spectrum of HIV-1-associated morbidity and mortality. Journal of Clinical Epidemiology. 2001;**54**(Suppl 1):S35-S43

[99] Richardson JK, Hurvitz EA. Peripheral neuropathy: A true risk factor for falls. The Journals of Gerontology. Series A, Biological Sciences and Medical Sciences. 1995;**50**:M211-M215

[100] Abe H, Mehraein P, Weis S. Degeneration of the cerebellar dentate nucleus and the inferior olivary nuclei in HIV-1-infected brains: A morphometric analysis. Acta Neuropathologica. 1996;**92**:150-155

[101] Anders KH et al. Multifocal necrotizing leukoencephalopathy with pontine predilection in immunosuppressed patients: A clinicopathologic review of 16 cases. Human Pathology. 1993;**24**:897-904

[102] Kinzel N, Strike D, Clark HB, Cavert W. Cerebellopontine degeneration as an immune restoration disease in HIV infection. AIDS. 2004;**18**:2348-2350

[103] Kuchelmeister K, Bergmann M, Gullotta F. Cellular changes in the cerebellar granular layer in AIDS-associated PML. Neuropathology and Applied Neurobiology. 1993;**19**:398-401

[104] Ruiz A, Post MJ, Bundschu CC. Dentate nuclei involvement in AIDS patients with CNS cryptococcosis: Imaging findings with pathologic correlation. Journal of Computer Assisted Tomography. 1997;**21**:175-182

[105] Tagliati M et al. Cerebellar degeneration associated with human immunodeficiency virus infection. Neurology. 1998;**50**:244-251

[106] Everall IP et al. Decreased expression of AMPA receptor messenger RNA and protein in AIDS: A model for HIV-associated neurotoxicity. Nature Medicine. 1995;**1**:1174-1178

[107] Scatliff JH et al. Postmortem MR imaging of the brains of patients with AIDS. Neuroimaging Clinics of North America. 1997;**7**:297-320

[108] Flowers CH et al. Encephalopathy in AIDS patients: Evaluation with MR imaging. AJNR. American Journal of Neuroradiology. 1990;**11**:1235-1245

[109] Klunder AD et al. Mapping cerebellar degeneration in HIV/AIDS. Neuroreport. 2008;**19**:1655-1659

[110] Burns S, Hernandez-Reif M, Jessee P. A review of pediatric HIV effects on neurocognitive development. Issues in Comprehensive Pediatric Nursing. 2008;**31**:107-121

[111] Webb KM, Mactutus CF, Booze RM. The ART of HIV therapies: Dopaminergic deficits and future treatments for HIV pediatric encephalopathy. Expert Review of Anti-Infective Therapy. 2009;**7**:193-203

[112] Willen EJ. Neurocognitive outcomes in pediatric HIV. Mental Retardation and Developmental Disabilities Research Reviews. 2006;**12**:223-228

[113] Horvath S. DNA methylation age of human tissues and cell types. Genome Biology. 2013;**14**:R115

[114] Hannum G et al. Genome-wide methylation profiles reveal quantitative views of human aging rates. Molecular Cell. 2013;**49**:359-367

[115] Jones MJ, Goodman SJ, Kobor MS. DNA methylation and healthy human aging. Aging Cell. 2015;**14**:924-932

[116] Zhang X et al. Epigenome-wide differential DNA methylation between HIV-infected and uninfected individuals. Epigenetics. 2016;**11**:750-760

[117] Youngblood B, Reich NO. The early expressed HIV-1 genes regulate DNMT1 expression. Epigenetics. 2008;**3**:149-156

[118] Fang JY, Mikovits JA, Bagni R, Petrow-Sadowski CL, Ruscetti FW. Infection of lymphoid cells by integration-defective human immunodeficiency virus type 1 increases de novo methylation. Journal of Virology. 2001;**75**:9753-9761

[119] Pion M, Jaramillo-Ruiz D, Martínez A, Muñoz-Fernández MA, Correa-Rocha R. HIV infection of human regulatory T cells downregulates Foxp3 expression by increasing DNMT3b levels and DNA methylation in the FOXP3 gene. AIDS. 2013;**27**:2019-2029

[120] Horvath S, Levine AJ. HIV-1 infection accelerates age according to the epigenetic clock. The Journal of Infectious Diseases. 2015;**212**:1563-1573

[121] Corley MJ et al. Comparative DNA methylation profiling reveals an immunoepigenetic signature of HIV-related cognitive impairment. Scientific Reports. 2016;**6**:33310

[122] Levine AJ et al. Accelerated epigenetic aging in brain is associated with pre-mortem HIV-associated neurocognitive disorders. Journal of Neurovirology. 2016;**22**:366-375

[123] Persengiev SP, Kondova II, Bontrop RE. The impact of MicroRNAs on brain aging and Neurodegeneration. Current Gerontology and Geriatrics Research. 2012;**2012**:359369

[124] Yamakuchi M, Ferlito M, Lowenstein CJ. miR-34a repression of SIRT1 regulates apoptosis. Proceedings of the National Academy of Sciences of the United States of America. 2008;**105**:13421-13426

[125] Brunet A et al. Stress-dependent regulation of FOXO transcription factors by the SIRT1 deacetylase. Science. 2004;**303**:2011-2015

[126] Zhan J et al. miR-34a is a common link in both HIV- and antiretroviral therapy-induced vascular aging. Aging (Albany NY). 2016;**8**:3298-3310

[127] Chang JR et al. HIV-1 Tat protein promotes neuronal dysfunction through disruption of microRNAs. The Journal of Biological Chemistry. 2011;**286**:41125-41134

[128] Mukerjee R et al. Deregulation of microRNAs by HIV-1 Vpr protein leads to the development of neurocognitive disorders. The Journal of Biological Chemistry. 2011;**286**:34976-34985

[129] Rippo MR et al. MitomiRs in human inflamm-aging: A hypothesis involving miR-181a, miR-34a and miR-146a. Experimental Gerontology. 2014;**56**:154-163

[130] Hackl M et al. miR-17, miR-19b, miR-20a, and miR-106a are down-regulated in human aging. Aging Cell. 2010;**9**:291-296

[131] Kou X et al. Swimming attenuates d-galactose-induced brain aging via suppressing miR-34a-mediated autophagy impairment and abnormal mitochondrial dynamics. Journal of Applied Physiology (1985). 2017;**122**:1462-1469

[132] Chandran R et al. Cellular calcium signaling in the aging brain. Journal of Chemical Neuroanatomy. 2017

[133] Khachaturian ZS. Calcium hypothesis of Alzheimer's disease and brain aging. Annals of the New York Academy of Sciences. 1994;**747**:1-11

[134] Khodr CE, Chen L, Al-Harthi L, Hu XT. Aging alters voltage-gated calcium channels in prefrontal cortex pyramidal neurons in the HIV brain. Journal of Neurovirology. 2018;**24**:113-118

[135] Nath A. Human immunodeficiency virus (HIV) proteins in neuropathogenesis of HIV dementia. The Journal of Infectious Diseases. 2002;**186**(Suppl 2):S193-S198

[136] Rom I et al. HIV-1 Vpr deregulates calcium secretion in neural cells. Brain Research. 2009;**1275**:81-86

[137] Haughey NJ, Mattson MP. Calcium dysregulation and neuronal apoptosis by the HIV-1 proteins Tat and gp120. Journal of Acquired Immune Deficiency Syndromes. 2002;**31**(Suppl 2):S55-S61

[138] Haughey NJ, Holden CP, Nath A, Geiger JD. Involvement of inositol 1,4,5-trisphosphate-regulated stores of intracellular calcium in calcium dysregulation and neuron cell death caused by HIV-1 protein tat. Journal of Neurochemistry. 1999;**73**:1363-1374

[139] Kruman II, Nath A, Mattson MP. HIV-1 protein Tat induces apoptosis of hippocampal neurons by a mechanism involving caspase activation, calcium overload, and oxidative stress. Experimental Neurology. 1998;**154**:276-288

[140] Gougeon ML. Alarmins and central nervous system inflammation in HIV-associated neurological disorders. Journal of Internal Medicine. 2017;**281**:433-447

[141] Buchanan JB, Sparkman NL, Chen J, Johnson RW. Cognitive and neuroinflammatory consequences of mild repeated stress are exacerbated in aged mice. Psychoneuroendocrinology. 2008;**33**:755-765

[142] Tonelli LH, Postolache TT. Tumor necrosis factor alpha, interleukin-1 beta, interleukin-6 and major histocompatibility complex molecules in the normal brain and after peripheral immune challenge. Neurological Research. 2005;**27**:679-684

[143] Reichenberg A et al. Cytokine-associated emotional and cognitive disturbances in humans. Archives of General Psychiatry. 2001;**58**:445-452

[144] Hilsabeck RC et al. Cognitive efficiency is associated with endogenous cytokine levels in patients with chronic hepatitis C. Journal of Neuroimmunology. 2010;**221**:53-61

[145] Rothenburg LS et al. The relationship between inflammatory markers and post stroke cognitive impairment. Journal of Geriatric Psychiatry and Neurology. 2010;**23**:199-205

[146] Gimeno D, Marmot MG, Singh-Manoux A. Inflammatory markers and cognitive function in middle-aged adults: The Whitehall II study. Psychoneuroendocrinology. 2008;**33**:1322-1334

[147] Rafnsson SB et al. Cognitive decline and markers of inflammation and hemostasis: The Edinburgh Artery Study. Journal of the American Geriatrics Society. 2007;**55**:700-707

[148] Oliveira MF et al. Early antiretroviral therapy is associated with lower HIV DNA molecular diversity and lower inflammation in cerebrospinal fluid but does not prevent the establishment of compartmentalized HIV DNA populations. PLoS Pathogens. 2017;**13**:e1006112

[149] Zhang G et al. Hypothalamic programming of systemic ageing involving IKK-β, NF-κB and GnRH. Nature. 2013;**497**:211-216

[150] Nitkiewicz J et al. HIV induces expression of complement component C3 in astrocytes by NF-κB-dependent activation of interleukin-6 synthesis. Journal of Neuroinflammation. 2017;**14**:23

[151] Godbout JP, Johnson RW. Interleukin-6 in the aging brain. Journal of Neuroimmunology. 2004;**147**:141-144

[152] Willette AA et al. Interleukin-8 and interleukin-10, brain volume and microstructure, and the influence of calorie restriction in old rhesus macaques. Age (Dordrecht, Netherlands). 2013;**35**:2215-2227

[153] Griffin WS, Mrak RE. Interleukin-1 in the genesis and progression of and risk for development of neuronal degeneration in Alzheimer's disease. Journal of Leukocyte Biology. 2002;**72**:233-238

[154] Ragin AB et al. Brain alterations within the first 100 days of HIV infection. Annals of Clinical Translational Neurology. 2015;**2**:12-21

[155] Walsh JG et al. Rapid inflammasome activation in microglia contributes to brain disease in HIV/AIDS. Retrovirology. 2014;**11**:35

[156] Tovar-y-Romo LB et al. Dendritic spine injury induced by the 8-hydroxy metabolite of efavirenz. The Journal of Pharmacology and Experimental Therapeutics. 2012;**343**:696-703

[157] Stauch KL, Emanuel K, Lamberty BG, Morsey B, Fox HS. Central nervous system-penetrating antiretrovirals impair energetic reserve in striatal nerve terminals. Journal of Neurovirology. 2017;**23**:795-807

[158] Funes HA et al. Neuronal bioenergetics and acute mitochondrial dysfunction: A clue to understanding the central nervous system side effects of efavirenz. The Journal of Infectious Diseases. 2014;**210**:1385-1395

[159] Jin J et al. HIV non-nucleoside reverse transcriptase inhibitor Efavirenz reduces neural stem cell proliferation in vitro and in vivo. Cell Transplantation. 2016;**25**:1967-1977

[160] Apostolova N, Blas-García A, Esplugues JV. Mitochondrial interference by anti-HIV drugs: Mechanisms beyond pol-γ inhibition. Trends in Pharmacological Sciences. 2011;**32**:715-725

[161] Saitoh A, Fenton T, Alvero C, Fletcher CV, Spector SA. Impact of nucleoside reverse transcriptase inhibitors on mitochondria in human immunodeficiency virus type 1-infected children receiving highly active antiretroviral therapy. Antimicrobial Agents and Chemotherapy. 2007;**51**:4236-4242

[162] Walker UA. Update on mitochondrial toxicity: Where are we now? Journal of HIV Therapy. 2003;**8**:32-35

[163] Anthony IC, Ramage SN, Carnie FW, Simmonds P, Bell JE. Influence of HAART on HIV-related CNS disease and neuroinflammation. Journal of Neuropathology and Experimental Neurology. 2005;**64**:529-536

[164] Uttara B, Singh AV, Zamboni P, Mahajan RT. Oxidative stress and neurodegenerative diseases: A review of upstream and downstream antioxidant therapeutic options. Current Neuropharmacology. 2009;**7**:65-74

[165] Beal MF. Aging, energy, and oxidative stress in neurodegenerative diseases. Annals of Neurology. 1995;**38**:357-366

[166] Turchan J et al. Oxidative stress in HIV demented patients and protection ex vivo with novel antioxidants. Neurology. 2003;**60**:307-314

[167] Mollace V et al. Oxidative stress and neuroAIDS: Triggers, modulators and novel antioxidants. Trends in Neurosciences. 2001;**24**:411-416

[168] Buhl R et al. Systemic glutathione deficiency in symptom-free HIV-seropositive individuals. Lancet. 1989;**2**:1294-1298

[169] Staal FJ et al. Intracellular glutathione levels in T cell subsets decrease in HIV-infected individuals. AIDS Research and Human Retroviruses. 1992;**8**:305-311

[170] Sacktor N et al. Novel markers of oxidative stress in actively progressive HIV dementia. Journal of Neuroimmunology. 2004;**157**:176-184

[171] Bandaru VV et al. Associative and predictive biomarkers of dementia in HIV-1-infected patients. Neurology. 2007;**68**:1481-1487

[172] Bonfoco E, Krainc D, Ankarcrona M, Nicotera P, Lipton SA. Apoptosis and necrosis: Two distinct events induced, respectively, by mild and intense insults with N-methyl-D-aspartate or nitric oxide/superoxide in cortical cell cultures. Proceedings of the National Academy of Sciences of the United States of America. 1995;**92**:7162-7166

[173] Dreyer EB, Kaiser PK, Offermann JT, Lipton SA. HIV-1 coat protein neurotoxicity prevented by calcium channel antagonists. Science. 1990;**248**:364-367

[174] Adamson DC et al. Immunologic NO synthase: Elevation in severe AIDS dementia and induction by HIV-1 gp41. Science. 1996;**274**:1917-1921

[175] Adamson DC, Kopnisky KL, Dawson TM, Dawson VL. Mechanisms and structural determinants of HIV-1 coat protein, gp41-induced neurotoxicity. The Journal of Neuroscience. 1999;**19**:64-71

[176] Ferrucci A, Nonnemacher MR, Cohen EA, Wigdahl B. Extracellular human immunodeficiency virus type 1 viral protein R causes reductions in astrocytic ATP and glutathione levels compromising the antioxidant reservoir. Virus Research. 2012;**167**:358-369

[177] Kowald A, Kirkwood TB. Evolution of the mitochondrial fusion-fission cycle and its role in aging. Proceedings of the National Academy of Sciences of the United States of America. 2011;**108**:10237-10242

[178] Villeneuve LM et al. HIV-1 transgenic rats display mitochondrial abnormalities consistent with abnormal energy generation and distribution. Journal of Neurovirology. 2016;**22**:564-574

[179] Fields JA et al. HIV alters neuronal mitochondrial fission/fusion in the brain during HIV-associated neurocognitive disorders. Neurobiology of Disease. 2016;**86**:154-169

[180] Rozzi SJ, Avdoshina V, Fields JA, Mocchetti I. Human immunodeficiency virus Tat impairs mitochondrial fission in neurons. Cell Death Discovery. 2018;**4**:8

[181] Mishra S, Mishra JP, Kumar A. Activation of JNK-dependent pathway is required for HIV viral protein R-induced apoptosis in human monocytic cells: Involvement of antiapoptotic BCL2 and c-IAP1 genes. The Journal of Biological Chemistry. 2007;**282**:4288-4300

[182] Jacotot E et al. The HIV-1 viral protein R induces apoptosis via a direct effect on the mitochondrial permeability transition pore. The Journal of Experimental Medicine. 2000;**191**:33-46

[183] Vieira HL et al. Permeabilization of the mitochondrial inner membrane during apoptosis: Impact of the adenine nucleotide translocator. Cell Death and Differentiation. 2000;**7**:1146-1154

[184] Sabbah EN, Roques BP. Critical implication of the (70-96) domain of human immunodeficiency virus type 1 Vpr protein in apoptosis of primary rat cortical and striatal neurons. Journal of Neurovirology. 2005;**11**:489-502

[185] Ferrucci A, Nonnemacher MR, Wigdahl B. Human immunodeficiency virus viral protein R as an extracellular protein in neuropathogenesis. Advances in Virus Research. 2011;**81**:165-199

[186] Wang Y et al. HIV-1 Vpr disrupts mitochondria axonal transport and accelerates neuronal aging. Neuropharmacology. 2017;**117**:364-375

[187] Frake RA, Ricketts T, Menzies FM, Rubinsztein DC. Autophagy and neurodegeneration. The Journal of Clinical Investigation. 2015;**125**:65-74

[188] Rubinsztein DC, Mariño G, Kroemer G. Autophagy and aging. Cell. 2011;**146**:682-695

[189] López-Otín C, Blasco MA, Partridge L, Serrano M, Kroemer G. The hallmarks of aging. Cell. 2013;**153**:1194-1217

[190] Madeo F, Zimmermann A, Maiuri MC, Kroemer G. Essential role for autophagy in life span extension. The Journal of Clinical Investigation. 2015;**125**:85-93

[191] Kyei GB et al. Autophagy pathway intersects with HIV-1 biosynthesis and regulates viral yields in macrophages. The Journal of Cell Biology. 2009;**186**:255-268

[192] Ojha CR et al. Interplay between autophagy, exosomes and HIV-1 associated neurological disorders: New insights for diagnosis and therapeutic applications. Viruses. 2017;**9**

[193] Alirezaei M, Kiosses WB, Fox HS. Decreased neuronal autophagy in HIV dementia: A mechanism of indirect neurotoxicity. Autophagy. 2008;**4**:963-966

[194] Dever SM, Rodriguez M, Lapierre J, Costin BN, El-Hage N. Differing roles of autophagy in HIV-associated neurocognitive impairment and encephalitis with implications for morphine co-exposure. Frontiers in Microbiology. 2015;**6**:653

[195] Campbell GR, Spector SA. Inhibition of human immunodeficiency virus type-1 through autophagy. Current Opinion in Microbiology. 2013;**16**:349-354

[196] Mehla R, Chauhan A. HIV-1 differentially modulates autophagy in neurons and astrocytes. Journal of Neuroimmunology. 2015;**285**:106-118

[197] Sardo L, Iordanskiy S, Klase Z, Kashanchi F. HIV-1 Nef blocks autophagy in human astrocytes. Cell Cycle. 2015;**14**:3781-3782

[198] Saribas AS, Khalili K, Sariyer IK. Dysregulation of autophagy by HIV-1 Nef in human astrocytes. Cell Cycle. 2015;**14**:2899-2904

[199] Fields J et al. HIV-1 Tat alters neuronal autophagy by modulating autophagosome fusion to the lysosome: Implications for HIV-associated neurocognitive disorders. The Journal of Neuroscience. 2015;**35**:1921-1938

[200] Liu Z, Xiao Y, Torresilla C, Rassart É, Barbeau B. Implication of different HIV-1 genes in the modulation of autophagy. Viruses. 2017;**9**

[201] Pandhare J, Dash S, Jones B, Villalta F, Dash C. A novel role of proline oxidase in HIV-1 envelope glycoprotein-induced neuronal autophagy. The Journal of Biological Chemistry. 2015;**290**:25439-25451

7

Human Immunodeficiency Virus-Hepatitis B Virus (HIV-HBV) Coinfection

Berthold Bivigou-Mboumba

Abstract

The global epidemics of hepatitis B and HIV have led to a new understanding of the complex interactions between these two viruses. Due to similar patterns of contamination, the high prevalence of HBV infection among the 33 million people living with HIV (PLHIV) across the world is about 10%. In highly endemic areas such as sub-Saharan Africa, this prevalence can be as high as 15% and leads us systematically to seek HIV/HBV co-infection. According to WHO, nearly 240 million people are chronically infected with HBV worldwide. Of these, 4 million are co-infected with HIV. Overall, co-infection rates range from 5 to 14% in areas of low prevalence of HBV infection and 5–73% in areas of high prevalence for HBV infection. Studies have revealed the complexity of the infection relationship between HIV and HBV. This complex relationship is thought to be responsible for greater morbidity and mortality of hepatic origin in co-infected patients than in mono-infected individuals. This chapter will highlight the following main points:

- Concomitant negative impact of HIV and HBV on their natural histories
- Implication of concomitant negative impact on the overall management of HIV-HBV coinfection
- Treatment and management.

Keywords: HIV, HBV, HIV-HBV coinfection, occult hepatitis B infection

1. Introduction

1.1. General information on HIV

The human immunodeficiency virus (HIV) is an enveloped RNA virus (two copies) belonging to the family of Retroviridae, genus Lentivirus. HIV infection and its natural evolution lead to a set of opportunistic, infectious, or tumoral manifestations, consequences of an immunodepression qualified as acquired immunodeficiency syndrome (AIDS). To date, there are two types of HIV: the first, called HIV-1, is responsible for the pandemic and HIV-2 is more common in West Africa [1].

1.2. Genomic structure and organization

Morphologically, HIV is a single spherical particle with a diameter ranging from 90 to 120 nm. The virion has a spiky envelope and a dense nucleocapsid, sometimes trapezoidal or bar-shaped.

Structurally it is described as follows (**Figure 1**).

The viral body comprises two identical RNA molecules; three viral enzymes (reverse transcriptase (p66/p51); protease (p10) and integrase (p32)]; and three internal proteins [24 kDa capsid protein (p24); the 7KDa nucleocapsid protein (p7) that is associated with the RNA molecules; and the outermost protein, associated with the viral protease, the 17 kDa matrix protein (p17)].

The viral envelope, emanation of the cellular cytoplasmic membrane, carries two viral glycoproteins (gp) essential in the virus-host cell interaction. This is the gp41 (41 kDa glycoprotein found in the transmembrane position) and the gp120 (120 kDa glycoprotein, lining the outer surface and thus allowing the attachment to its cellular receptor, the CD4 molecule) [1].

HIV has gag, pol, and env as structural genes that encode internal proteins, viral enzymes, and envelope glycoproteins, respectively [2], and it has six regulatory genes: tat, rev, nef, alive, vpr, vpu (for HIV-1), and vpx (for HIV-2) [1] (**Figure 2**).

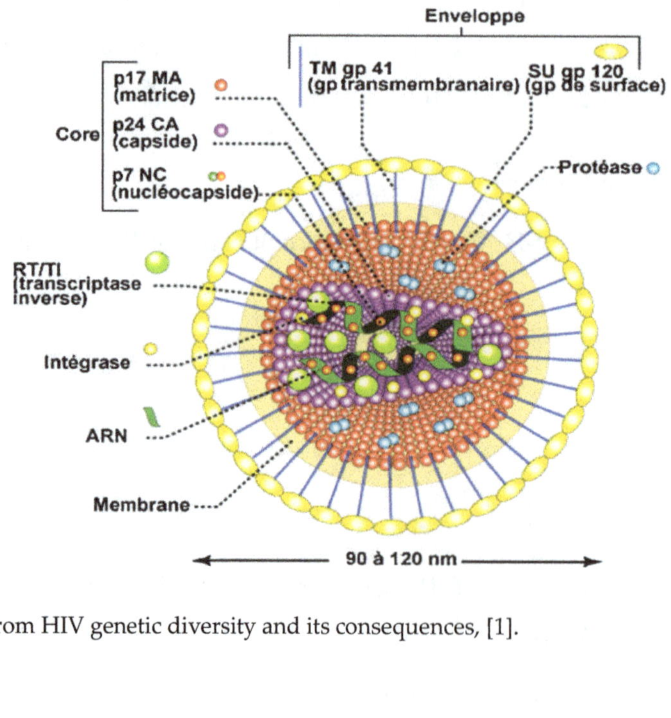

Figure 1. HIV structure (from HIV genetic diversity and its consequences, [1].

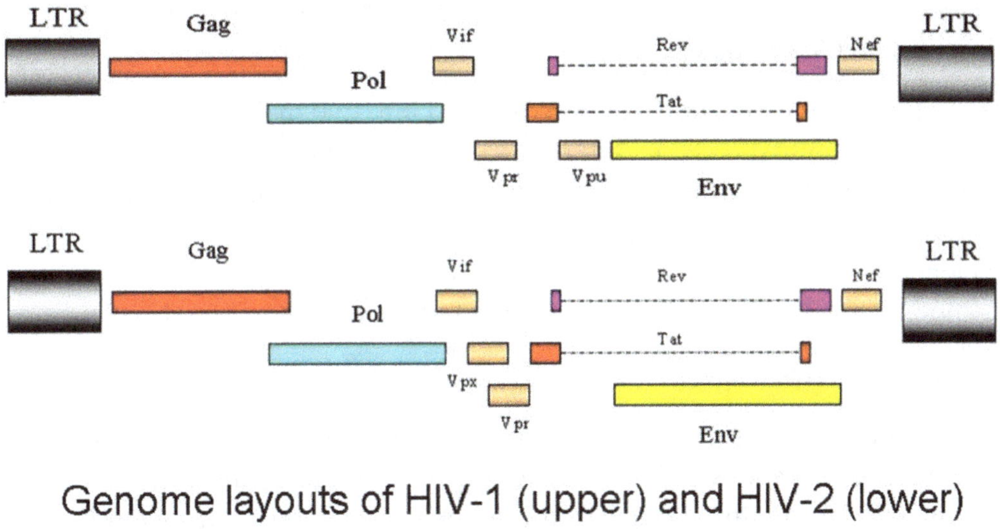

Figure 2. Genomic organisation of HIV-1 and HIV-2 [2].

The reverse transcriptase (RT) allows the viral genome (RNA) to be retro-transcribed into DNA, thus promoting integration into the chromosomal DNA of the host cell: at this stage, the HIV is called "provirus." In its proviral form, HIV is flanked on both sides by repetitive sequences, strongly implicated in the transcription and integration of the virus. These sequences are called LTR for long terminal repeat and consist of three non-coding regions (U3, R, and U5), allowing the integration of double-stranded DNA into the chromosomal DNA of the host cell. These regions contain, at the 5 'ends of the LTRs, promoters that control the initiation and regulation of viral genome transcription, under the influence of viral and cellular factors [2].

1.3. Prevalence of HIV in the world

In 2015, the number of HIV-related deaths ranged from 930,000 to 1,300,000 worldwide [3]. According to Global AIDS in 2016, approximately, 37 million people live with HIV and 21 million are under treatment.

The distribution of HIV infection is not equitable in the world, sub-Saharan Africa is the most affected region. In 2015, it alone counted 25,600,000 people living with HIV (PLHIV) or nearly 70% of the world's PLHIV. The overall prevalence in this part of the world is 5.0% (95% CI, 4.7–5.2), with 1,900,000 new infections per year.

1.4. Pathophysiology

Infection caused by HIV is responsible for the progressive destruction of the immune system, primarily by the removal of CD4 T-cells. These are the targets of the virus to ensure its replication. Lymphocyte homeostasis, which allows proliferation of lymphocyte cells, is gradually becoming ineffective. The immune system thus weakened leads to the appearance of so-called "opportunistic" infections. Eventually, the infected subject dies as a result of this generalized immunosuppression (AIDS stage).

The natural history of HIV infection has been divided into two major phases. The seroconversion stage occurs in the first 6 weeks after infection, a period between the time of infection and the appearance of antibodies. In some patients this phase is accompanied by an influenza state. During this phase, viral replication is intense (every day 1 billion viruses are produced), where viral load levels up to more than 1 million copies per mL of plasma [4], and the patient is very infectious. CD4 T-cell level drops transient but usually returns to baseline.

The chronic phase has two stages.

Asymptomatic phase: This is the clinical latency phase. The immune system continuously destroys the viruses to keep the viral load low (no virological latency). At the same time the CD4 count will gradually decrease. This phase may persist for several years (up to 15 years).

Symptomatic phase: It lasts from a few months to several years. The immune system begins to weaken and no longer effectively controls viral replication. The number of CD4 T lymphocytes then decreases significantly. The lymphoid organs no longer compensate for this destruction. Opportunistic infections make their appearance, defining the AIDS stage.

Much progress has been made in the fight against the HIV pandemic. Antiretroviral treatment (ART) is based on the use of three molecules (triple therapy) interacting with HIV on its different targets. ART aims to achieve and maintain undetectable plasma viral load. It must restore immunity, measurable by measuring the level of CD4. Finally, it significantly reduces the risk of transmission in patients controlling viral replication [5].

TAR blocks viral multiplication by acting on the replicative cycle stages of HIV by interference. Currently there are six classes of antiretrovirals for five targets located in the replicative cycle:

- Three enzymatic targets: nucleos(t)idic and non-nucleos(t)idic reverse transcriptase inhibitors (NRTIs and NNRTIs), protease inhibitors (PIs), and integrase inhibitors (IINs);
- One protein target: fusion inhibitor (IF); and
- One cell target: antagonist of the CCR5 co-receptor.

Nucleoside inhibitors of reverse transcriptase (NIRT)
Abacavir (ABC)
Stavudine (D4T)
Ténofovir (TDF)
Lamivudine (3TC)
Didanosine (DDI)
Zidovudine (AZT)
Emtricitabine (FTC)

Non-nucleosidic inhibitors of reverse transcriptase (NNIRT)

Efavirenz(EFV)

Etravirine (ETR)

Névirapine (NVP)

Rilpivirine (RPV)

Protease inhibitor (PI)

Atazanavir/r (ATV/r)

Darunavir/r (DRV/r)

Fosamprenavir/r (FPV/r)

Indinavir/r (IDV/r)

Lopinavir/r (LPV/r)

Nelfinavir (NFV)

Saquinavir/r (SQV/r)

Tipranavir/r (TPV/r)

Integrase inhibitors

Dolutégravir (DTG)

Elvitégravir (EVG)

Raltégravir (RAL)

Fusion inhibitor

Enfuvirtide (ENF ou T20)

CCR5 antagonist

Maraviroc (MRC)

The new 2015 WHO guidelines stipulate that anyone infected with HIV should be systematically put on ART, regardless of CD4 T-cell level or viral load.

2. General information on HIV-HBV coinfection

The global epidemics of hepatitis B and HIV have led to a new understanding of the complex interactions between these two viruses. Due to similar patterns of contamination (bloodstream, sexual pathway, and mother-to-child transmission), the high prevalence of HBV infection among the 33 million people living with HIV (PLHIV) across the world is about 10% [6]. In highly endemic areas such as the sub-Saharan Africa, this prevalence can be as high as 15% and leads us systematically to seek HIV/HBV coinfection.

According to the WHO, nearly 240 million people are chronically infected with HBV worldwide. Of these, 4 million are coinfected with HIV. Overall, coinfection rates range from 5 to

14% in areas of low prevalence of HBV infection and 5–73% in areas of high prevalence for HBV infection [7–9].

2.1. Concomitant negative impact of HIV and HBV on their natural histories

2.1.1. HIV impact

Studies have revealed the complexity of the infection relationship between HIV and HBV. This complex relationship is thought to be responsible for greater morbidity and mortality of hepatic origin in co-infected patients than in mono-infected individuals [10, 11].

The natural history of HBV infection has changed in people living with HIV, where the immune system is weakened by the destruction of HIV-infected CD4 T-cells [12]. The risk of developing chronic hepatitis B after contracting HBV is six times more common in HIV-infected people than in non-HIV-infected people [13]. Indeed, immunosuppression caused by HIV is associated with a change in the time of occurrence of each event in the natural history of HBV infection. The evolution of acute HBV infection is altered in PLHIV with serological, biochemical, immunological and molecular consequences:

Focus on the serological markers, the rates of anti-HBs and HBsAg loss and/or seroconversion might be higher in HIV-HBV coinfected patients compared with patients who are HBV monoinfected [14]. So occult hepatitis B infection, reactivation (reverse seroconversion) of chronic HBV infection and fulminate hepatitis, appears mainly in HIV virologic failure [15]. In PLHIV and those chronically infected by HBV, the related rate of hepatitis B e antigen (HBeAg) clearance is five times lower than in HBV-infected individuals alone [13]. Diminution of HBsAg quantity may be responsible for its non-detection by immunochromatographic tests, in cases of patients with HBV active replication.

2.1.2. Fulminant hepatitis B (HBF)

A syndrome produced by the major dysfunction of certain functions of the liver, fulminant hepatitis occurs in less than 1% of cases of acute jaundice hepatitis. It may be due to isolated acute hepatitis B or coinfection with hepatitis delta virus. More rarely, fulminant hepatitis occurs in chronic HBV carriers due to spontaneous or chemo-induced reactivation or super-infection with HDV [16]. It is characterized by a reduction of more than 50% of coagulation factors of hepatic origin. The liver is no longer able to destroy the neurotoxic substances produced; they are found in the bloodstream and migrate to the brain where they cause hepatic encephalopathy. All this is in the absence of an underlying liver pathology [17]. Typically, HBV DNA and HBeAg become undetectable rapidly, while hepatocellular insufficiency occurs. The simultaneous presence of HBsAg and anti-HBs in immune complexes is implicated in the severity of the clinical picture.

2.1.3. Occult hepatitis B (HBO)

The Taormina conference held in Italy in 2008 defined occult hepatitis B (HBO) as "the presence of HBV DNA in the liver, detectable or undetectable in serum, in individuals tested negative for HBsAg by an internationally validated serological test" [18]. It is a chronic infection, therefore persistent over time with low-noise viral replication: It is described as a silent infection. In fact, in most cases, the HBV CV associated with these infections is very low (<200 IU/mL), but it can vary to reach high levels [19]. Serologically, occult infections known as seronegative are characterized by the absence of anti-HBs and anti-HBc and are distinguished from occult infections called seropositive that are associated with the seroconversion of anti-HBs and/or anti-HBc. Numerous studies have shown that the presence of isolated anti-HBc antibodies is closely correlated with the occult status of HBV infection [18, 20]. However, in 20% of patients with occult infection, no serologic marker of HBV infection is observed [21]. The prevalence of HBOs varies from 1 to 87% [22], depending on the population studied, the sensitivity of the diagnostic tests, and the nature of the sample used [23, 24]. Studies also show that HBO is significantly associated with the endemicity of HBV infection but is not limited to hyper-endemic countries for HBV [23–26]. The actuality of this problem is related to the fact that HBO can be transmitted during blood transfusions, provoke the reactivation of chronic hepatitis B in immunocompromised persons, and facilitate the development of hepatic cirrhosis and hepatocellular carcinoma. In most cases, occult infection goes unnoticed, which poses significant health problems, such as the transmission of the virus through blood transfusions and transplants [27–30].

This type of hepatitis B also has the distinction of being the cause of fulminant hepatitis but also of promoting cirrhosis of the liver, HCC, and treatment failure in the case of coinfection with HCV [31, 32].

Variations in the genome including mutations in the major antigenic loop, mutations in viral polymerase, modifications resulting from alternative splicing, and mutations in the pre-S region have been associated with occult hepatitis B.

Studies have shown that HBV DNA is detected more often in people living with HIV than in non-HIV people [33, 34]. The severity and persistence of immunosuppression play an important role in reactivating HBO.

On the biochemical point of view, interaction between HIV and HBV, it is observed that Alanine aminotransferase (ALT) enzyme levels are often greater than 5 times the upper limit of the normal range (ALT normal range: 1–22 IU/L) [35]. This has consequences on physiopathology, by increasing the risk of liver-related morbidity and mortality compared to HIV monoinfected individuals. However, normal transaminase levels should not be interpreted to mean that there is no underlying hepatic fibrosis.

On the immunological point of view, HIV has been shown to directly infect hepatocytes, hepatic stellate cells (HSC), or Kupffer cells, which are implicated on intrahepatic injury. HIV can also significantly affect the integrity of the gastrointestinal tract leading to elevated levels of LPS. LPS can directly activate Kupffer cells and HSC leading to increased intrahepatic inflammation and fibrosis [36].

On the molecular point of view, in PLHIV, HBV DNA replication may be diminished due to hepatocytes' direct infection by HIV in competition with HBV.

HBV resistance mutations are more common in HIV patients than in non-HIV patients. This is linked to the massive consumption of reverse transcriptase inhibitors (active against both HIV and HBV) with a low genetic barrier, such as 3TC.

HBV reactivation is more prevalent in HIV-HBV co-infected individuals than in HBV mono-infected individuals. This reactivation is particularly found in patients with an isolated anti-HBc profile [37, 38].

HIV accelerates the risk of cirrhosis and HCC. HIV/HBV patients have higher HBV CVs and therefore more frequent cirrhosis compared to HBV-only patients [11, 39, 40].

HBV is not directly cytopathic and the physiopathogenesis of its infection is immunomodulated. Hepatic lesions are recorded due to inflammation and lysis of infected cells that express HBsAg on their surface as a consequence of an immune response of the host.

The evolution of the infection is thus conditioned by the intensity, the efficiency, and the speed of the activation of the immune response. Healing is easily associated with an early and effective immune response. On the other hand, viral persistence is associated with a defective immune response. Cells such as macrophages, neutrophils, NK, and NKT cells provide a nonspecific and early immune response, causing necroinflammatory lesions [41].

The fact that HIV attaches to the surface of hepatocytes using co-receptors CCR5 and CXCR4 and Kupffer cells (hepatic stellate cells, HSC) causes a direct cytopathic effect of HIV on the liver tissue. This results in the triggering of cellular apoptosis by TNF-α (TRAIL: TNF-α-related apoptosis-inducing ligand) [42, 43]. Moreover, by infecting HSCs, HIV increases myofibroblastic differentiation and leads to the acceleration of the fibrosis process [44]. Finally, there is the hepatotoxicity of HIV treatment taken on a continuous basis.

2.1.4. HBV impact

Likewise, HBV infection would have a negative impact on the natural history of HIV infection. Permanent activation of the immune system in patients chronically infected with HBV would result in the increased viral replication of HIV [45]. Other studies have shown that HBV can induce continuous replication of HIV due to the action of HBV gene X expression in synergy with the Kappa B cell enhancer and T cell activators on the cell [46, 47].

HBV has also been indexed in reducing CD4 levels, although the mechanism is not clearly known [9, 48]. In sum, studies indicate that the risk of progression to AIDS and/or dying is 3.6–6.8 times higher in coinfection (HIV-HBV) than in HIV mono-infection [49, 50].

Finally, HBV, by destroying hepatocytes, the regulator of toxins in the body, increases the risk of antiretroviral toxicity [51].

2.2. Implication of concomitant negative impact on the overall management of HIV-HBV coinfection

The goal of HBC treatment is to improve the quality of life and survival of infected people by preventing progression of cirrhosis, complications of chronic hepatitis B infection (HBF, HBO, reactivation…), and the hepatocellular carcinoma (HCC) [52, 53].

Therapeutic management of HBV infection was clearly defined in the WHO guidelines in 2015. It is therefore stipulated that in HIV-HBV co-infected individuals, antiretroviral therapy

(ART) should be introduced. For all those who have evidence of chronic hepatitis, regardless of the stage of hepatitis, specifically, for adults, adolescents, and children 3 years of age and older, the TDF + 3TC/FTC + EFV fixed-dose combination is recommended to begin antiretroviral therapy [54].

It is therefore imperative that the diagnosis be made. In case of resistance to 3TC, the addition of TDF to antiretroviral therapy including 3TC or FTC is the solution of choice [55].

It is true that the current WHO recommendations are "test and treat". However, as these measures are not yet universally adopted, the previous recommendations of the WHO and the European AIDS Clinical Society (EACS) will be proposed here for the global management of HIV-HBV coinfection.

These recommendations stem from the management of patients who are mono-infected with HBV. They take into account three parameters required to initiate treatment against HBV: (a) the level of serum HBV DNA (>2000 IU/ml), (b) the elevation of ALT to more than two times the normal rate, and (c) liver histological lesions following the METAVIR score (activity expressed as grade ≥A2 and/or fibrosis level expressed as ≥F2) [56].

The therapeutic choice is based on two elements: (i) the indication or not of an antiretroviral treatment and (ii) the possible presence of cirrhosis.

In cases where HIV treatment is not indicated, that is, in patients with CD4 greater than 500 cells/mm^3, dual activity HIV and HBV molecules should not be used to avoid the resistance of HIV against these molecules [56] (**Figure 3**).

Surveillance and treatment include HBV viral load and ALT level. (1) The high rate of DNA is correlated with the risk of progression to cirrhosis and hepatocellular carcinoma, the analyses continue before treatment. (2) METAVIR score ≥A2 and/or APRI score ≥F2. (3) Treatment duration is 48 weeks for Peg IFN and nucleoside or nucleotide analogues may be discontinued 6 months after seroconversion HBs and/or Hbe. (4) The use of telbivudine and adefovir in this situation is difficult because of potential anti-HIV activity [55].

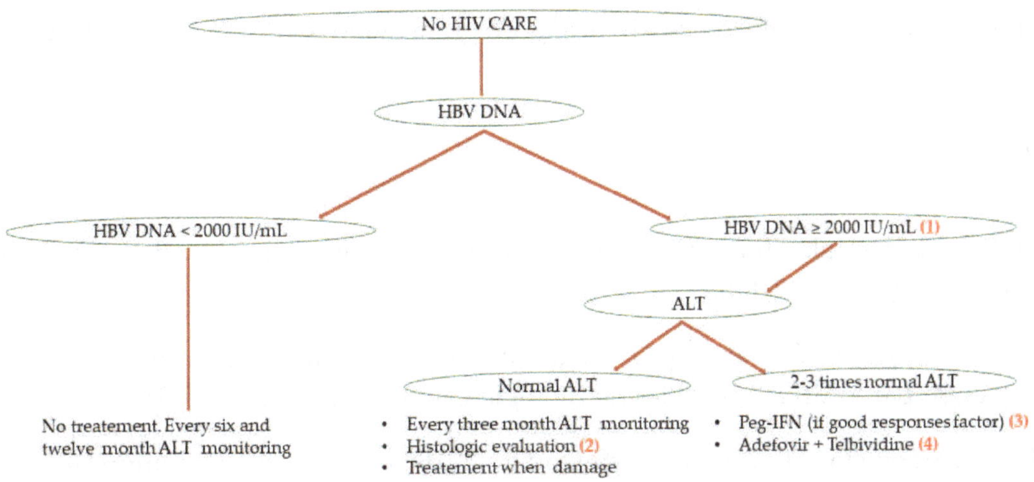

Figure 3. Therapeutic strategy in patients without indication of HIV treatment [56].

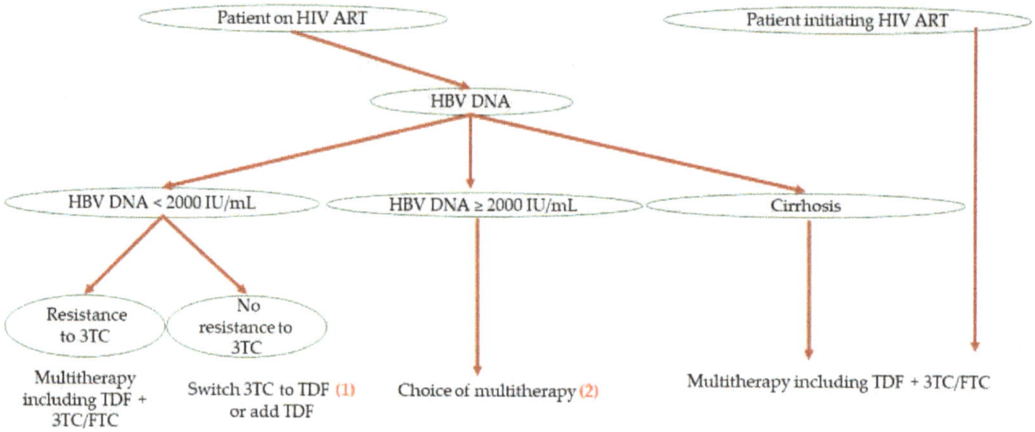

Figure 4. Therapeutic strategy in patients with indication of HIV treatment [56].

In cases where HIV treatment is recommended, the following pattern is adapted (**Figure 4**) [56]. HIV-infected patients should be routinely screened for HBV infection. In highly endemic areas, in patients with elevated transaminase levels, HBV DNA should be sought for the evidence of HBO.

Monitoring and treatment include HBV viral load, presence or absence of cirrhosis, and resistance to 3TC. TDF is the molecule with the highest genetic barrier; therefore, it is strongly recommended in all combinations against HIV-HBV coinfection: (1): if feasible and appropriate for maintaining control of HIV replication and (2): some experts recommend systematically including tenofovir plus emtricitabine/lamivudine if antiretroviral therapy is indicated, even if HBV treatment is not indicated [55].

Author details

Berthold Bivigou-Mboumba

Address all correspondence to: bivigou.berthold@gmail.com

Centre International de Recherches Médicales de Franceville (CIRMF), Libreville, Gabon

References

[1] Roquebert B et al. HIV genetic diversity and its consequences. Pathologie Biologie (Paris). 2009;**57**(2):142-148

[2] Lazrek M et al. Différentes approches de vaccination thérapeutique dans le traitement de l'infection par le VIH-1. Annales de Biologie Clinique. 2005;**63**:581-588

[3] UNAIDS Secretariat. Global-AIDS-Update-2016. Geneva, Switzerland: Unaids; 2016. Available online on june 2018 the 20th: http://www.unaids.org/en/resources/documents/2016/Global-AIDS-update-2016

[4] Mayaphi SH et al. Detection of acute and early HIV-1 infections in an HIV hyper-endemic area with limited resources. PLoS One. 2016;**11**(10):e0164943

[5] Bartlett JA et al. An updated systematic overview of triple combination therapy in antiretroviral-naive HIV-infected adults. AIDS. 2006;**20**(16):2051-2064

[6] Kourtis AP et al. HIV-HBV coinfection—A global challenge. The New England Journal of Medicine. 2012;**366**(19):1749-1752

[7] Agyeman AA, Ofori-Asenso R. Prevalence of HIV and hepatitis B coinfection in Ghana: A systematic review and meta-analysis. AIDS Research and Therapy. 2016;**13**:23

[8] Alter MJ. Epidemiology of viral hepatitis and HIV co-infection. Journal of Hepatology. 2006;**44**(1 Suppl):S6-S9

[9] Li YJ, Wang HL, Li TS. Hepatitis B virus/human immunodeficiency virus coinfection: Interaction among human immunodeficiency virus infection, chronic hepatitis B virus infection, and host immunity. Chinese Medical Journal. 2012;**125**(13):2371-2377

[10] Attia KA. Co-infection VIH-VHB au sud du Sahara: Données épidémiologiques, cliniques et thérapeutiques. Journal Africain d'Hépato-Gastroentérologie. 2007;**1**:51-53

[11] Thio CL et al. HIV-1, hepatitis B virus, and risk of liver-related mortality in the multicenter cohort study (MACS). Lancet. 2002;**360**(9349):1921-1926

[12] McGovern BH. The epidemiology, natural history and prevention of hepatitis B: Implications of HIV coinfection. Antiviral Therapy. 2007;**12**(Suppl 3):H3-H13

[13] Bodsworth NJ, Cooper DA, Donovan B. The influence of human immunodeficiency virus type 1 infection on the development of the hepatitis B virus carrier state. The Journal of Infectious Diseases. 1991;**163**(5):1138-1140

[14] Biggar RJ, Goedert JJ, Hoofnagle J. Accelerated loss of antibody to hepatitis B surface antigen among immunodeficient homosexual men infected with HIV. The New England Journal of Medicine. 1987;**316**(10):630-631

[15] Rouphael NG, Talati NJ, Rimland D. Hepatitis B reverse seroconversion in HIV-positive patients: Case series and review of the literature. AIDS. 2007;**21**(6):771-774

[16] Fafi-Kremer S, Zarski JP. What tests should be prescribed in HBs-positive patients. Gastroentérologie Clinique et Biologique. 2005;**29**(4):364-368

[17] Petrosillo N et al. Molecular epidemiology of an outbreak of fulminant hepatitis B. Journal of Clinical Microbiology. 2000;**38**(8):2975-2981

[18] Raimondo G et al. Statements from the Taormina expert meeting on occult hepatitis B virus infection. Journal of Hepatology. 2008;**49**(4):652-657

[19] Chemin I et al. Close monitoring of serum HBV DNA levels and liver enzymes levels is most useful in the management of patients with occult HBV infection. Journal of Hepatology. 2009;**51**(4):824-825

[20] Zaaijer HL et al. HBsAg-negative mono-infection with hepatitis B virus genotype G. Journal of Viral Hepatitis. 2011;**18**(11):815-819

[21] Torbenson M, Thomas DL. Occult hepatitis B. The Lancet Infectious Diseases. 2002;**2**(8): 479-486

[22] Makvandi M. Update on occult hepatitis B virus infection. World Journal of Gastroenterology. 2016;**22**(39):8720-8734

[23] Hu KQ. Occult hepatitis B virus infection and its clinical implications. Journal of Viral Hepatitis. 2002;**9**(4):243-257

[24] Schmeltzer P, Sherman KE. Occult hepatitis B: Clinical implications and treatment decisions. Digestive Diseases and Sciences. 2010;**55**(12):3328-3335

[25] Chemin I, Trepo C. Clinical impact of occult HBV infections. Journal of Clinical Virology. 2005;**34**(Suppl 1):S15-S21

[26] Zhu HL et al. Genetic variation of occult hepatitis B virus infection. World Journal of Gastroenterology. 2016;**22**(13):3531-3546

[27] Allain JP, Candotti D. Diagnostic algorithm for HBV safe transfusion. Blood Transfusion. 2009;**7**(3):174-182

[28] Brechot C et al. Persistent hepatitis B virus infection in subjects without hepatitis B surface antigen: Clinically significant or purely "occult"? Hepatology. 2001;**34**(1):194-203

[29] Ceneli O et al. Hepatitis B-related events in autologous hematopoietic stem cell transplantation recipients. World Journal of Gastroenterology. 2010;**16**(14):1765-1771

[30] Shetty K et al. Prevalence and significance of occult hepatitis B in a liver transplant population with chronic hepatitis C. Liver Transplantation. 2008;**14**(4):534-540

[31] Fernandez-Rodriguez CM et al. Influence of occult hepatitis B virus infection in chronic hepatitis C outcomes. World Journal of Gastroenterology. 2011;**17**(12):1558-1562

[32] Raffa G et al. Analysis of occult hepatitis B virus infection in liver tissue of HIV patients with chronic hepatitis C. AIDS. 2007;**21**(16):2171-2175

[33] Pol S. Co-infection HIV/HBV. Gastroentérologie Clinique et Biologique. 2002;**26**(5):518-521

[34] Hofer M et al. Frequent chronic hepatitis B virus infection in HIV-infected patients positive for antibody to hepatitis B core antigen only. Swiss HIV Cohort Study. European Journal of Clinical Microbiology & Infectious Diseases. 1998;**17**(1):6-13

[35] Burnett RJ et al. Hepatitis B virus and human immunodeficiency virus co-infection in sub-Saharan Africa: A call for further investigation. Liver International. 2005;**25**(2):201-213

[36] Singh KP et al. HIV-hepatitis B virus coinfection: Epidemiology, pathogenesis, and treatment. AIDS. 2017;**31**(15):2035-2052

[37] Chamorro AJ et al. Reactivation of hepatitis B in an HIV-infected patient with antibodies against hepatitis B core antigen as the only serological marker. European Journal of Clinical Microbiology & Infectious Diseases. 2005;**24**(7):492-494

[38] Clark SJ et al. Reactivation of latent hepatitis B virus infection with HIV-related immunosuppression. International Journal of STD & AIDS. 2006;**17**(1):67-69

[39] Colin JF et al. Influence of human immunodeficiency virus infection on chronic hepatitis B in homosexual men. Hepatology. 1999;**29**(4):1306-1310

[40] Sun HY et al. Hepatitis B virus coinfection in human immunodeficiency virus-infected patients: A review. World Journal of Gastroenterology. 2014;**20**(40):14598-14614

[41] Dienes HP et al. Immunoelectron microscopic observations on the inflammatory infiltrates and HLA antigens in hepatitis B and non-A, non-B. Hepatology. 1987;**7**(6):1317-1325

[42] Babu CK et al. HIV induces TRAIL sensitivity in hepatocytes. PLoS One. 2009;**4**(2):e4623

[43] Kong F et al. The enhanced expression of death receptor 5 (DR5) mediated by HBV X protein through NF-kappaB pathway is associated with cell apoptosis induced by (TNF-alpha related apoptosis inducing ligand) TRAIL in hepatoma cells. Virology Journal. 2015;**12**:192

[44] Tuyama AC et al. Human immunodeficiency virus (HIV)-1 infects human hepatic stellate cells and promotes collagen I and monocyte chemoattractant protein-1 expression: Implications for the pathogenesis of HIV/hepatitis C virus-induced liver fibrosis. Hepatology. 2010;**52**(2):612-622

[45] Israel N et al. Tumor necrosis factor stimulates transcription of HIV-1 in human T lymphocytes, independently and synergistically with mitogens. Journal of Immunology. 1989;**143**(12):3956-3960

[46] Gomez-Gonzalo M et al. The hepatitis B virus X protein induces HIV-1 replication and transcription in synergy with T-cell activation signals: Functional roles of NF-kappaB/NF-AT and SP1-binding sites in the HIV-1 long terminal repeat promoter. The Journal of Biological Chemistry. 2001;**276**(38):35435-35443

[47] Twu JS, Chu K, Robinson WS. Hepatitis B virus X gene activates kappa B-like enhancer sequences in the long terminal repeat of human immunodeficiency virus 1. Proceedings of the National Academy of Sciences of the United States of America. 1989;**86**(13):5168-5172

[48] Peters MG. Diagnosis and management of hepatitis B virus and HIV coinfection. Topics in HIV Medicine. 2007;**15**(5):163-166

[49] Chun HM et al. Hepatitis B virus coinfection negatively impacts HIV outcomes in HIV seroconverters. The Journal of Infectious Diseases. 2012;**205**(2):185-193

[50] Scharschmidt BF et al. Hepatitis B in patients with HIV infection: Relationship to AIDS and patient survival. Annals of Internal Medicine. 1992;**117**(10):837-838

[51] Wandeler G et al. Hepatitis B virus infection is associated with impaired immunological recovery during antiretroviral therapy in the Swiss HIV cohort study. The Journal of Infectious Diseases. 2013;**208**(9):1454-1458

[52] European Association for the Study of the Liver. EASL clinical practice guidelines: Management of chronic hepatitis B virus infection. Journal of Hepatology. 2012;**57**(1):167-185

[53] Terrault NA et al. AASLD guidelines for treatment of chronic hepatitis B. Hepatology. 2016;**63**(1):261-283

[54] WHO. Hépatite B. Centre des Medias. 2017. Available online on june 2018 the 20th: http://www.who.int/en/news-room/fact-sheets/detail/hepatitis-b

[55] Pais R, Benhamou Y. Long-term therapy for chronic hepatitis B in HIV co-infected patients. Gastroentérologie Clinique et Biologique. 2010;**34**(Suppl 2):S136-S141

[56] Rockstroh JK et al. European AIDS Clinical Society (EACS) guidelines for the clinical management and treatment of chronic hepatitis B and C coinfection in HIV-infected adults. HIV Medicine. 2008;**9**(2):82-88

8

Neurological Manifestations of HIV

Girish Modi, Andre Mochan and Mala Modi

Abstract

Neurological manifestations of human immunodeficiency virus (HIV) infection are common in certain regions of the world, notably Sub-Saharan Africa. The chapter highlights the neurotropism and neurovirulence of HIV underlying its direct neuropathology. The high frequency of neurological HIV disease is discussed in respect with the different viral clades. Sub-Saharan Africa is highlighted as bearing the brunt of the HIV pandemic. An approach to neurological HIV disease is given with a sensible classification system of manifestations and complications according to the level of immune suppression, primary HIV-related versus secondary opportunistic conditions, and other metabolic, drug induced, nutritional, or unrelated causes. Major manifestations of neuro-HIV are aseptic meningitis, HIV-associated neurocognitive disorders, HIV myelopathies and pediatric HIV-associated CNS disease; these are discussed in detail, and reference is made to the discrepancy of available data and literature between the so-called developed and developing countries. The role of antiretroviral treatment and its potential limitation in reaching the CNS compartment is stressed.

Keywords: HIV, neurology, pathophysiology, central and peripheral effects, special effects of HIV in childhood

1. Introduction

The human immunodeficiency virus (HIV) has a predilection to infect the nervous system. It is therefore neurotropic [1–3]. This correlates clinically with the fact that neurological symptoms occur commonly and during all stages of HIV infection [2, 3]. Between 40 and 70% of people infected with HIV will develop clinically symptomatic neurology, and at autopsy, 90% have neurological disease [2].

HIV-1, once it enters the human body, spreads hematogenously. The entry into the brain compartment is through blood-derived macrophages. The mechanisms are not completely understood but are proposed to involve cell trafficking across the blood brain barrier. The blood-derived infected macrophages or lymphocytes adhere to the vascular endothelium and then are thought to pass through it by EMPERIPOLESIS [2]. The trafficking-infected cell then transmits the virus to microglial cells or perivascular macrophages on the brain side of the blood brain barrier, a "Trojan horse" type of mechanism. The virus in these infected microglia then undergo productive replication and infects other microglia spreading the infection. Astrocytes are likewise infected but replication within these cells is incomplete or nonproductive and forms a reservoir. Neurons and oligodendrocytes are not directly infected by the virus and damage to these cells occurs by chemokines and cytokines released from the infected microglia and astrocytes [2, 3].

The essential mediators of HIV-related CNS disease are the microglial soluble mediators, including quinolinic acid, TNF-alpha, IL-1 beta (**Figure 1**). Quinolinic acid binds to the NMDA receptor and increases calcium uptake with resultant activation of apoptotic mechanisms. TNF-alpha damages myelin and IL-1 beta stimulates astrocytes. Astrocytes produce nitric oxide and colony stimulating factors that feed back on microglia [2, 3].

The net result of this inflammatory cascade is an encephalitis, which is pathologically characterized by white matter pallor, neuronal loss, and astroglial reaction. This initiates and is the basis of primary HIV disease or as is commonly referred to as direct HIV infection of the nervous system.

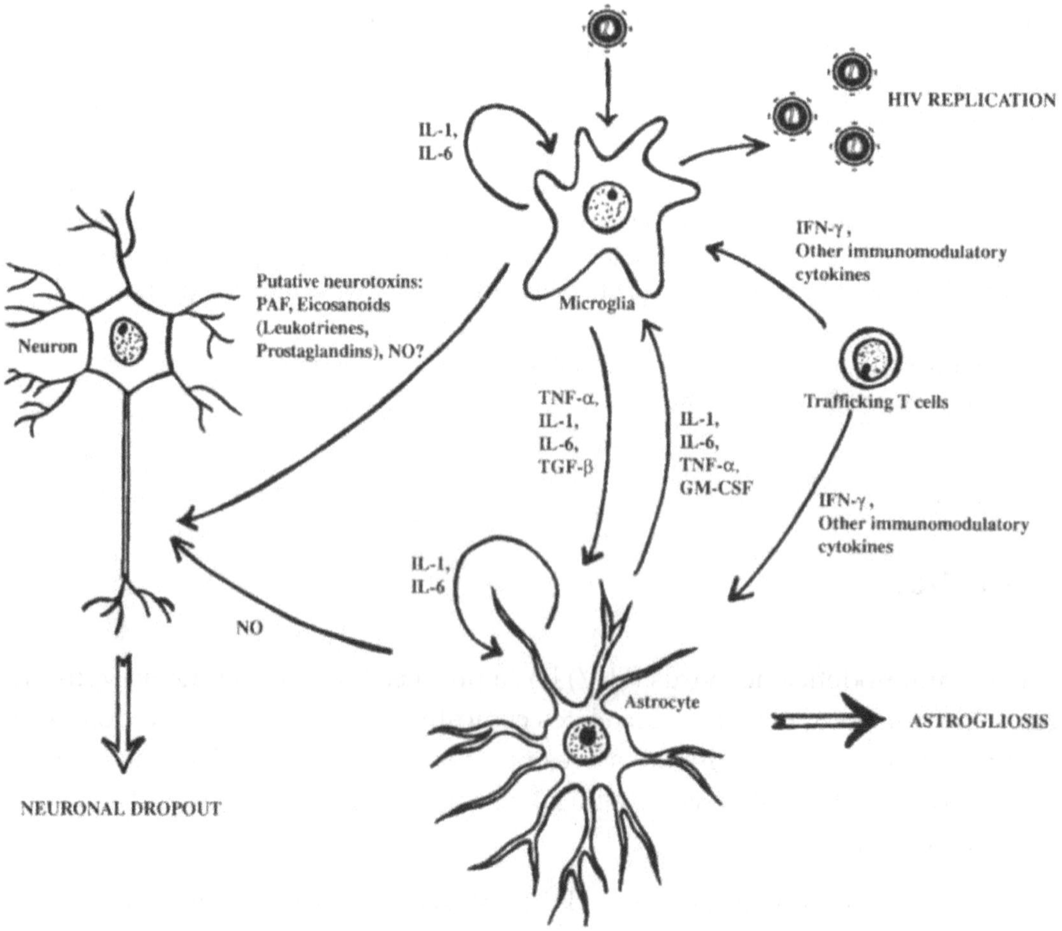

Figure 1. Neuropathophysiology of HIV infection in the Brain.

The nervous system is also affected by HIV through indirect mechanisms that involve immunosuppression-related opportunistic disease and metabolic complications of systemic HIV infection and treatment with antiretroviral agents [1–3].

2. Neurological disease classification

The spectrum of HIV related or associated neurological disorders is broad and any part of the neural axis may be affected. Neurological complications of HIV are very *stage-specific* and relate to altered immune responses and deficiencies of cell mediated immunity–*dysregulation of immunity* [1, 2].

Metabolic diseases that result from dysfunction of other organ systems and *toxic* complications of drugs used to treat the HIV infection and its complications also cause neurological complications, especially in late stage HIV infection [1–3].

Dysregulation of immunity is caused by:

1. impairment of protective defenses with reduction in CD4 lymphocytes and macrophages. This occurs with late infection and is the most important determinant of neurological disease in HIV
2. elaboration of certain cytokines also determine neurological disease in late infection
3. autoimmune reactions in early HIV infection determine some neurological disorders

2.1. Immune dysregulation

1. Autoimmune disease (early and middle phases of HIV infection)

   Acute phase encephalitis, neuropathies (AIDP)

   Subacute and chronic inflammatory neuropathies

   Acute disseminated encephalomyelitis (ADEM)

2. Immunosuppression: opportunistic infections/neoplasms (late phase HIV infection)

   Cerebral toxoplasmosis

   Primary CNS lymphoma (PCNSL)

   CMV encephalitis

   Cryptococcal meningitis

   Progressive multifocal leukoencephalopathy (PML)

3. HIV driven

   HIV-related neurocognitive disorders (HAND)

   Distal sensory polyneuropathy

Vacuolar myelopathy

HIV myopathy

2.2. Secondary conditions

1. Metabolic

   Hypoxic encephalopathies

   Narcotic overdose

   Nucleoside neuropathies

   Zidovudine myopathy

2. Psychiatric disorders

   Reactive anxiety, depression

3. Other

   Nutritional and metabolic disorders

   Drug toxicity

   Cerebrovascular complication

3. Epidemiology of neurological HIV disease

Studies on the prevalence of HIV among neurologic patients are sparse. The most often quoted study is the CDC study of 195,000 patients in 20 acute-care US hospitals, which found a seroprevalence of 0–13%. This was highly correlated with the seroprevalence among all patients in the hospitals [2]. The study data was difficult to interpret as almost two-thirds of the HIV patients were previously undiagnosed. In a hospital-based study that audited HIV manifestations in medical inpatients in South Africa, the frequency of neurological involvement was 75%, with 11% pure neurological disease, and 64% neurological and non-neurological disease combined [4].

The paucity of this type of data is in stark contrast to established data on the global prevalence of HIV from the Joint United Nations Programme on HIV/AIDS (UNAIDS). In 2016, the WHO estimated that 36.7 million people worldwide are infected with HIV. Sub-Saharan Africa bears the brunt of the HIV epidemic with 25.5 million infected individuals (a prevalence of 6% and 69% of all persons with HIV globally). Asia and the Pacific have 5.1 million infected people, and Latin America has 1.6 million infected people [5].

There are two principal subtypes of HIV, namely HIV-1 and HIV-2:

HIV-1, the predominant subtype is spread worldwide. HIV-2 was found predominantly in West Africa with scattered cases reported in the Americas and Western Europe. Both are associated with the clinical development of progressive immunological impairment with some differences in incubation and transmission properties. HIV-1 is the major cause of AIDS in humans [6].

There are several different HIV-1– clades based on phylogenetic data from the diverse HIV strains. Group M ("main") is responsible for the majority of infections worldwide, and is further divided into at least 10 distinct subtypes or clades A, B, C, D, F1, F2, G, H, J, and K. Group O ("out-group") is a relatively rare group currently found in Cameroon, Gabon, and France [6].

The different clades of HIV-1 are not distributed evenly throughout the world. Clade B dominates in North America and Europe. Clade C virus predominates in parts of Sub-Saharan Africa and Asia. Globally, clade C virus is responsible for an estimated 50% of infections and is linked to the rapidly growing epidemics in Sub-Saharan Africa and some parts of Asia, mainly in India and China [6, 7].

The effect of the different clades in different populations on the pathological spectrum of HIV infection in these populations is not known. The majority of published data on HIV-associated neurological disease relates mainly to clade B, which is found in North America, Europe, and Australia. Information from regions where clade C dominates is emerging and seems to indicate that there is no effect of the clade on the spectrum of neurological manifestations [4].

4. HIV-associated neurological HIV disease

4.1. Aseptic meningitis

4.1.1. Introduction

Aseptic meningitis is a clinicopathological syndrome, and the cardinal symptoms of which are headache, fever, and meningism. Pathologically, it is characterized by serous, nonpyogenic inflammation of the meninges. The defining cerebrospinal fluid (CSF) findings include a mononuclear pleocytosis, normal, or mildly raised protein and normal glucose levels [1]. Aseptic meningitis occurs with an annual incidence rate of 11–27 cases per 100,000 population. The causes are mainly viral infections. Of these, enteroviruses (Echo and Coxsackie) make up 80% of cases followed by mumps, HSV-2, lymphocytic choriomeningitis, and adenovirus. Uncommon causes include infectious mononucleosis, cytomegalovirus (CMV), leptospirosis, HSV-1, mycoplasma, arboviruses (in epidemics mainly in the United States and Europe) and rarely during the icteric phase of infectious hepatitis. In the majority of instances, a causative agent cannot be established (exceptions include enteroviruses, mycoplasma, leptospirosis, and Lyme borreliosis) [1]. The aseptic meningitis in most of these conditions is a self-limiting illness and rarely is of sufficient severity to produce pathological changes in the brain that can be visualized with imaging modalities (CT or MRI).

It is important to recognize that an aseptic meningitis syndrome can occur in the course of other infectious and noninfectious inflammatory granulomatous and vasculitic and autoimmune illnesses. This is well described with respect to partially treated bacterial meningitis, so-called neighborhood infections, fungal, mycobacterial, spirochetal, and parasitic meningitis, malignant meningitis, and other noninfectious inflammatory diseases such as sarcoidosis, Behçet's disease, Wegener's granulomatosis, and granulomatous angiitis of the nervous system [1, 2].

4.1.2. Aseptic meningitis in HIV

Aseptic meningitis in HIV may be caused by HIV itself or by an opportunistic viral infection (CMV and JCV), mycobacterial infection, noninfectious inflammatory processes (immune reconstitution inflammatory syndrome, IRIS) or CNS neoplasia (lymphoma) [2]. In terms of direct infection, HIV has been identified in the CSF by polymerase chain reaction (PCR) or viral culture techniques throughout the course of HIV infection, and especially during late stage disease. Often despite extensive investigations, the causative infection or agent is not identified. In these latter situations, the aseptic meningitis is presumed to be due to HIV itself.

HIV-associated aseptic meningitis occurs in several different settings: at the time of seroconversion, during the course of the disease, and with highly active antiretroviral treatment (HAART) where it can be an IRIS-related manifestation [2, 3].

The aseptic meningitis in these HIV-related settings presents as an acute self-limiting illness (often with a cranial neuropathy, e.g., facial nerve palsy), an acute symptomatic meningitis or a chronic asymptomatic meningitis. Pleocytosis or elevated CSF protein has been described in almost two-thirds of asymptomatic HIV seropositive persons [2].

4.1.3. Epidemiology

Aseptic meningitis is the second commonest type of meningitis in HIV positive patients, the commonest being cryptococcal meningitis, which is described to affect between 5 and 7% of patients with AIDS [3].

The incidence or prevalence of aseptic meningitis in HIV cannot be accurately determined because it is most often asymptomatic (up to two-thirds of patients) and rarely symptomatic. Frequencies of 0.5–1% have been reported. No gender, ethnic, geographical, or clade-related differences have been described. The non-HIV conditions that can manifest as aseptic meningitis include cryptococcal meningitis, tuberculous meningitis, parasitic meningitis, and CNS neoplasms (lymphoma). Progressive multifocal leukoencephalopathy (PML) caused by JC virus can also mimic the CSF findings of an aseptic meningitis syndrome [2]. The relative frequencies with which these occur are related to the prevalence of infections in the environment and in this regard geographical and clade related differences have been described. Cryptococcal meningitis occurs with frequencies of 6% in South Africa (clade C), 3% in India (clade C), 1% in the United States (clade B), 1% in Brazil (clade B), 7% in Uganda (clades A and D), and 2% in Thailand (clade E). Tuberculous meningitis, on the other hand, occurs in 6% of HIV-infected South Africans, 3% of Indians, 1% of US citizens, 1% of Brazilians, 7% of Ugandans, and in 2% of Thai HIV-infected patients [4]. The frequencies of CMV and the other opportunistic pathogens causing HIV-associated aseptic meningitis are not well documented. The non-HIV viral infections described above that cause an aseptic meningitis syndrome have not been systematically studied in HIV-infected patients.

4.1.4. Pathophysiology

HIV enters the nervous system at any stage of infection in particular during the primary viremia that accompanies seroconversion. The mechanisms by which this process occurs are now better understood. Peripheral blood-infected monocytes carry HIV to the blood brain barrier and induce a macrophage tropism of tissue invasion. This HIV tropism for macrophages is determined by the V3 domain of the viral envelope glycoprotein. The infected macrophage releases adhesion molecules (intracellular or VCAMs), which cause adherence of the infected macrophage to the vascular endothelium. This triggers an immunological reaction involving inflammatory cytokines as well as matrix metalloproteinases that result in trafficking into the nervous system compartment. HIV may also penetrate the brain as free viral particles when there is a disrupted blood brain barrier. The subsequent events after invasion or trafficking are largely immunological and include activation of various cytokines with macrophage proliferation, microglial infection, and other processes that constitute so-called neurotropism and neurovirulence.

Meningeal inflammation occurs as a result of HIV breaching the meningeal blood-CSF barrier or from autoimmune processes causing an inflammatory response. Meningeal invasion occurs by hematogenous spread or via neurotropic mechanisms. Meningeal irritation produces reflex neck stiffness and causes headache and cranial nerve lesions.

4.1.5. Clinical presentation

The illness takes typically a biphasic course with initial nonspecific constitutional symptoms then followed by the classical features usually associated with meningitis, namely, headache, malaise, fever, neck stiffness, rigors, photophobia, nausea, and vomiting. Skin rash like the eruptions of varicella zoster (VZV) may appear concurrently. Other less common manifestations are cranial neuropathies, confusion, decreased level of consciousness and seizures.

4.1.6. Investigations

As described above, an aseptic meningitis syndrome is suspected when the CSF profile of a moderately raised protein with predominantly lymphocytic pleocytosis is identified. The crucial investigation is therefore CSF analysis. The subsequent investigations on the spinal fluid are performed to exclude conditions that mimic aseptic meningitis and in some instances to identify specific viral etiologies. In this regard, the following studies are useful:

- Biochemistry, microscopy, and cellular counts
- Gram stain, bacterial culture, and sensitivity
- Acid-fast bacilli
- India ink and cryptococcal antigen
- Specific and nonspecific syphilis serology
- PCR for HSV, VZV, Epstein-Barr virus (EBV), and CMV

The typical CSF profile in aseptic meningitis is that of a lymphocytic pleocytosis of less than 500 cells per mm^3, normal or mildly elevated protein, normal glucose concentration, and negative bacterial antigen tests. Early CSF analysis may reveal a neutrophil predominance. An important differential diagnosis of this CSF constellation is partially treated bacterial meningitis especially in the presence of a history of recent antimicrobial therapy. Latex agglutination tests for bacterial antigens may be helpful in this setting. Aseptic meningitis due to noninfectious inflammatory diseases like sarcoid, Behçet's disease, uveo-meningeal syndromes usually have a more complicated course and always must be considered because they may respond to specific treatments [2, 3].

4.1.7. Imaging

CT or MRI may help to exclude suspected structural disease like parameningeal infectious foci, but is generally not necessary. A Chest X-ray may be indicated when tuberculosis is suspected as an underlying cause of aseptic meningitis.

4.1.8. Treatment

Management is symptomatic (fluids, analgesics, anti-inflammatories, antipyretics, antiemetics) with hospitalization often not required. If bacterial or partially treated bacterial meningitis is suspected, empiric antibiotics should be commenced. Acyclovir is used for HSV-1 or HSV-2, or severe EBV and VZV infections; antiretrovirals can be considered for HIV. Corticosteroids are not recommended because of their inhibitory effect on immune responses [1].

Hyponatremia as a consequence of infection-induced syndrome of inappropriate antidiuretic hormone secretion (SIADH) needs to be recognized and managed.

4.1.9. Prognosis

The outcome following aseptic viral meningitis is generally excellent with full recovery in 5–14 days after onset of symptoms. Rarely headaches, lightheadedness, and fatigue may persist for longer in some patients. The natural history of aseptic meningitis is determined by the natural history of the HIV infection and its effects on immunity. It is not clear whether the aseptic meningitis syndrome in HIV is a prelude to dementia, CNS neoplasia, or focal brain lesions [1, 2].

5. HIV-associated neurocognitive disorder

5.1. Introduction

Cognitive dysfunction in HIV infection is either due to the virus itself or caused by opportunistic disease resulting from progressive immunosuppression like CNS infections (cryptococcal meningitis, toxoplasma encephalitis, and progressive multifocal leukoencephalopathy) and neoplasia (lymphoma) [8].

Primary HIV-related neurocognitive disease is a result of direct infection by the virus, due to its predilection to invade (neurotropism) and cause disease (neurovirulence) in the CNS [9]. It is now identified worldwide as the commonest preventable and treatable neurocognitive illness in people below the age of 50 years [10].

Clinically, HIV neurocognitive illness comprises a spectrum ranging from mild asymptomatic neurocognitive impairment (ANI) through moderate mild neurocognitive disorder (MND) to severe HIV associated dementia (HAD) cognitive deficits [10]. The cardinal manifestations are a triad of cognitive, behavioral, and motor dysfunction.

5.2. Epidemiology

The HIV epidemic can be described in three phases. The first of these is the illness prior to the introduction of antiretrovirals, followed by the era of monotherapy with zidovudine (AZT), and now more recently, the era of highly active antiretroviral therapy (HAART) or combination antiretroviral therapy (cART).

Before the introduction of antiretrovirals dementia was a common manifestation of late disease occurring in over 50% of AIDS patients prior to death. That phase was characterized by a rapid turnover of prevalent dementia cases due to high incidence rates combined with high mortality rates resulting from AIDS-related complications (opportunistic infections and neoplasms). With the availability of monotherapy like zidovudine dementia rates and overall mortality decreased, but prolonged survival and incomplete recovery of prevalent cases has led to a relative increase of patients with the milder forms of HIV neurocognitive impairment (MCMD and NPI). This phenomenon has been enhanced more recently during the current era of HAART.

This scenario however only applies to the developed regions mainly of North America and Europe, where HAART is the standard of management. These regions are largely dominated by the clade B strain of HIV-1.

Clade C virus is responsible for an estimated 50% of infections globally and associated with the epidemics in Sub-Saharan Africa, and parts of Asia, particularly India and China. How the different clades in different populations may influence the pathological and clinical spectrum of HIV infection is poorly documented [4]. Relatively little data is available on HIV-related neurocognitive impairment from non-clade B regions. In these developing regions, HIV neurocognitive deficits were either poorly documented or thought to be a minor problem compared to the overwhelming burden of opportunistic infections. The apparently low prevalence of dementia was explained by possible under-diagnosis and underreporting, short life expectancy and short survival of HIV infected patients due to fatal opportunistic infections. Subsequent research has found the frequency to be higher than previously suspected with reported figures of 38% in South Africa (clade C), up to 35% in India (clade C), and 31% in Uganda (clades A and D), indicating that the influence of clade subtype on the spectrum of cognitive dysfunction is probably minimal if at all [4, 11].

5.3. Pathophysiology

HIV enters the brain during the initial viremia following infection. This occurs through infected macrophage/monocyte lineage cells crossing the blood–brain barrier, the so-called "Trojan horse" mechanism or directly across the blood brain barrier [3].

In the brain parenchyma, mainly monocyte-derived cells (microglia and macrophages), and to a lesser extent astrocytes, can be infected by HIV. Penetration of microglial cells is via the cellular surface CD4 receptor in conjunction with the chemokine receptors CCR5 and CCR3 leading to productive infection ultimately resulting in cell death. The exact mechanism of viral entry into astrocytes is unknown as these cells lack both CD4 and chemokine receptors. Following an initial productive phase of astrocyte infection, the virus enters a latent or restrictive, noncytopathic phase. This phase can persist long term and accounts for the latent virus escaping antiretrovirals currently in use.

Once the virus is within the brain parenchyma, it distributes selectively with the highest concentrations being found in the basal ganglia, subcortical frontal white matter and frontal cortex. This regionally preferential distribution within the brain may relate to viral entry through CSF pathways, to patterns of monocyte trafficking within the brain, or to possibly selective vulnerability of particular neuronal populations or anatomical brain regions. The neuropathology of these changes is white matter pallor, microglial nodules, multinucleated giant cells and gliosis; this pathological constellation is termed HIV encephalitis (HIVE). The extent of damage to synaptic and dendritic structures dominates over fairly mild neuronal loss. *Histopathological damage and clinical severity correspond poorly, which implies that biochemical and immunological factors of host-virus interactions are determinants of the clinical dementia picture rather than structural changes.* Neurotoxicity is thought to occur directly from viral proteins (gp 120, gp 41, tat, nef), or indirectly from macrophage factors (quinolinic acid, prostaglandins, leukotrienes), cytokines, and chemokines (TNF alpha, IL-1, IL-6, IL-10, interferons). In addition, disruption of the blood–brain barrier promotes access of neurotoxins from the systemic to the extracellular CNS compartment. Excitotoxicity through activation of NMDA receptors is the putative final common pathway resulting in neuronal dysfunction from disrupted cell energy metabolism and membrane integrity, with calcium influx leading to apoptosis [8, 11, 12].

5.4. Clinical features

HIV-associated cognitive impairment and dementia manifest over a period of weeks to months with the triad of cognitive decline, behavioral abnormalities, and motor dysfunction indicative of subcortical frontal lobe and basal ganglia involvement.

5.5. Cognitive decline

The early affected cognitive domains are verbal and visual memory retrieval, complex sequencing, and mental flexibility with the inability to sustain attention as the underlying phenomenon. The clinical effects are poor short-term memory, impaired concentration and executive dysfunction with mental slowing and flawed judgement. Patients present with increasing forgetfulness (appointments, medication schedules, and telephone numbers) and lose track of conversations and plots; the more complex daily tasks become difficult to complete timeously [11].

5.6. Behavioral abnormalities

These include lack of interest and drive, loss of libido, irritability, blunting of emotional responses, and waning engagement in work and hobbies, ultimately leading to social withdrawal, apathy, and inertia. Early subtle symptoms can easily be diagnosed as depression. Frank psychiatric presentations with delirium, mania, and psychosis can be presenting features in up to 10% of cases [8, 11].

5.7. Motor dysfunction

Difficulties with fine finger movements and subtle balance problems are early motor features, manifesting with deterioration handwriting and a tendency to appear clumsy. Subtle gait difficulties may resemble the loss of quick righting reflexes as seen in patients with extrapyramidal disease. During these early stages, the neurological examination is normal except for mild slowing of repetitive movements (e.g., finger tapping), and increased deep tendon reflexes. Spasticity (especially of the lower limbs) with clonus, ataxia, frontal release reflexes, tremor, and sphincter disturbance evolve with progression of the disease. Seizures and myoclonus may appear late in the course. In advanced dementia signs of co-occurring myelopathy and/or peripheral neuropathy may contribute to the abnormal motor findings [8, 11, 12]. The presence of clear focal neurological signs like hemiplegia, hemianopia, hemisensory impairment, and cortical deficits such as apraxia, agnosia, or aphasia is suggestive of other or associated pathologies [11].

In advanced HIV-associated dementia (HAD), the picture becomes global with mutism, abulia, and incontinence followed by a vegetative state where all intellectual and social interaction is lost.

5.8. Diagnostic criteria for HIV associated cognitive impairment

- Seropositivity for HIV
- History of progressive alterations in cognition and behavior
- Demonstrated impairment in at least two domains of neuropsychological performance
- Absence of
    - Focal neurological signs
    - Intoxication or withdrawal (alcohol or other substance)
    - Metabolic derangement
    - CNS opportunistic infection or neoplastic lesions

Asymptomatic neuropsychological impairment (ANI), minor neurocognitive disorder (MND), and HIV associated dementia (HAD) form part of a continuum, where activities of daily living are unaffected in ANI and MND, and are impaired to varying degrees in HAD. Since there are no globally accepted measurements of a patient's degree of impairment in work, social, or other daily activities, determining this degree of impairment caused by cognitive dysfunction is largely based on clinical judgement [11].

HIV-associated neurocognitive impairment is a clinical diagnosis, made after exclusion of other potential causes. The presence of commonly occurring comorbidities like substance use disorders, major depression, and hepatitis B or C infection does not exclude the diagnosis [10].

5.9. Investigations

No single or combination of laboratory tests or parameters can reliably establish the diagnosis of HIV-associated cognitive impairment. Ancillary blood and CSF investigations and neuroimaging studies are necessary and useful to exclude other potential causes of cognitive changes in HIV infection. The main differential diagnostic considerations include delirium secondary to drugs and metabolic derangements, encephalopathies due to substance abuse or head injury, CNS opportunistic disease (meningitis and focal brain lesions), and primary psychiatric conditions. Hepatic and renal failure can cause metabolic encephalopathy directly or via impaired drug clearance.

5.10. Blood tests

Full blood count, electrolytes, urea and creatinine, liver and thyroid functions, Vitamin B12 level, syphilis serology, CD4 count and viral load should be evaluated.

5.11. Cerebrospinal fluid

This can be normal but is usually abnormal. Patients with HIV-associated cognitive impairment have CSF abnormalities, typical of a lymphocytic pleocytosis with mildly elevated protein and detectable viral RNA (aseptic meningitis syndrome). Similar abnormalities however can be found in the CSF of neurologically normal HIV patients and are thus nonspecific and unhelpful in confirming a diagnosis of dementia. CSF analysis helps to exclude other etiologies, in particular cryptococcal and tuberculous meningitis, neurosyphilis, CMV encephalitis, and PML [2, 3, 11].

High CSF viral load titers loosely correlate with worsening cognitive performance in patients with advanced disease (CD4 counts below 200 cells/mm^3), but since the introduction of HAART and the resultant viral suppression attained by most patients, CSF viral load is no longer useful as a potential marker of CNS infection. Molecular CSF markers of immunological activation like beta2–microglobulin, neopterin, and quinolinic acid are not useful in routine clinical practice due to lack of sensitivity and specificity [11].

5.12. Neuroimaging

Structural imaging with computed tomography (CT) or magnetic resonance imaging (MRI) is integral to the diagnostic evaluation of patients with suspected HIV associated cognitive impairment ruling out any opportunistic processes. In HAD, cerebral atrophy with ex vacuo ventriculomegaly is the respective radiological finding. The subcortical tissue loss with resultant increase in ventricular size mirrors progressive clinical deterioration. On T2-weighted or T2 FLAIR MRI sequences this appears as patchy and later confluent high intensity white matter signal change, more prominently involving frontal white matter with a characteristic sparing of the subcortical U fibers [11].

Functional imaging techniques (magnetic resonance spectroscopy, MRS; single photon emission computed tomography, SPECT; and positron emission tomography, PET) remain research tools at this stage.

5.13. Neuropsychological testing

This type of testing, when available, can be used for screening purposes in high-risk asymptomatic or early symptomatic patients, and for follow-up evaluation in patients with established cognitive impairment. Useful neuropsychological tests include those that examine psychomotor speed, verbal and nonverbal learning, and sustained attention [10]. Performance in these tests is interpreted by comparing patients' results to a normative control database and can be influenced by differences in racial, ethnic, cultural, and social background. Appropriate normative standards are not available for large parts of the developing world. The value of standard neuropsychological testing in these regions is questionable [4].

5.14. Treatment/management

The use of HAART has led to a decreased frequency of HIV dementia. This is due to the effect of HAART improving cognitive performance in some patients with already established deficits and delaying or even preventing the onset of symptoms in others. HAART is therefore the suggested standard treatment for patients with HIV-associated cognitive impairment. Despite this, there are no specific consensus treatment guidelines. Current evidence and recommendations support the commencement of HAART at diagnosis of seropositivity. HAART should be initiated at the earliest stage of neurocognitive impairment irrespective of the immunological stage as the severity of the impairment at the initiation of HAART is the strongest predictor of persistent cognitive deficits.

CNS penetration of antiretrovirals across the blood–brain barrier has become an important consideration in the planned selection of drugs for CNS-targeted treatment. In this respect, protein binding capacities, lipophilic properties and CSF virological responses are the pharmacological parameters that determine which particular drugs achieve better bioavailability within the CNS compartment. Such putative neuro-active antiretrovirals would theoretically be superior in dementia-targeted treatment. However, clinical trials have failed to consistently confirm such a benefit [11].

Clinical trials of neuroprotective therapies like the NMDA antagonist memantine, and the antioxidant and selective monoamino-oxidase B inhibitor selegiline, targeting pathophysiological mechanisms beyond viral suppression, have to date not yielded conclusive results. Their use in routine clinical practice is not recommended, but remains a subject of further research.

Symptomatic treatment of depression, anxiety, psychosis or mania in patients with HIV neurocognitive impairment remains an integral part of their management.

6. HIV-associated myelopathies

6.1. Introduction

HIV-associated myelopathies are less frequent manifestations than encephalopathies. The etiologies of HIV myelopathy include mainly infections and neoplasms. Vacuolar myelopathy (VM) is a manifestation of primary HIV infection as is HIV transverse myelitis. Opportunistic infectious etiologies include CMV, HSV1 and 2, VZV, HTLV1, measles, JC virus, tuberculosis (TB), pseudomonas, syphilis, nocardia, cryptococcus, aspergillus, and *Toxoplasma gondii*. Neoplastic myelopathy in HIV occurs with primary CNS lymphoma (PCNSL), metastatic lymphoma, astrocytoma, and plasmacytoma. Vascular myelopathy is described in the context of necrotizing vasculitis and disseminated intravascular coagulation (DIC) [12, 13].

6.2. Epidemiology

Myelopathy in HIV/AIDS occurs with a frequency of 5–10%, compared with HAD frequencies of 15–30% and distal sensory polyneuropathy (DSP) frequencies of 15–50%. These are US based data; in the South African Black population the myelopathy frequency is 3% [4]. Little data is available from elsewhere.

In the US, the vacuolar myelopathy accounts for 5–10% of HIV-related neurological disease (or 20–55% of HIV myelopathy). VM accounts for 4% of HIV neurological disease in Japan (clade B), 1% in Brazil (clade B), and 2% in South Africa (clade C) [4].

The commonest cause of myelopathy in HIV in South Africa is TB (18–50%) [4].

6.3. Pathophysiology

The pathological hallmark of VM is patchy vacuolization, occurring mainly in the thoracic region and predominantly affecting the lateral and dorsal columns. Axonal degeneration is a secondary phenomenon. There is no significant inflammatory infiltrate.

The exact pathogenesis of VM is unknown. HIV-infected macrophages, microglia, and astrocytes secrete myelin toxic immunoactive substances like TNF α, IL 1, and 6. TNF α causes oligodendrocyte and myelin damage via reactive oxygen species. This oxidative stress to oligodendrocyte membranes causes increased consumption of antioxidants (e.g., glutathione) and methyl groups, which are essential in myelin maintenance. In HIV patients with VM, S-adenosylmethionine (SAM), the universal methyl group donor is decreased like in patients with vitamin B12 deficiency, accounting for the striking pathological similarities, namely the vacuolar change. It is postulated that cytokines released by HIV infected macrophages lead, via SAM depletion to a metabolic disorder that causes the white matter vacuolization in VM. Co-occurrence of SAM depletion and macrophage activation in immune suppressed HIV negative individuals (hematological malignancies, organ transplantation) can produce a clinically and pathologically identical myelopathy [12–14].

6.4. Clinical features

VM clinically manifests as a subacute, gradually progressive dorsolateral thoracic spinal cord syndrome presenting with spastic paraparesis, hyperreflexia, and extensor plantar responses. Sensory ataxia (30%) and a co-existent distal sensory neuropathy (53%) are present while a crisp sensory level is rare (13%). Bladder sphincter disturbance can occur. VM has been observed to co-occur with HAD and DSP as a possible distinctive syndrome [4].

Tuberculosis can cause a transverse myelitis (often longitudinally extensive), spinal meningitis and Pott's disease of the spine leading to cord compression. The latter is characterized by back pain, spinal tenderness and fever are characteristic features. Presentation is with para- or tetraplegia. TB myelopathy is common in endemic areas and is not HIV stage specific [4].

HSV 1 and 2, CMV, and VZV are other viral myelitides associated with HIV infection.

Co-infection of HIV and HTLV-1 has been reported in HTLV-1 endemic regions.

Toxoplasma gondii uncommonly causes myelitis in isolation or in conjunction with focal cerebral lesions.

6.5. Investigations

CSF findings in VM are nonspecific and nondiagnostic (raised protein with lymphocytic pleocytosis). MRI in VM is often normal, but thoracic high signal changes during progression and cord atrophy in the chronic phase may be observed. Increased T2 cord signal, meningeal, and nerve root enhancement have been described in viral or post viral myelitides, in particular with CMV. In TB of the spine vertebral body and intervertebral disc involvement appears as low signal on T1- and high signal on T2-weighted images; irregular endplates and enhancing paraspinal collections have been documented. Lymphoma shows focal areas of low signal on T1 and high signal on T2 with patchy contrast enhancement.

6.6. Treatment

There is no treatment for VM. Unlike with HAD, VM has not shown to respond to HAART. Vitamin B12 supplementation, although theoretically beneficial, has not shown any effect. Symptomatic treatment of spasticity and sensory symptoms is pragmatically indicated.

CMV spinal cord disease can improve with the use of ganciclovir alone or in combination with cidofavir. Herpes simplex myelitis requires high dose intravenous acyclovir.

HTLV-1-associated myelopathy responds temporarily to intravenous corticosteroids.

TB spine responds well to standard treatment.

Early diagnosis of a *Toxoplasma gondii* myelitis and therapy with sulfadiazine and pyrimethamine or Bactrim produce a good response.

Primary CNS lymphoma may respond to chemotherapy.

7. HIV associated CNS disorders: children

7.1. Introduction

AIDS in pediatric medicine and child health has been recognized and described since the early 1980s after the identification of the virus itself. It is now a leading cause of childhood morbidity and mortality [15].

Pediatric HIV is mainly acquired through vertical mother-to-child transmission. This occurs either transplacentally during fetal development in utero; peripartum during passage of the fetus through the birth canal; or postnatally from contaminated breast milk. Other routes of infection include horizontal transmission through sexual abuse or transfusion of contaminated blood products. Adolescent HIV infection follows the same modes of transmission seen in adults, that is, sexual exposure and intravenous drug use.

Pediatric HIV-related CNS disease is primarily caused by the virus itself affecting all components of the neural axis, but with particular predilection for the brain. The clinical manifestations described below are thus varied with the commonest being progressive HIV encephalopathy (PHE). This selective vulnerability of the brain may in part be due to the effect of HIV on an immature brain (see below).

CNS opportunistic infections and malignancies on the other hand do not contribute significantly to HIV associated CNS disorders in childhood [15].

7.2. Epidemiology

The available data shows that approximately 2.3 million children worldwide are living with HIV/AIDS with nearly 2000 new infections and 1500 deaths occurring daily. These figures refer mainly to the developing world, and in particular Sub-Saharan Africa, dominated by the clade C strain of HIV. In these regions less than 10% of HIV positive pregnant women have access to appropriate measures to prevent mother-to-child transmission. In the developed world (clade B virus), pediatric HIV has ceased to be a significant problem as a result of effective use and delivery of antiretrovirals during pregnancy, elective cesarean section and infant formula feeding.

In the United States and Europe, highly active antiretroviral therapy (HAART) has reduced the rate of PHE from 9 to 35% in the early years of the HIV epidemic to 0–2% currently. Few studies from Sub-Saharan Africa report cognitive and motor developmental delay affecting 15–40% of HIV-infected children. There is no published data on the effects of HAART in this population. PHE occurs in 32–36% of HIV positive children in Latin America. Opportunistic CNS infections were relatively frequent at 34% in a Brazilian hospital-based study and at 12% in a study from Argentina. The latter study documented a remarkable reduction of severity and frequency of PHE after the introduction of HAART [15].

7.3. Pathophysiology

The CNS is affected early during the course of HIV infection. Neuro-invasion and pathogenesis are similar to that described in adults with HIV associated cognitive impairment.

The interaction between fetal astrocytes and endothelial cells is central to the development of the blood–brain barrier (BBB). This happens in early gestation. HIV interferes with healthy BBB development by restricted or nonproductive CD4 receptor independent infection of the astrocytes. The consequently impaired or disrupted BBB has increased susceptibility to neuro-invasion. In the immature brain this leads to the encephalopathy (PHE). The restricted infection of astrocytes causes neuronal dysfunction via loss of supporting growth factors and impaired neurotransmitter re-uptake with resultant excitotoxicity. Macrophages, microglia, and multinucleated giant cells are involved in productive HIV infection with viral replication. The consequent inflammatory cascade leads to production of neurotoxic cytokines. Neuronal loss in PHE occurs from these processes as an indirect result of HIV infection. Active infection of neurons or neuronal progenitor cells remains controversial, but may occur in children at low levels [15].

The pathophysiological mechanisms in pediatric HIV-associated CNS disorders reflect the complex interactions between HIV a maturing brain.

7.4. Clinical features

7.4.1. Progressive HIV encephalopathy (PHE)

Clinically well-defined triad of:

1. Acquired microcephaly due to impaired brain growth.
2. Progressive motor dysfunction.
3. Loss, plateau or delay of neurodevelopmental milestones.

Acquired microcephaly: The diagnosis is made with stagnating or decreasing serial measurements of head circumference in children below 2 years of age. In the older child with closed skull sutures, the impaired brain growth correlates with parenchymal atrophy on neuroimaging.

Progressive motor dysfunction: The motor deficit in PHE children typically results from pyramidal tract abnormalities and presents with impaired fine motor function and ultimately loss of gross motor skills. Tone is often spastic. Motor milestones are either not achieved or can be lost. Extrapyramidal dysfunction with parkinsonian features of rigidity, drooling, and hypomimic facies may occur; cerebellar involvement is unusual. Advanced disease leads to a spastic, bedridden state.

These motor features are symmetrical. The occurrence of focal deficits should alert to possible underlying structural brain involvement by a mass lesion or infarction.

Neurodevelopmental decline: Neurodevelopmental deterioration involves global cognitive deficit with language and visuospatial, attention, concentration, and executive function problems. Delayed language milestones especially of expressive language often herald other cognitive and motor impairments. The delay is more easily observed in school-age children, but may often be attributed to other causes like nutritional, environmental, and psychosocial factors. Other symptoms include behavioral problems such as social withdrawal, apathy, mood disorders, and impulsiveness.

The clinical disease pattern of PHE varies widely with respect to age of onset, rate of progression, and domain(s) of functional impairment. Onset of PHE is most common in the first year of life with incidence rates of 9.9% in the first, 4.2% in the second year and less than 1% thereafter. Rates of progression vary widely with rapid decline over few months or a gradual deterioration. Early disease onset, especially when accompanied by advanced immune suppression predicts a more rapid and aggressive course with high mortality [15].

7.4.2. Static encephalopathy

A static encephalopathy with nonprogressive deficit or neurodevelopmental delay is also described. In contrast to PHE, there is no regression and there may be spontaneous improvement. This encephalopathy may be directly due to the HIV infection or secondary to other neurological insults, for example, premature birth, pre-natal exposure to toxins or infectious agents, genetic factors or head injury.

7.4.3. CNS infections

HIV positive children are prone to CNS infections caused by common and opportunistic organisms. Congenital CNS infections (toxoplasmosis, CMV) have been documented albeit infrequently. The commonest reported opportunistic infections (OIs) are CMV encephalitis, *Candida albicans* meningitis and micro-abscesses secondary to septicemia. OIs and their spectrum and occurrence in developing countries are not well described in the literature. Endemic infections like tuberculosis may play a bigger role than in developed countries [4]. Malaria and HIV co-infection may contribute to neurodevelopmental delay in affected children [15].

The frequency of OIs overall is low in children compared to adults, where reactivation of previously acquired infections (toxoplasmosis, JC virus) is common.

7.4.4. Cerebrovascular disease:

Strokes, both cerebral infarction and intracranial hemorrhage have been described in HIV-infected children. The frequency is lower than that seen in adults. Hemorrhage can occur into a tumor or be due to thrombocytopenia. Cerebral infarction may result from the vasculitis accompanying meningitis, or from cardio-embolic disease secondary to cardiomyopathy. HIV aneurysmal vasculopathy has been described in pediatric AIDS cases with fusiform aneurysms affecting the arteries around the circle of Willis.

7.4.5. Seizures

HIV infected children are more prone to seizures than their HIV negative counterparts. Seizures, especially if focal/partial in onset should prompt a search for underlying localized cerebral pathology.

7.4.6. Neoplasms

Primary CNS lymphoma and metastatic lymphoma to the CNS have been described. The clinical presentation may be with seizures, focal neurological signs, or deteriorating mental function.

7.4.7. Myelopathy

Spinal cord syndromes are rare in children and due to reactivated infections, for example, CMV. Vacuolar myelopathy, a frequent manifestation in adults with HIV is rarely seen in children.

7.5. Investigations

7.5.1. Cerebrospinal fluid

The CSF findings in patients with PHE are often normal, even in florid disease. Equally common are nonspecific changes including a slightly raised protein and lymphocytic pleocytosis. Intrathecal antibody production, oligoclonal bands and other markers of immune-activation may be present in PHE children, but also in neurologically intact patients. HIV viral RNA is typically present in the CSF and may loosely correlate with PHE severity. Suppression of CSF viral load is utilized as a marker of response to treatment.

CSF findings can be helpful in establishing the diagnosis of certain common or opportunistic infections (pyogenic, tuberculous and cryptococcal meningitis; toxoplasmosis; CMV encephalitis) and neoplasm (CNS lymphoma).

7.5.2. Neuroimaging

Computed tomography (CT) scans of the brain reveal varying degrees of cerebral atrophy with corresponding ventriculomegaly and white matter hypodensities. Bilateral symmetrical basal ganglia calcifications are commonly seen. Magnetic resonance imaging (MRI) is sensitive to detect white matter changes, but not the calcifications. Serial imaging studies might assist to document progression, but quantitative and volumetric studies have not yet been standardized to be useful surrogate markers for early diagnosis or disease progression in clinical practice. Emerging functional neuroimaging techniques like magnetic resonance spectroscopy (MRS), functional MRI (fMRI), and positron emission tomography (PET) may become future tools in early disease detection and monitoring of disease progression or response to treatment.

7.5.3. Psychometric testing

Neuropsychological and neurobehavioral assessment tools can be useful to document the neurodevelopmental deficit and its progression, but require careful and skilled interpretation. Many factors other than HIV may influence a child's performance on testing. In addition, HIV positive children are more likely to be exposed to poor socio-economic circumstances and low levels of maternal education, and are more likely to suffer from compounding illnesses like birth asphyxia, anemia, and malnutrition leading to a multitude of biological and psychosocial confounders.

Standard psychometric testing remains to children in most developing countries. Such assessment tools still need to be validated in regions outside the US and Europe and in a greater variety of languages and cultural settings.

7.5.4. Treatment/management

Implementation of public health systems preventing mother to child transmission effectively can eradicate pediatric HIV altogether.

Once PHE has set in HAART should be initiated. The ideal timing of commencement and choice of regimen is yet to be determined. However, this is not a cure as it fails to completely eradicate the virus from the CNS reservoir.

8. Conclusion

Neurological HIV disease remains a common and often serious reality, particularly in developing countries. Both adult and pediatric populations are at risk; it is important for the physician to be able to recognize and treat both the common and uncommon manifestations.

Opportunistic infections continue to dominate the picture in the developing world, where the locally endemic infections like tuberculosis stand out as underlying etiologies.

Despite advances in antiretroviral therapies the CNS remains at risk due to its sanctuary status protected by the blood brain barrier and the potential of viral escape in this compartment. However, antiretroviral treatment has started and will continue to moderate and improve neurological HIV disease.

Author details

Girish Modi*, Andre Mochan and Mala Modi

*Address all correspondence to: gmodicns@mweb.co.za

Division of Neurology, Department of Neurosciences, School of Clinical Medicine, Faculty of Health Sciences, University of the Witwatersrand, Johannesburg, South Africa

References

[1] Victor M, Ropper AH. Adams and Victor's Principles of Neurology. New York: McGraw-Hill; 2001

[2] Berger JR, Levy RM. AIDS and the Nervous System. Philadelphia: Lippincott-Raven; 1997

[3] Gendelman HE, Lipton SA, Epstein L, Swindells S. The Neurology of AIDS. New York: Chapman & Hall; 1998

[4] Modi G, Hari K, Modi M, Mochan A. The frequency and profile of neurology in black south African HIV infected (clade C) patients – A hospital-based prospective audit. Journal of the Neurological Sciences. 2007;**254**:60-64

[5] Available from: www.unaids.org/en/resources/documents/2017/2017_data_book

[6] Kandathil AJ, Ramalingam S, Kannangai R, David S, Sridaran G. Molecular epidemiology of HIV. The Indian Journal of Medical Research. 2005;**121**:333-334

[7] Bures R, Morris L, Williamson C, Ramjee G, Deers M, Fiscus SA, Abdool-Karim S, Montefiori DC. Regional clustering of shared neutralization determinants on primary isolates of clade C human immunodeficiency virus type 1 from South Africa. Journal of Virology. 2002;**76**:2233-2244

[8] Ances BM, Ellis RJ. Dementia and neurocognitive disorders due to HIV-1 infection. Seminars in Neurology. 2007;**27**:86-92

[9] Mcguire D, So YT. Neurological dysfunction: Overview. In: Cohen PT, Sande MA, Volberding PA, editors. The AIDS Knowledge Base. 2nd ed. Boston: Mass, Little Brown & Co; 1994. pp. 5.6-1-5.6-2

[10] Antinori A, Arendt G, Becker TJ, Brew BJ, Byrd DA, et al. Updated research nosology for HIV-associated neurocognitive disorders. Neurology. 2007;**69**(18):1789-1799

[11] Clifford DB, Ances BM. HIV-associated neurocognitive disorder (HAND). The Lancet Infectious Diseases. 2013;**13**(11):976-986

[12] Tan SV, Guiloff RJ. Hypothesis on the pathogenesis of vacuolar myelopathy, dementia and peripheral neuropathy in AIDS. Journal of Neurology, Neurosurgery, and Psychiatry. 1998;**65**:23-28

[13] Shankar SK, Mahadevan A, Satishchandra P, Uday Kumar R, Yasha TC, Santosh V, Chandramuki A, Ravi V, Nath A. Neuropathology of HIV/AIDS with an overview of the Indian scene. The Indian Journal of Medical Research. 2005;**121**:468-488

[14] Gray F, Gherardi R, Scaravilli F. The neuropathology of the acquired immune deficiency syndrome (AIDS) – A review. Brain. 1998;**111**:245-266

[15] Van Rie A, Harrington PR, Dow A, Robertson K. Neurologic and neurodevelopmental manifestations of paediatric HIV/AIDS. European Journal of Paediatric Neurology. 2007;**11**:1-9

9

HIV-Associated Cardiovascular Disease

Hadil Saad and Ntobeko A.B. Ntusi

Abstract

Currently, 17 million people worldwide are receiving antiretroviral therapy (ART) for human immunodeficiency viral (HIV) infection. There has been a dramatic decline in mortality from HIV infection in the last decade due to increased availability of ART. HIV-associated cardiac failure is on the increase, with more cases of diastolic dysfunction reported in the ART era. HIV increases the risk of CVD, because of longer survival on ART, ongoing subclinical inflammation, traditional cardiovascular risk factors and the complications of chronic ART use. HIV-associated CVD encompasses a wide spectrum of heterogeneous clinical entities, which include diastolic dysfunction, asymptomatic left ventricular dysfunction, cardiomyopathy, myocarditis, heart failure, myocardial fibrosis, myocardial steatosis, pulmonary hypertension, peripheral arterial disease, cerebrovascular disease, infective endocarditis, coronary artery disease and cardiac neoplasms (e.g. Kaposi sarcoma and B-cell immunoblastic lymphoma). In this chapter, we review the complex association of HIV infection and CVD. We describe important recent developments and perspectives based on a systematic analysis of the important advances in this field published in the last decade.

Keywords: HIV, heart failure, cardiovascular disease, inflammation, cardiomyopathy

1. Introduction

By end of 2017, about 37 million people worldwide were living with the human immunodeficiency virus (HIV) [1]. Sub-Saharan Africa (SSA) is the region of the world most severely affected by HIV infection, where 69% of the global population of people living with HIV reside [2]. South Africa has the largest population of HIV infected persons: an adult prevalence of 18.9% and an estimated 7.1 million people living with HIV in 2016 [2]. At the end of 2016, the country had 270,000 new infections while 110,000 South Africans died from AIDS-related illnesses [3].

The connection between HIV infection and cardiovascular disease (CVD) was established quite early in the history of the AIDS pandemic [4]. Early studies in Africans with HIV infection reported that CVD, involving predominantly the myocardium and pericardium, occurred in up to 60% of patients studied [5]. The frequency and pattern of CVD in HIV infected persons is determined by geography, access to combination antiretroviral therapy (ART) and degree of immunosuppression [6]; and several studies have reported the incidence of HIV-associated CVD to be much higher in SSA compared to high-income countries [7, 8].

The risk of CVD in HIV infected individuals is influenced not only by traditional cardiovascular risk factors, genetics and family history, but also by the effect of ART and the effect of HIV itself [9]. Common HIV-associated CVD manifestations include HIV-associated cardiomyopathy (38%), pericardial disease (13%) and pulmonary hypertension (8%) [10]. Approximately 50% of asymptomatic HIV infected persons without known CVD have been found to have diastolic dysfunction on echocardiography [11]. Studies from Africa have found the prevalence of diastolic dysfunction in HIV infected patients to be much higher and to be more severe in patients with AIDS at autopsy, where up to 40% of HIV infected patients were found to have histological evidence of interstitial fibrosis [12]. Despite effective suppression of viral replication, treated HIV infection is associated with persistent inflammation, tissue fibrosis, suboptimal immune recovery and organ damage [13].

2. Heart failure

Heart failure, a regular consequence of cardiac disease, appears to be more common among HIV patients. The global prevalence of heart failure in HIV infected patients in the pre-ART era was between 4 and 5 million cases [13]. Heart failure remains a significant problem in HIV infected patients; the incidence of HIV/AIDS related heart failure is on increase, and current evidence suggests that diastolic, rather than systolic dysfunction is the predominant form of heart failure in the era of ART [14, 15]. Risk factors for systolic dysfunction included elevated high-sensitivity C-reactive protein, tobacco use and prior myocardial infarction (MI); for diastolic dysfunction, risk factors were hypertension and older age [16–18]. In 2242 HIV infected patients on ART from 11 contemporaneous studies, systolic and diastolic dysfunction were in 8.3% and 43.4% of study subject, respectively [16].

2.1. Pathogenesis of HIV-associated heart failure

Several mechanisms may be responsible HIV-associated heart failure, as shown in **Figure 1**, including direct HIV infection, toxicity of HIV components and ART, opportunistic infections and abnormal autoimmune responses to viral infection [19, 20]. HIV associated myocarditis, malignancy, myocardial fibrosis, myocardial steatosis, arterial stiffness, endothelial dysfunction capillary leak syndrome and abnormal coagulation have been considered in the pathogenesis [21–27]. Also, traditional risk factors such as hypertension, diabetes, dyslipidaemia and smoking are more common in HIV infected people [28].

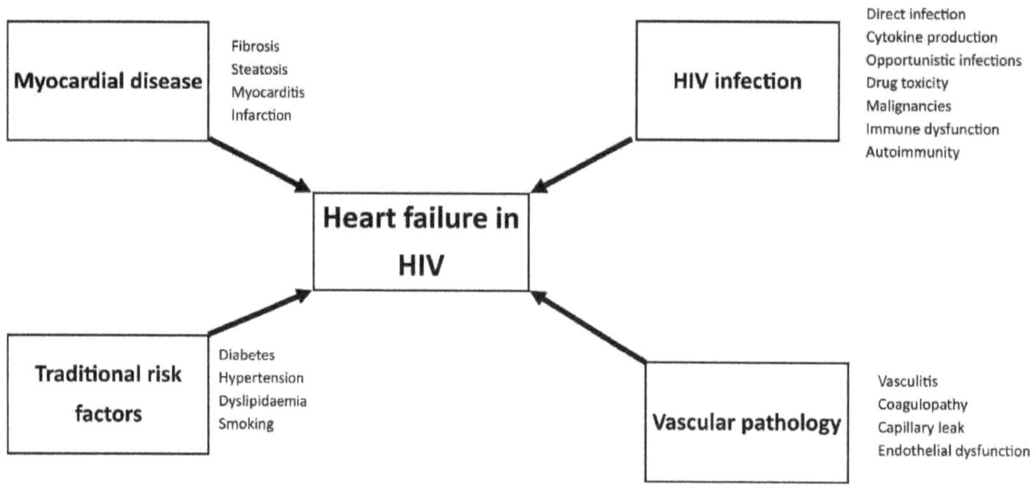

Figure 1. Mechanisms of cardiovascular involvement in HIV infection.

2.2. Myocarditis in HIV

At autopsy, myocarditis was reported in up to 50% of AIDS patients who had not died from cardiac reasons [29]. Direct invasion of cardiomyocytes by HIV has been described, however, the virus affects the myocardial cells in a haphazard fashion with no clear association between viral load and extent of myocardial involvement [30]. The invasion of cardiomyocytes in HIV infection can be through other microorganisms, including fungi (Candida, *Histoplasma capsulatum* [31], *Cryptococcus neoformans* [32], Aspergillus [32]); viruses (*Herpes simplex* [33], cytomegalovirus [30], Coxsackievirus B3 [34], Parvovirus [33]); bacteria (*Mycobacterium tuberculosis* [35], *Mycobacterium avium* [36]) and parasites (*Toxoplasma gondii* [37]).

Myocarditis with lymphocytic infiltration was reported in 40–52% of patients who died of AIDS in the pre-ART era, although no specific pathogen was reported in most affected patients and clinical presentation was heterogeneous with most remaining asymptomatic despite ongoing subclinical myocardial oedema and inflammation (**Figure 2**) [30]. In different study of HIV-associated cardiomyopathy, endomyocardial biopsy (EMB) of almost cases revealed myocarditis with cardiotropic viral infections [38]. The prevalence of myocarditis and cardiotropic viral genomes in HIV-associated cardiomyopathy, HIV uninfected idiopathic dilated cardiomyopathy (DCM) patients and orthotopic heart transplant recipients was compared using EMB and the immunohistological criteria of the World Heart Federation in 33 patients. Myocarditis was present in 44% of HIV-associated cardiomyopathy, 36% of heart transplant recipients and 25% of participants with idiopathic DCM. Multiple viruses were identified in most cases. Cardiotropic viral infection was present in all HIV-associated cardiomyopathy patients, with HIV-associated cardiomyopathy, heart transplant recipients and idiopathic DCM patients having an average of 2.5, 2.2 and 1.1 viruses per individual, respectively [39].

Viral and opportunistic infections trigger myocarditis in the setting of uncontrolled HIV infection. Direct invasion of cardiac myocytes by cardiotropic viruses, including HIV, leads to a local cytokine release and subsequent infiltration of the myocardium with clonal expansion

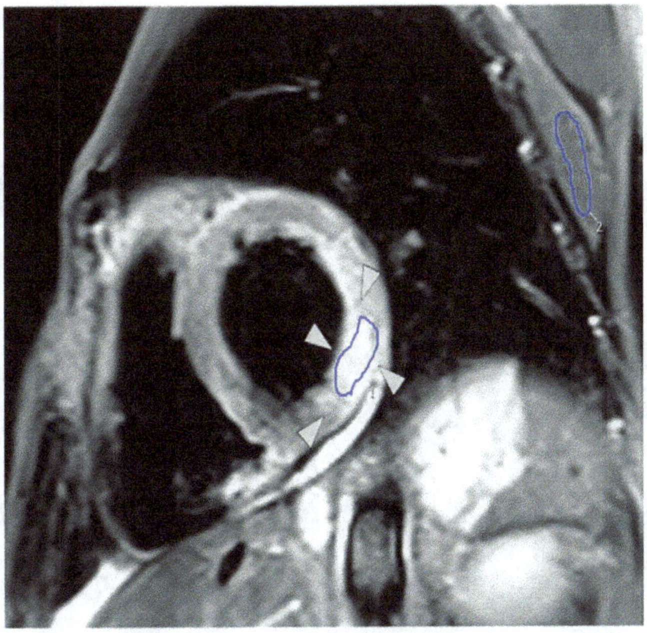

Figure 2. CMR T2-weighted short-tau inversion recovery image showing elevated myocardial: Skeletal muscle signal intensity ratio of the lateral wall (white arrows) in a patient with HIV-associated acute myocarditis. Regions of interest drawn in blue.

of B cells [40]. Reduction in opportunistic infections in patients on ART may be responsible for the impressive drop in myocarditis rates and declining prevalence of HIV-associated cardiomyopathy [15, 41, 42].

2.3. Cardiomyopathy and systolic dysfunction in HIV

The most commonly reported cardiac manifestations of HIV/AIDS in SSA are cardiomyopathy, pericardial disease (related to tuberculosis), and pulmonary hypertension [10]. Initial descriptions of HIV-associated cardiomyopathy have evolved since the 1980s [43]. The pathogenesis of HIV-associated cardiomyopathy is multifactorial and can be direct action of HIV on myocardial tissue or from proteolytic enzymes and cytokine mediators induced by HIV alone or in conjunction with cardiotropic viruses [44]. There has been a marked reduction in incidence of HIV-associated cardiomyopathy after the introduction of ART [15, 26, 41].

HIV-associated cardiomyopathy was showed manifestations of systolic dysfunction associated with a dilated left ventricle and indicated a poor prognosis [4]. The clinical presentation of HIV-associated cardiomyopathy is similar to that of DCM in HIV uninfected persons, and pathological features include dilated cardiac chambers with endocardial fibrosis and mural thrombus (**Figure 3**) [45]. Histologically, it manifests as myocyte hypertrophy and degeneration with increased interstitial and endocardial fibrin collagen and evidence of prior myocarditis [45]. However, more recent reports indicate that HIV-associated cardiomyopathy more commonly manifests with subclinical diastolic dysfunction, particularly in individuals with well controlled HIV infection [46]. Contemporaneous series of significant systolic dysfunction in treated HIV infection have been associated with prior myocardial infarction [47].

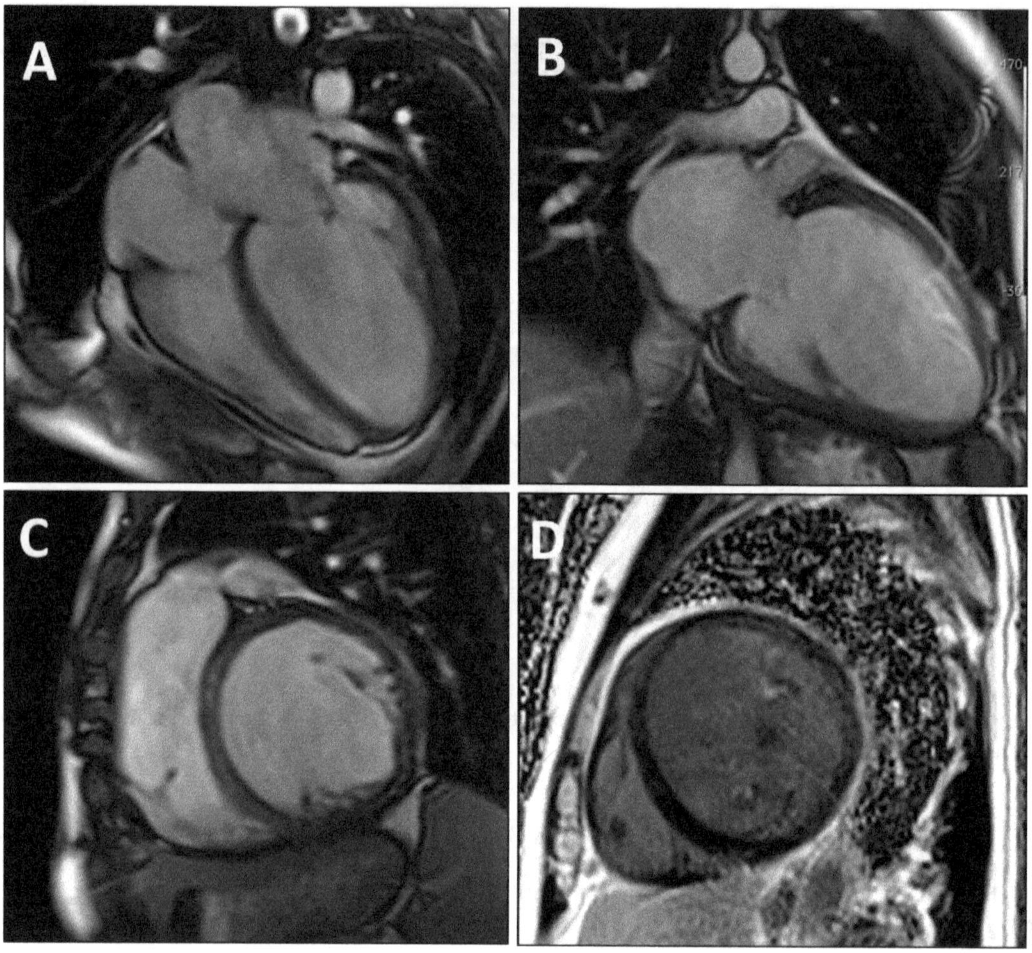

Figure 3. CMR balanced steady state free precession images showing (A) 4-chamber view, (B) 2-chamber view, and (C) a mid-ventricular short-axis image; and (D) late gadolinium enhancement image showing linear mid-wall enhancement in a patient diagnosed with HIV-associated cardiomyopathy.

A phenotype of HIV-associated heart muscle disease with normal chamber size and mildly impaired systolic function increases risk of heart failure, even in the absence of coronary artery disease [48].

2.4. Diastolic dysfunction in HIV

Left ventricular dysfunction associated with HIV is often clinically silent but may progress to symptomatic heart failure. Many studies have reported high incidence of diastolic dysfunction in HIV (**Figure 4**) [11, 12, 16–18, 22, 23, 47, 49, 50]. In addition, diastolic dysfunction is considered an early marker of coronary artery disease in HIV uninfected patients without cardiac symptoms and preserved systolic function [51]. Diastolic dysfunction in HIV is associated with longer duration of HIV infection, higher body mass index and exposure to zidovudine [52, 53]. In different echocardiographic screening studies of asymptomatic HIV infected individuals, diastolic dysfunction was seen in 26–48% [46, 47, 49, 54]. In these studies, diastolic dysfunction has been associated with elevated body mass, total cholesterol, hypertension, smoking and viral load.

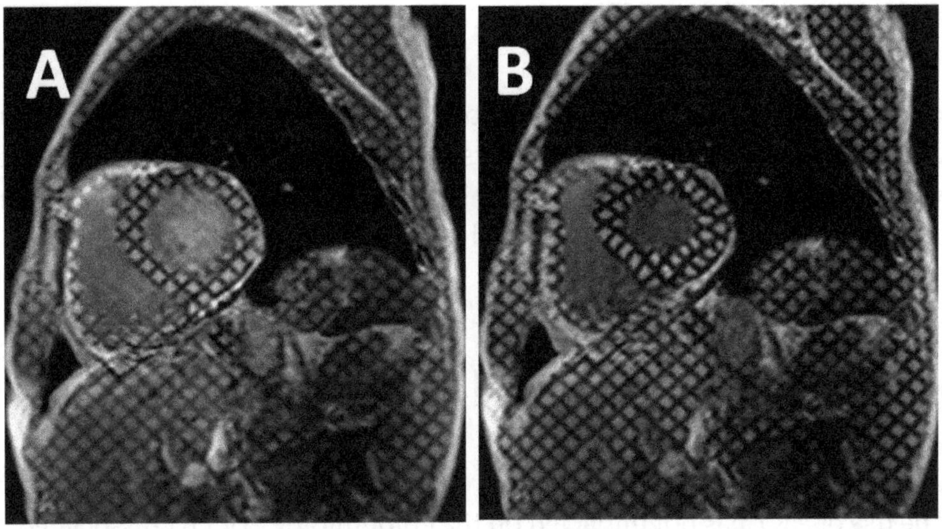

Figure 4. CMR cine tagging using spatial modulation of magnetisation in a short axis image through the mid left ventricle at end-diastole (a) and at end-systole (B) in a patient infected with HIV. Tagging for strain and strain rate imaging in circumferential, longitudinal and radial directions is one of the main techniques for assessment of diastolic dysfunction with CMR.

3. Myocardial fibrosis in HIV

Myocardial fibrosis an important reason of development and progression systolic and diastolic cardiac failure [55]. There is histological evidence of interstitial fibrosis at autopsy in 40% of subjects with HIV infection [29]. CMR studies have demonstrated a prevalence of focal fibrosis in asymptomatic HIV infected individuals of close to 80% (**Figure 5**) [22, 23, 25, 56]. Diffuse myocardial fibrosis estimated by extracellular volume (ECV) calculation was also found to be elevated in HIV infected individuals [56].

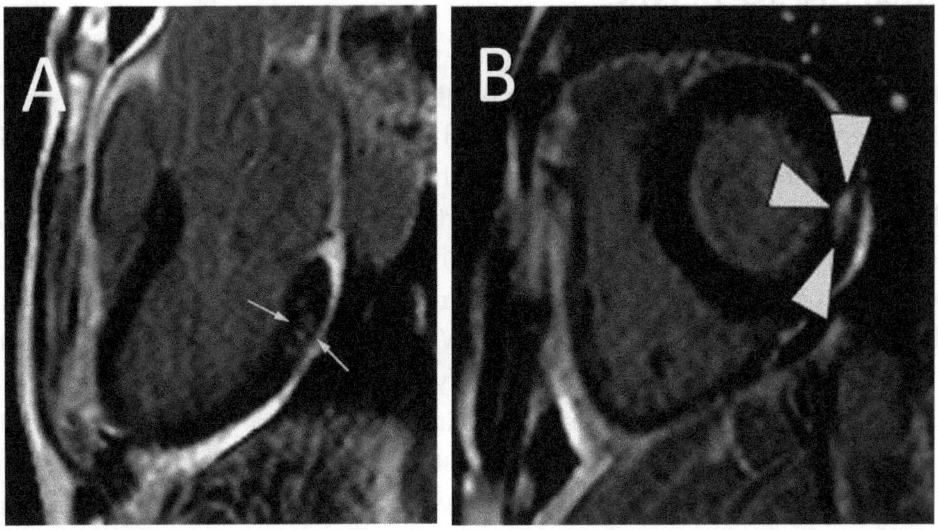

Figure 5. Late post gadolinium images showing mid-wall focal fibrosis in the basal inferolateral wall in (a) 3-chamber view and in the lateral wall in (B) short-axis (white arrows depict the fibrosis).

4. Myocardial steatosis in HIV

Cardiovascular magnetic resonance spectroscopy studies have reported increased incidence of myocardial lipidosis in HIV infected patients receiving ART, even in the absence of cardiovascular symptoms [22, 25]. In these studies, steatosis was associated with elevated serum lipid levels, duration of ART use and impaired strain.

5. HIV-associated pulmonary arterial hypertension

Primary pulmonary arterial hypertension is rare in HIV infected persons, with a prevalence of 0.5% [57]. The use of ART has not impacted on the epidemiology of HIV-associated pulmonary arterial hypertension [58]. There is no correlation between HIV-associated pulmonary arterial hypertension and CD4 cell count, HIV viremia, or duration since HIV diagnosis [47]. The pathogenesis of HIV-associated pulmonary arterial hypertension is poorly understood, with inflammatory and genetic factors both implicated [59]. Pulmonary hypertension in HIV occurs without documented thromboembolic disease, intravenous drug use or pulmonary infections [57, 58]. In a study of 47 patients in the Swiss Cohort Study, patients receiving ART had a significantly decreased median right ventricular systolic pressure over right atrial pressure gradient compared to patients who did not receive ART [60]. ART has also been reported to improve the 6 minute walk test in HIV infected patients with pulmonary hypertension, but with no effect on haemodynamic parameters [61]. Histologically, HIV-associated pulmonary arterial hypertension manifests most commonly as a plexogenic pulmonary arteriopathy, but thrombotic pulmonary arteriopathy and pulmonary veno-occlusive disease also described [62].

6. Pericardial disease in HIV

Pericardial effusion and pericarditis are encountered frequently in patients with HIV infection. The prevalence of symptomatic pericardial effusions before the advent of ART was up to 11% of patients with AIDS [63]. However, in the ART era, the incidence of pericardial effusions in HIV is much less: in a multicentre cohort study of treated HIV patients, only 2 of 872 HIV infected patients had pericardial effusions, neither clinically important [64]. Using CMR with greater resolution, our group has demonstrated the prevalence of small, asymptomatic pericardial effusions to be much higher [23]. While generally nonspecific, pericardial effusions may indicate active inflammation and may be associated with subclinical myocarditis or disseminated tuberculosis, particularly in patients with low CD4 cell counts. In patients with large pericardial effusions, *Mycobacterium tuberculosis* is likely pathogen, especially in tuberculosis endemic regions [65]. In prospective study of patients with a large pericardial effusion, tuberculosis was identified as cause in 85% of cases [66]. In HIV, tuberculous pericarditis is commonly associated with heart failure [67]. HIV is associated with reduced incidence of pericardial constriction [68].

Mortality of pericardial effusions in HIV-infected patients is based on the severity and aetiology of the disease, especially if associated with tuberculosis [69]. We have demonstrated more frequent myocardial fibrosis in HIV-associated pericardial constriction when compared to those without HIV infection [35]. Prednisone does not reduce mortality in tuberculous pericarditis, but has been shown to be associated with reduced hospitalisation and constriction, but with increased risk of malignancies in those with HIV infection [70]. Other causes of pericarditis and pericardial effusions in HIV include HIV itself, bacterial infections, Kaposi's sarcoma and lymphoma [71, 72].

7. Infective endocarditis in HIV

The epidemiology and clinical profile of infective endocarditis in HIV infection are the same as in uninfected individuals [73]. The one setting where HIV is associated with increased risk of infective endocarditis is intravenous drug abuse. *Staphylococcus aureus, Streptococcus viridans* and Salmonella species are the most common organisms and the tricuspid valve is most involved in intravenous drug users developing infective endocarditis [74, 75]. Nonbacterial (marantic) endocarditis has been described in HIV, usually clinically silent and manifests with large, friable, sterile vegetations on the cardiac valves, which can lead to pulmonary embolization [75]. Patients with low CD4 counts have a poorer prognosis when they develop infective endocarditis [76]. Rates of infective endocarditis have decreased with the advent of ARV therapy [76]. When intravenous drug use is excluded, HIV infection has not been shown to be a risk factor for infective endocarditis [77].

8. Coronary artery disease in HIV

HIV-infected patients are known to be at risk for premature coronary artery disease (CAD) [78]. Different factors related to HIV can lead to development atherosclerosis, including immune dysfunction, proliferation of T-cells, inflammation, endothelial dysfunction, and lipid abnormalities [79, 80]. During atherogenesis, HIV promotes monocyte penetration of the vascular intima to promote secretion of cytokines and expression of endothelial cell adhesion molecules [81]. The process of endothelial dysfunction in HIV patients may be driven by HIV transcription factors [82]. Increased risk of CVD in HIV infected patients is directly related to lower CD4 T-cell counts [83]. Higher number of activated CD8 T-cells is observed in relation to increased rates of coronary artery plaque and carotid artery stiffness [84].

In the early stage of HIV infection both total cholesterol and high-density lipoprotein cholesterol are decreased [85]. Lower levels of apolipoprotein B and smaller low-density lipoprotein cholesterol have been reported in more advanced stages of HIV infection [86]. In addition, deleterious metabolic effects such as dyslipidaemia and insulin resistance after exposure to certain ART treatments have been reported [79]. Recent studies observed that HIV infected patients presented with large thrombus burden than atherosclerotic plaques suggesting *de novo* arteriothrombosis and thrombophilia as possible causes of CAD events [87, 88].

9. Cardiovascular malignancy in HIV

Cardiac malignancy usually manifests late in HIV disease. Kaposi's sarcoma and cardiac lymphoma are the main malignancies associated with HIV [89]. Non-Hodgkin lymphoma occurs 25–60 times more in HIV infected patients [90]. Cardiac lymphoma can infiltrate the myocardium, the subendocardial layer or be located within pericardial effusion [90]. Clinical features include dyspnoea, right-sided heart failure, heart failure, chest pain and arrhythmia. Presentations range from asymptomatic to cardiac tamponade, myocardial infarction, heart failure or conduction abnormalities [91].

In the pre-ART era, the prevalence of Kaposi's sarcoma from autopsy studies ranged from 12 to 28%, however, cardiac sarcomas were rare [6, 62]. In Kaposi's sarcoma, the coronary arteries are not affected. The incidence of non-Hodgkin lymphoma is not related to the level of immunosuppression and has not changed with ART use [92].

10. Conclusion

Two third of those infected with HIV reside in SSA. Currently, 17 million people globally receive ART for HIV infection. This widespread use of ART has been associated with a dramatic reduction in HIV-related mortality. CVD and heart failure are on the increase in HIV: the mechanisms responsible for HIV-associated CVD are manifold and incompletely understood. Diastolic dysfunction has emerged as the dominant form of HIV-associated CVD in the era of ART. HIV-associated CVD encompasses heterogeneous disorders and has the propensity to involve every segment of the cardiovascular axis. We have described important recent developments and perspectives based on a systematic analysis of the important advances in this field.

Conflicts of interest

None.

Funding

This manuscript is not funded. Dr. Ntusi gratefully acknowledges support from the American Heart Association, the National Institutes of Health/National Heart, Lung, and Blood Institute,

National Research Foundation and the Medical Research Council of South Africa, as well as the Harry Crossley Foundation.

Abbreviations

AIDS	acquired immunodeficiency syndrome
ART	antiretroviral therapy
CAD	coronary artery disease
CD	cluster of differentiation
CMR	cardiovascular magnetic resonance
CVD	cardiovascular disease
DCM	dilated cardiomyopathy
EMB	endomyocardial biopsy
HIV	human immunodeficiency syndrome
SSA	sub-Saharan Africa

Author details

Hadil Saad and Ntobeko A.B. Ntusi*

*Address all correspondence to: ntobeko.ntusi@uct.ac.za

Department of Medicine, Faculty of Health Sciences, University of Cape Town, Cape Town, South Africa

References

[1] UNAIDS: 2012 Report on the Global AIDS Epidemic. UNAIDS. http://www.unaids.org. [Accessed: 07-Feb-2018]

[2] UNAIDS. Ending AIDS: Progress towards the 90-90-90 Targets. UNAIDS. http://www.unaids.org/en/resources/documents/2017/20170720_Global_AIDS_update_2017. [Accessed: 12-Feb-2018]

[3] UNAIDS. HIV Prevalence in South Africa. UNAIDS. http://www.unaids.org/en/regionscountries/countries/southafrica. [Accessed: 14-Aug-2017]

[4] Lewis W. Cardiomyopathy in AIDS: A pathophysiological perspective. Progress in Cardiovascular Diseases. 2000;**43**(2):151-170

[5] Hakim JG, Matenga JA, Siyiza S. Myocardial dysfunction in human immunodeficiency virus infection: An echocardiographic study of 157 patients in hospital in Zimbabwe. Heart. 1996;**76**(2):161-165

[6] Ntsekhe M, Mayosi BM. Cardiac manifestations of HIV infection: An African perspective. Nature Clinical Practice. Cardiovascular Medicine. 2009;**6**(2):120-127

[7] Magula N, Mayosi BM. Cardiac involvement in HIV-infected people living in Africa: A review. Cardiovascular Journal of South Africa. 2003;**14**(5):231-237

[8] Ntsekhe M, Hakim J. Impact of human immunodeficiency virus infection on cardiovascular disease in Africa. Circulation. 2005;**112**(23):3602

[9] Friis-Møller N, Thiébaut R, Reiss P, Weber R, Monforte AD, et al. Predicting the risk of cardiovascular disease in HIV-infected patients: The data collection on adverse effects of anti-HIV drugs study. European Journal of Cardiovascular Prevention and Rehabilitation. 2010;**17**(5):491-501

[10] Sliwa K, Carrington MJ, Becker A, Thienemann F, Ntsekhe M, Stewart S. Contribution of the human immunodeficiency virus/acquired immunodeficiency syndrome epidemic to de novo presentations of heart disease in the heart of Soweto study cohort. European Heart Journal. 2012;**33**(7):866-874

[11] Hsue PY, Hunt PW, Ho JE, Farah HH, Schnell A, et al. Impact of HIV infection on diastolic function and left ventricular mass. Circulation. Heart Failure. 2010;**3**(1):132-139

[12] Longo-Mbenza B, Seghers LV, Vita EK, Tonduangu K, Bayekula M. Assessment of ventricular diastolic function in AIDS patients from Congo: A Doppler echocardiographic study. Heart. 1998;**80**(2):184-189

[13] Lipshultz SE, Easley KA, Orav EJ, Kaplan S, Starc TJ, et al. Cardiac dysfunction and mortality in HIV-infected children: The prospective P2C2 HIV multicenter study. Pediatric pulmonary and cardiac complications of vertically transmitted HIV infection (P2C2 HIV) study group. Circulation. 2000;**102**(13):1542-1548

[14] Al-Kindi SG, ElAmm C, Ginwalla M, Mehanna E, Zacharias M, et al. Heart failure in patients with human immunodeficiency virus infection: Epidemiology and management disparities. International Journal of Cardiology. 2016;**218**:43-46

[15] Ntusi NAB, Ntsekhe M. Human immunodeficiency virus-associated heart failure in sub-Saharan Africa: Evolution in the epidemiology, pathophysiology, and clinical manifestations in the antiretroviral era. ESC Heart Failure Journal. 2016;**3**(3):158-167

[16] Cerrato E, D'Ascenzo F, Biondi-Zoccai G, Calcagno A, Frea S, et al. Cardiac dysfunction in pauci symptomatic human immunodeficiency virus patients: A meta-analysis in the highly active antiretroviral therapy era. European Heart Journal. 2013;**34**(19):1432-1436

[17] Onur I, Ikitimur B, Oz F, Ekmekci A, Elitok A, et al. Evaluation of human immunodeficiency virus infection-related left ventricular systolic dysfunction by tissue Doppler strain echocardiography. Echocardiography. 2014;**31**(10):1199-1204

[18] Reinsch N, Kahlert P, Esser S, Sundermeyer A, Neuhaus K, et al. Echocardiographic findings and abnormalities in HIV-infected patients: Results from a large, prospective, multicenter HIV-heart study. American Journal of Cardiovascular Disease. 2011;**1**(2): 176-184

[19] Grody WW, Cheng L, Lewis W. Infection of the heart by the human immunodeficiency virus. The American Journal of Cardiology. 1990;**66**(2):203-206

[20] Currie PF, Boon NA. Immunopathogenesis of HIV-related heart muscle disease: Current perspectives. AIDS. 2003;**17**(Suppl 1):S21-S28

[21] Grinspoon S, Mulligan K, Department of Health and Human Services Working Group on the Prevention and Treatment of Wasting and Weight Loss. Weight loss and wasting in patients infected with human immunodeficiency virus. Clinical Infectious Diseases. 2003;**36**(Suppl 2):S69-S78

[22] Holloway CJ, Ntusi N, Suttie J, Mahmod M, Wainwright E, et al. Comprehensive cardiac magnetic resonance imaging and spectroscopy reveal a high burden of myocardial disease in HIV patients. Circulation. 2013;**128**(8):814-822

[23] Ntusi N, O'Dwyer E, Dorrell L, Wainwright E, Piechnik S, et al. HIV-1-related cardiovascular disease is associated with chronic inflammation, frequent pericardial effusions, and probable myocardial edema. Circulation. Cardiovascular Imaging. 2016;**9**(3):e004430

[24] Rider OJ, Asaad M, Ntusi N, Wainwright E, Clutton G, et al. HIV is an independent predictor of aortic stiffness. Journal of Cardiovascular Magnetic Resonance. 2014;**16**:57

[25] Thiara DK, Liu CY, Raman F, Mangat S, Purdy JB, et al. Abnormal myocardial function is related to myocardial steatosis and diffuse myocardial fibrosis in HIV-infected adults. The Journal of Infectious Diseases. 2015;**212**(10):1544-1551

[26] Lipshultz SE, Mas CM, Henkel JM, Franco VI, Fisher SD, Miller TL. HAART to heart: Highly active antiretroviral therapy and the risk of cardiovascular disease in HIV-infected or exposed children and adults. Expert Review of Anti-Infective Therapy. 2012;**10**(6):661-674

[27] Gresele P, Falcinelli E, Sebastiano M, Baldelli F. Endothelial and platelet function alterations in HIV-infected patients. Thrombosis Research. 2012;**129**(3):301-308

[28] Triant VA, Lee H, Hadigan C, Grinspoon SK. Increased acute myocardial infarction rates and cardiovascular risk factors among patients with human immunodeficiency virus disease. The Journal of Clinical Endocrinology and Metabolism. 2007;**92**(7):2506-2512

[29] d'Amati G, di Gioia CR, Gallo P. Pathological findings of HIV-associated cardiovascular disease. Annals of the New York Academy of Sciences. 2001;**946**:23-45

[30] Barbaro G, Di Lorenzo G, Grisorio B, Barbarini G. Cardiac involvement in the acquired immunodeficiency syndrome: A multicenter clinical-pathological study. Gruppo Italiano per lo Studio Cardiologico dei pazienti affetti da AIDS Investigators. AIDS Research and Human Retroviruses. 1998;**14**(12):1071-1077

[31] Hofman P, Drici MD, Gibelin P, Michiels JF, Thyss A. Prevalence of toxoplasma myocarditis in patients with the acquired immunodeficiency syndrome. British Heart Journal. 1993;**70**(4):376-381

[32] Kinney EL, Monsuez JJ, Kitzis M, Vittecoq D. Treatment of AIDS-associated heart disease. Angiology. 1989;**40**(11):970-976

[33] Freedberg RS, Gindea AJ, Dieterich DT, Greene JB. Herpes simplex pericarditis in AIDS. New York State Journal of Medicine. 1987;**87**(5):304-306

[34] Barbaro G, Di Lorenzo G, Soldini M, Giancaspro G, Grisorio B, et al. Intensity of myocardial expression of inducible nitric oxide synthase influences the clinical course of human immunodeficiency virus-associated cardiomyopathy. Gruppo Italiano per lo studio Cardiologico Dei pazienti affetti da AIDS (GISCA). Circulation. 1999;**100**(9):933-939

[35] Ntusi NAB, Palkowski G, Samuels P, Moosa S, Ntsekhe M, et al. Cardiovascular magnetic resonance characterisation of pericardial and myocardial involvement in patients with tuberculous pericardial constriction with and without HIV co-infection. Journal of Cardiovascular Magnetic Resonance. 2016;**8**(Suppl 1):Q29

[36] Barbaro G. Cardiovascular manifestations of HIV infection. Journal of the Royal Society of Medicine. 2001;**94**(8):384-390

[37] Adair OV, Randive N, Krasnow N. Isolated toxoplasma myocarditis in acquired immune deficiency syndrome. American Heart Journal. 1989;**118**(4):856-857

[38] Herskowitz A, Wu TC, Willoughby SB, Vlahov D, Ansari AA, et al. Myocarditis and cardiotropic viral infection associated with severe left ventricular dysfunction in late-stage infection with human immunodeficiency virus. Journal of the American College of Cardiology. 1994;**24**(4):1025-1032

[39] Shaboodien G, Maske C, Wainwright H, Smuts H, Ntsekhe M,et al. Prevalence of myocarditis and cardiotropic virus infection in Africans with HIV-associated cardiomyopathy, idiopathic dilated cardiomyopathy and heart transplant recipients: A pilot study: Cardiovascular topic. Cardiovascular Journal of Africa. 2013;**24**(6):218-223

[40] Magnani JW, Dec GW. Myocarditis: Current trends in diagnosis and treatment. Circulation. 2006;**113**(6):876-890

[41] Pugliese A, Isnardi D, Saini A, Scarabelli T, Raddino R, Torre D. Impact of highly active antiretroviral therapy in HIV-positive patients with cardiac involvement. The Journal of Infection. 2000;**40**(3):282-284

[42] Barbaro G, Barbarini G. Human immunodeficiency virus & cardiovascular risk. The Indian Journal of Medical Research. 2011;**134**(6):898-903

[43] Cohen IS, Anderson DW, Virmani R, Reen BM, Macher AM, et al. Congestive cardiomyopathy in association with the acquired immunodeficiency syndrome. The New England Journal of Medicine. 1986;**315**(10):628-630

[44] Pozzan G, Pagliari C, Tuon FF, Takakura CF, Kauffman MR, Duarte MI. Diffuse-regressive alterations and apoptosis of myocytes: Possible causes of myocardial dysfunction in HIV-related cardiomyopathy. International Journal of Cardiology. 2009;**132**(1):90-95

[45] Barbaro G. Evolution of the involvement of the cardiovascular system in HIV infection. Advances in Cardiology. 2003;**40**:15-22

[46] Remick J, Georgiopoulou V, Marti C, Ofotokun I, Kalogeropoulos A, Lewis W, Butler J. Heart failure in patients with human immunodeficiency virus infection: Epidemiology, pathophysiology, treatment, and future research. Circulation. 2014;**129**(17):1781-1789

[47] Mondy KE, Gottdiener J, Overton ET, Henry K, Bush T, et al. High prevalence of echocardiographic abnormalities among HIV-infected persons in the era of highly active antiretroviral therapy. Clinical Infectious Diseases. 2011;**52**(3):378-386

[48] Butt AA, Chang CC, Kuller L, Goetz MB, Leaf D, et al. Risk of heart failure with human immunodeficiency virus in the absence of prior diagnosis of coronary heart disease. Archives of Internal Medicine. 2011;**171**(8):737-743

[49] Cardoso JS, Moura B, Martins L, Mota-Miranda A, Rocha Gonçalves F, Lecour H. Left ventricular dysfunction in human immunodeficiency virus (HIV)-infected patients. International Journal of Cardiology. 1998;**63**(1):37-45

[50] Schuster I, Thöni GJ, Edérhy S, Walther G, Nottin S, et al. Subclinical cardiac abnormalities in human immunodeficiency virus–infected men receiving antiretroviral therapy. The American Journal of Cardiology. 2008;**101**(8):1213-1217

[51] Nayak G, Ferguson M, Tribble DR, Porter CK, Rapena R, et al. Cardiac diastolic dysfunction is prevalent in HIV-infected patients. AIDS Patient Care and STDs. 2009;**23**(4):231-238

[52] Luo L, Ye Y, Liu Z, Zuo L, Li Y, et al. Assessment of cardiac diastolic dysfunction in HIV-infected people without cardiovascular symptoms in China. International Journal of STD & AIDS. 2010;**21**(12):14-18

[53] Blaylock JM, Byers DK, Gibbs BT, Nayak G, Ferguson M, et al. Longitudinal assessment of cardiac diastolic function in HIV-infected patients. International Journal of STD & AIDS. 2012;**23**(2):105-110

[54] Kelly KM, Tarwater PM, Karper JM, Bedja D, Queen SE, et al. Diastolic dysfunction is associated with myocardial viral load in simian immunodeficiency virus-infected macaques. AIDS. 2012;**26**(7):815-823

[55] Krenning G, Zeisberg EM, Kalluri R. The origin of fibroblasts and mechanism of cardiac fibrosis. Journal of Cellular Physiology. 2010;**225**(3):631-637

[56] Luetkens JA, Doerner J, Schwarze-Zander C, Wasmuth JC, Boesecke C, et al. Cardiac magnetic resonance reveals signs of subclinical myocardial inflammation in asymptomatic HIV-infected patients. Circulation. Cardiovascular Imaging. 2016;**9**(3):e004091

[57] Janda S, Quon BS, Swiston J. HIV and pulmonary arterial hypertension: A systematic review. HIV Medicine. 2010;**11**(10):620-634

[58] Cicalini S, Almodovar S, Grilli E, Flores S. Pulmonary hypertension and human immunodeficiency virus infection: Epidemiology, pathogenesis, and clinical approach. Clinical Microbiology and Infection. 2011;**17**(1):25-33

[59] Pellicelli AM, Palmieri F, Cicalini S, Petrosillo N. Pathogenesis of HIV-related pulmonary hypertension. Annals of the New York Academy of Sciences. 2001;**946**:82-94

[60] Zuber JP, Calmy A, Evison JM, Hasse B, Schiffer V, et al. Pulmonary arterial hypertension related to HIV infection: Improved hemodynamics and survival associated with antiretroviral therapy. Clinical Infectious Diseases. 2004;**38**(8):1178-1185

[61] Degano B, Guillaume M, Savale L, Montani D, Jaïs X, et al. HIV-associated pulmonary arterial hypertension: Survival and prognostic factors in the modern therapeutic era. AIDS. 2010;**24**(1):67-75

[62] Klatt E. Cardiovascular pathology in AIDS. In: Barbardo G, editor. HIV and the Cardiovascular System. Adv Cardiol. Vol. 40. Basel: Karger; 2003. pp. 21-48

[63] Heidenreich PA, Eisenberg MJ, Kee LL, Somelofski CA, Hollander H, Schiller NB, et al. Pericardial effusion in AIDS. Incidence and survival. Circulation. 1995;**92**(11):3229-3234

[64] Lind A, Reinsch N, Neuhaus K, Esser S, Brockmeyer NH, et al. Pericardial effusion of HIV-infected patients? Results of a prospective multicenter cohort study in the era of antiretroviral therapy. European Journal of Medical Research. 2011;**16**(11):480-483

[65] Mayosi BM, Wiysonge CS, Ntsekhe M, Volmink JA, Gumedze F, et al. Clinical characteristics and initial management of patients with tuberculous pericarditis in the HIV era: The investigation of the Management of Pericarditis in Africa (IMPI Africa) registry. BMC Infectious Diseases. 2006;**6**:2

[66] Reuter H, Burgess LJ, Doubell AF. Epidemiology of pericardial effusions at a large academic hospital in South Africa. Epidemiology and Infection. 2005;**133**(3):393-399

[67] Syed FF, Ntsekhe M, Gumedze F, Badri M, Mayosi BM. Myopericarditis in tuberculous pericardial effusion: Prevalence, predictors and outcome. Heart. 2014;**100**(2):135-139

[68] Ntsekhe M, Wiysonge CS, Gumedze F, Maartens G, Commerford PJ, et al. HIV infection is associated with a lower incidence of constriction in presumed tuberculous pericarditis: A prospective observational study. PLoS One. 2008;**3**(6):e2253

[69] Mayosi BM, Wiysonge CS, Ntsekhe M, Gumedze F, Volmink JA, et al. Mortality in patients treated for tuberculous pericarditis in sub-Saharan Africa. South African Medical Journal. 2008;**98**(1):36-40

[70] Mayosi BM, Ntsekhe M, Bosch J, Pandie S, Jung H, et al. Prednisolone and *Mycobacterium indicus pranii* in tuberculous pericarditis. The New England Journal of Medicine. 2014;**371**(12):1121-1130

[71] Gowda RM, Khan IA, Mehta NJ, Gowda MR, Sacchi TJ, Vasavada BC. Cardiac tamponade in patients with human immunodeficiency virus disease. Angiology. 2003;**54**(4):469-474

[72] Stotka JL, Good CB, Downer WR, Kapoor WN. Pericardial effusion and Tamponade due to Kaposi's sarcoma in acquired immunodeficiency syndrome. Chest. 1989;**95**(6):1359-1361

[73] Vasudev R, Shah P, Bikkina M, Shamoon F. Infective endocarditis in HIV. International Journal of Cardiology. 2016;**214**:216-217

[74] Fisher SD, Kanda BS, Miller TL, Lipshultz SE. Cardiovascular disease and therapeutic drug-related cardiovascular consequences in HIV-infected patients. American Journal of Cardiovascular Drugs. 2011;**11**(6):383-394

[75] Miró JM, del Río A, Mestres CA. Infective endocarditis and cardiac surgery in intravenous drug abusers and HIV-1 infected patients. Cardiology Clinics. 2003;**21**(2):167-184

[76] Gebo KA, Burkey MD, Lucas GM, Moore RD, Wilson LE. Incidence of, risk factors for, clinical presentation, and 1-year outcomes of infective endocarditis in an urban HIV cohort. Journal of Acquired Immune Deficiency Syndromes. 2006;**43**(4):426-432

[77] Sudano I, Spieker LE, Noll G, Corti R, Weber R, Lüscher TF. Cardiovascular disease in HIV infection. American Heart Journal. 2006;**151**(6):1147-1155

[78] d'Arminio A, Sabin CA, Phillips AN, Reiss P, Weber R, et al. Cardio- and cerebrovascular events in HIV-infected persons. AIDS. 2004;**18**(13):1811-1817

[79] DAD Study Group, Friis-Møller N, Reiss P, Sabin CA, Weber R, et al. Class of antiretroviral drugs and the risk of myocardial infarction. The New England Journal of Medicine. 2007;**356**(17):1723-1735

[80] Hazenberg MD, Stuart JW, Otto SA, Borleffs JC, Boucher CA, et al. T-cell division in human immunodeficiency virus (HIV)-1 infection is mainly due to immune activation: A longitudinal analysis in patients before and during highly active antiretroviral therapy (HAART). Blood. 2000;**95**(1):249-255

[81] Park IW, Wang JF, Groopman JE. HIV-1 tat promotes monocyte chemoattractant protein-1 secretion followed by transmigration of monocytes. Blood. 2001;**97**(2):352-358

[82] Kaplan RC, Sinclair E, Landay AL, Lurain N, Sharrett AR, et al. T cell activation predicts carotid artery stiffness among HIV-infected women. Atherosclerosis. 2011;**217**(1):207-213

[83] Hsue PY, Deeks SG, Hunt PW. Immunologic basis of cardiovascular disease in HIV-infected adults. The Journal of Infectious Diseases. 2012;**205**(Suppl 3):S375-S382

[84] Kaplan RC, Sinclair E, Landay AL, Lurain N, Sharrett AR, et al. T cell activation and senescence predict subclinical carotid artery disease in HIV-infected women. The Journal of Infectious Diseases. 2011;**203**(4):452-463

[85] Calza L, Manfredi R, Verucchi G. Myocardial infarction risk in HIV-infected patients: Epidemiology, pathogenesis, and clinical management. AIDS. 2010;**24**(6):789-802

[86] Riddler SA, Smit E, Cole SR, Li R, Chmiel JS, et al. Impact of HIV infection and HAART on serum lipids in men. JAMA. 2003;**289**(22):2978-2982

[87] Becker AC, Jacobson B, Singh S, Sliwa K, Stewart S, et al. The thrombotic profile of treatment-naive HIV-positive black south Africans with acute coronary syndromes. Clinical and Applied Thrombosis/Hemostasis. 2011;**17**(3):264-272

[88] Becker AC, Sliwa K, Stewart S, Libhaber E, Essop AR,et al. Acute coronary syndromes in treatment-naïve black south Africans with human immunodeficiency virus infection. Journal of Interventional Cardiology. 2010;**23**(1):70-77

[89] Ioachim HL, Cooper MC, Hellman GC. Lymphomas in men at high risk for acquired immune deficiency syndrome (AIDS). A study of 21 cases. Cancer. 1985;**56**(12):2831-2842

[90] Nishikawa Y, Akaishi M, Handa S, Nakamura Y, Hori S, Ogata K, Hosoda Y. A case of malignant lymphoma simulating acute myocardial infarction. Cardiology. 1991;**78**:357-362

[91] Llitjos JF, Redheuil A, Puymirat E, Vedrenne G, Danchin N. AIDS-related primary cardiac lymphoma with right-sided heart failure and high-grade AV block: Insights from magnetic resonance imaging. Annales de cardiologie et d'angéiologie (Paris). 2014;**63**(2): 99-101

[92] Zoufaly A, Stellbrink HJ, Heiden MA, Kollan C, Hoffmann C, van Lunzen J, Hamouda O, ClinSurv Study Group. Cumulative HIV viremia during highly active antiretroviral therapy is a strong predictor of AIDS-related lymphoma. The Journal of Infectious Diseases. 2009;**200**(1):79-87

10

Achieving 90-90-90: A Focus on Sero-Discordant Couples

Jacqueline Mthembu, Gadija Khan and
Thabile Manengela

Abstract

The South African Department of Health adopted numerous strategies to manage the HIV epidemic. Recently, the global 90-90-90 HIV treatment strategy was adopted. This strategy hope to ensure that 90% of people living with HIV will know their status, 90% of those testing HIV positive will receive sustained antiretroviral therapy and 90% of those receiving antiretroviral therapy will reach and maintain viral suppression by 2020. With a focus on literature, policies and implementation interventions, this chapter aims to provide an overview on current strategies used to reach the 90-90-90 goals and discusses how these strategies can be strengthened among sero-discordant couples within the South African public health system.

Keywords: sero-discordance, couples-counselling and testing, safe conception, behavioural interventions, treatment and adherence, gender norms, sexual health rights

1. Introduction

The burden of HIV has long plagued Sub-Saharan Africa [1]. Since the start of the epidemic, three decades ago, the country has made significant progress in managing the disease [2]. Over the last 10 years South Africa has successfully implemented HIV prevention and treatment strategies, informed by empirical research. Despite the gains made, incidence continues to increase given several socio-behavioural factors associated with HIV transmission [3–5]. Additionally, with an estimated 469,000 new infections noted in 2012, an increase in sero-discordant relationships can be anticipated [4]. It is therefore imperative to strengthen sero-discordant interventions as a response to managing the HIV epidemic among couples that goes beyond couple testing [6].

2. Definition and prevalence of sero-discordance globally, SADC and SA

In sub-Saharan Africa, sero-discordance is a critical factor for the transmission of HIV [7]. Sero-discordance, refers to couples with a mixed HIV status. In such relationships one partner has a known HIV positive status while his or her partner is HIV negative [8, 9]. Hence, for the purpose of this chapter, we define a sero-discordant couple as two individuals who are in a current sexual relationship in which both partners are aware of the other's HIV status. Some authors have argued that sero-discordant sexual relationships are high risk as HIV transmission is more likely to happen in longer-term relationships [10–12].

Despite the misconception that a greater proportion of men are likely to be the index partner, through a systematic review Eyawo et al. [13] established that nearly half (47%) of the index partners were women. This indicates that men and women are equally likely to be the index partner in sero-discordant couples in the sub-Saharan African region. These findings also speak to the prevention and marketing strategies that are meant to be gender balanced in heterosexual sero-discordant couples.

In regions with high HIV prevalence, proportions of sero-discordant intra-couple transmission range from 13.0 to 55% of new HIV infections [14]. For South Africa, the estimated proportion of sero-discordant couples is unclear, however, transmission among longer-term couples were estimated above 10.0% per year [15]. Thus the prevention of intra-couple HIV transmission may delay the progression of the epidemic. As such, sero-discordant couples are a key target population in the context of HIV prevention.

3. Policies and policy implementation

South Africa has been very vigilant in the fight against HIV. For the last 20 years policy adoption and implementation has been at the foreground of HIV management. This section provides an overview of policy strategies that guide HIV management and discuss how these strategies influence the well-being of sero-discordant couples.

Since the start of the new millennium, the management of HIV was spearheaded by comprehensive, multi-sectorial action orientated National Strategic Plans for HIV/AIDS and Sexually Transmitted Infections [15]. Over the last 18 years, many gains have been made in curbing the HIV epidemic. Initiated by the health ministry in 1999 the NSP 2000–2005, in partnership with governmental and non-governmental organisations, as well as, community- and faith-based organisations priority areas related to HIV management were identified. The outcome of this discussion produced four key focus areas.

These included a focus on:

- Prevention;
- Treatment, care and support;
- Research, monitoring, and surveillance;
- Human rights and access to justice.

In essence, the NSP 2000–2005 garnered immense progress in the fight against HIV, but aetiological differences regards the epidemic between the government and civil society posed numerous challenges that curbed the progress [15]. Informed by the successes and limitations of the NSP 2000–2005, in addition to, the progress of the disease and the gains made in terms of biomedical advances, the NSP 2007–2011 continued to focus on improving prevention; treatment, care and support; research, monitoring, and surveillance; human rights and access to justice. Some primary goals were attached to each of these key priority areas. In terms of prevention, the goal was to decrease new infections by 50% with a focus on the 15–24 age year group. Even though this goal was not attained, the mother-to-child transmission was significantly reduced [16]. The treatment focused goal aimed to facilitate access to the appropriate HIV treatment to 80% of PLHIV by the end of the 5 year period. With some challenges regarding implementation, monitoring and evaluation, the decrease in the general adult mortality rates could be accredited to the increase in treatment access [16]. The third and fourth priority areas were reportedly riddled with implementation barriers and therefore did not reach all its goals. It can therefore be established that the second NSP (2007–2011) made some gains in managing HIV, but much more needs to be done at the structural level to ensure greater success.

The NSP 2012–2016, introduced a comprehensive response, which included goals and targets, linked to treatment, prevention, human rights and TB. While many goals were achieved during the 2012–2016 period, gaps were also identified. For instance, notable declines were reported in terms of reducing new HIV and TB infections, but the goal to reduce new HIV infections and new TB infections by at least 50% has not been achieved. What has become evident is that reducing incidence and stabilising prevalence, will require the scale-up of HIV/TB prevention, testing, linkage to care and life-long adherence strategies, with a particular focus on high risk populations.

Two years prior to the end of the NSP 2012–2016 term, South Africa adopted the global 90-90-90 treatment strategy. With its focus on treatment, the strategy targets aims to facilitate the necessary processes so that 90% of people living with HIV can know their status, 90% of those who tested HIV positive can receive sustained antiretroviral therapy and that 90% of those receiving antiretroviral therapy reach and maintain viral suppression by 2020 (see **Figure 1**).

According to Bain et al. [17] the success of the strategy would "… result in 73% of people with HIV achieving viral suppression, a crucial step in ending the AIDS epidemic by 2030 "(p. 1). With this strategy in place, the South African National AIDS Council (SANAC) [18] recently

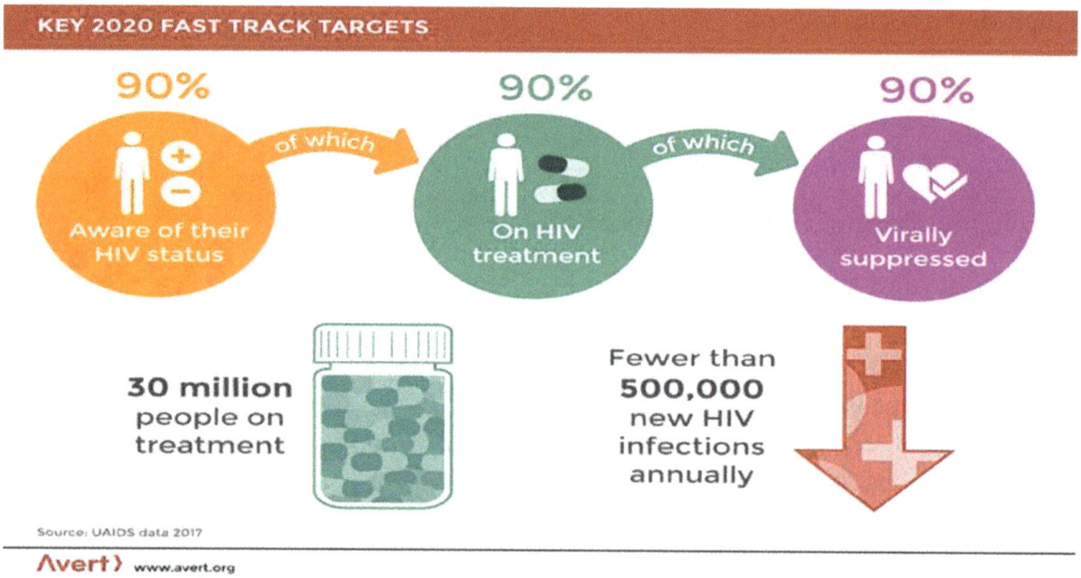

Figure 1. Key targets of the 90-90-90 HIV treatment strategy.

reported that among adults aged 15–59 years old, 86.0% were aware of their HIV status, of those 65.0% were currently on treatment, while of those who are on treatment 81% were virally suppressed (see **Figure 2**).

The current 2017–2022 NSP proposes a focus on social and behavioural aspects of HIV/AIDS and TB that prioritises a research agenda. This includes a commitment to having dedicated research funding for these health issues, build capacity to conduct research, and to identify better ways to collect and disseminate research findings. In addition, the plan acknowledges that we cannot simply treat our way out of the HIV epidemic, but that prevention strategies would offer the best response to curbing the HIV and TB epidemic.

While the NSP 2017–2022 stipulates the importance of Social Science and Humanities research in the 5 year plan, the proposed research foci continue to hover around understanding the

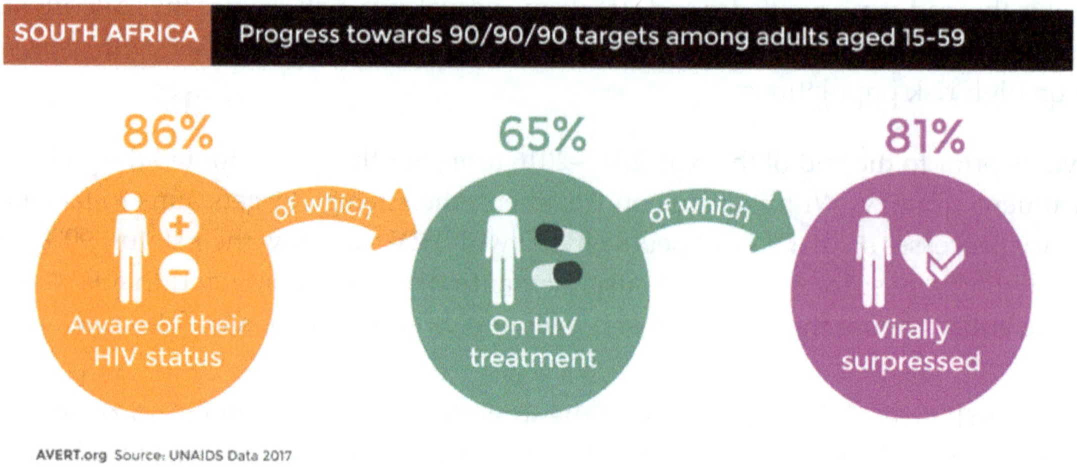

Figure 2. Progress towards the 90-90-90 HIV treatment strategy.

social determinants of HIV and TB. Because of the changing nature of the epidemics, research on social determinants will always be relevant. However, at this stage in the fight against HIV and TB, developing and testing robust behavioural intervention models should be at the foreground of our national HIV/TB response. Furthermore, what the current NSP lacks is a clear strategy that marries bio-medical and socio-behavioural models to improve the HIV/TB-related outcomes for the country.

For instance, with 6.8 mil PLHIV, more comprehensive work should be prioritised. An example of such work could include a socio-behavioural intervention among sero-discordant couples. The NSP highlights a focus on family, but fail to clearly define possible intervention entry points that could help achieve the 90-90-90 goals within the family. A family- or couple-focused intervention may include encouraging home-based testing, family participation in achieving adherence and ultimately viral suppression.

4. Existing prevention interventions for sero-discordant couples

This section provides an overview of existing prevention and intervention programmes, that are implemented in the public and private health care systems as well as those implemented by civil society organisations.

4.1. Current couple-centred HIV prevention services

The prevalence of sero-discordance among romantic relationships is growing in South Africa for various reasons [6]. What is concerning is the fact that, in the country and globally, it has been documented that HIV is most commonly transmitted between partners who are in a committed relationship [6]. This ultimately raises important issues including the risk of infection, reproductive choices and stress and change in the relationship dynamics. Despite the salience of couple relationships, existing HIV prevention interventions mainly focus on individuals instead of couples as a unit [19]. This negates the significant influence that couples play on each other's behaviour. There is growing agreement on the fact that prevention interventions and research should be aimed at couples as a unit to bring about change and maintain discordance. Couples-focused programs could concurrently include both dyad members, target each member separately and alone, in other instances might involve a combination of both modalities. The World Health Organisation has set out specific prevention interventions for couples with respect to their sero-status [20]. **Figure 3** lists the interventions that are specific for sero-discordant couples be it whether the male or female is the index partner.

4.1.1. Case identification through HIV testing services (HTS) for couples

Paying closer attention to literature pertaining to HIV Testing Services, couples counselling and testing are especially important for identifying HIV sero-discordant status among couples. Many men and women who are in relationships with a partner who is HIV positive do not know their own HIV status let alone their partner's [21]. In settings with a generalised HIV epidemic, research shows that in the context of sero-discordant relationships women

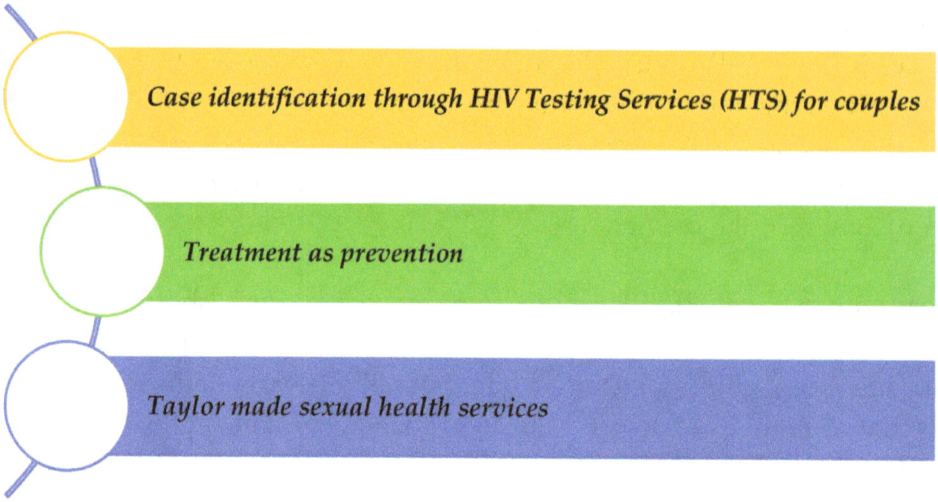

Figure 3. Prevention strategies to reduce the risk of HIV transmission for sero-discordant couples.

are especially more vulnerable to contracting the virus, due to their biological susceptibility as well as the infidelity of men [21]. A study conducted in a rural setting within South Africa, however found that HIV transmission was high among migrant men as well as migrant women returning to their partners. This finding suggest that there is a need to reconsider the premise that HIV transmission within stable relationships is attributed to extra marital sexual activity by men.

With this being said, HIV counselling and testing has mainly been individual based and sex-specific. In regard to individual based prevention strategies, Jones et al. [22] implemented a couples HIV risk reduction intervention (called Partner Project) that included HIV Counselling and Testing program in 6 urban community health clinics in Lusaka, Zambia. The researchers found that the use sexual barrier indicators was achieved among the intervention group. The results also showed that there was a reduction in intimate partner violence (IPV) for the entire sample. IPV commonly inhibits discussions among partners regarding HIV testing, sero-status disclosure and condom use. Hence there should be an essential component of HIV prevention services that also target the reduction of IPV.

4.1.2. Treatment as prevention

In the contexts of sero-discordant couples, two broad prevention strategies with ARVs can be considered. Namely: antiretroviral treatment (ART) for the HIV-positive partner and pre-exposure prophylaxis (PrEP) for the HIV-negative partner.

4.1.2.1. Antiretroviral treatment (ART) for the HIV-positive partner

The WHO HIV treatment guidelines [20, 23] recommend initiation of lifelong ART for individuals with a CD4 counts of 350/mm^3 or lower. More recently, the WHO guidelines in 2013 recommended ART for all patients regardless of their CD4 count. Furthermore, for those who are in relationships with an HIV negative partner, the discordant partner is also recommended to initiate treatment [24]. The utilisation of ARV to prevent HIV transmission thus transformed the field of comprehensive care for couples, particularly when the existing foundation was primarily the promotion of condom use. In an analysis conducted by Lasry et al. [25] who assessed the plausibility of a combination of strategies to reduce risk among sero-discordant couples. They established that ART initiation was the most protective strategy employed. To demonstrate the effectiveness of the use of ARVs in reducing the risk of HIV transmission Hallal et al. [26] cites the Partners in Prevention project, among various other studies in their systemic review. The study was conducted across seven African countries namely Botswana, Kenya, Rwanda, South Africa, Tanzania, Uganda, and Zambia. The sample comprised of 3400 sero-discordant couples who were followed for a period of 24 months. A total of 349 (10.0%) started on HAART. The findings of the study showed that there was substantial (92.0%) reduction of HIV risk transmission through the utilisation of HAART [27]. An emerging trend is to employ strategies in combination with ART to expand the possibilities of interventions for sero-discordant couples [26]. In a rural setting in KwaZulu-Natal, South Africa, Oldenburg et al. [28] estimated the effect of ART in reducing the acquisition of HIV in sero-discordant couples in a HIV-hyperendemic and resource constrained setting. In the study, ART was delivered through primary care clinics that were primarily staffed and led by nurses. The researchers found that ART is highly effective in reducing HIV acquisition in sero-discordant couples, this is despite the constrained resources in the public health system.

4.1.2.2. Pre-exposure prophylaxis (PrEP) for the HIV-negative partner

A breakthrough for the extremely high infection rates in the SADC region is PrEP, where ARVs are administered to those individuals who are at risk of sexually acquiring the virus [29]. In the contexts of sero-discordant couples, PrEP is usually administered to the HIV-negative partner, before possible HIV exposure, which inadvertently reduces the risk of HIV acquisition [23]. In various forms PrEP has been tested (i.e. oral tablets, vaginal/rectal microbicides) or being developed as long-acting vaginal rings and intramuscular injectables [30]. In regard to oral PrEP, findings from the Partners PrEP Study showed that daily oral consumption of Tenofovir Disoproxil Fumarate/emtricitabine (TDF/FTC) reduced the acquisition of HIV-1 by 75.0% and HSV-2 by 33.0% in heterosexual sero-discordant couples from Uganda and Kenya [26, 31]. Two PrEP trials, namely the FemPrEP and Vaginal and Oral Interventions to Control the Epidemic (VOICE), were stopped prematurely due to the futility associated with poor adherence [29]. An active arm of the VOICE trial also established no prevention benefit for oral TDF/FTC owing to poor levels of adherence [29].

In regard to vaginal gels, the CAPRISA 004 study assessed the effectiveness and safety of 1.0% Tenofovir gel for the prevention of HIV infection in among 889 women (aged 18–40 years, who were sexually active with a sero negative status) from urban and rural KwaZulu-Natal [31, 32]. The researchers investigated the reduction of HIV incidence against varying degrees of adherence. The findings of the study demonstrated that HIV incidence reduction was 54.0% for high adherence (gel adherence >80%), the HIV incidence was 38.0% and 28.0% lower for intermediate adherence (gel adherence 50–80%) and low adherence (gel adherence <50%) respectively. Overall, the HIV infection was reduced with Tenofovir gel at an estimated 39.0%.

4.1.3. Tailor-made sexual health services

4.1.3.1. Voluntary medical male circumcision (VMMC) for HIV-negative male partners

VMMC has been recommended by PEPFAR and WHO, as an HIV prevention method to reduce the risk of HIV acquisition in generalised epidemics [30]. Evidence from South African, population-based data, demonstrates that there were lower HIV prevalence and incidence (55.0 and 65.0% lower, respectively) among circumcised men compared to uncircumcised men [29, 32]. Voluntary medical male circumcision is recommended, within heterosexual sero-discordant couples in the case where the male is the HIV-negative partner [31]. It is an excellent HIV prevention method, because it offers lifelong partial protection against female-to-male sexual transmission of HIV. However, it is not recommended for HIV-positive males within heterosexual relationships or men who have sex with men [31]. To help increase coverage of VMMC, WHO recommended that all HIV-negative men in sero-discordant or concordant negative couples be routinely counselled about and linked to VMMC services [30].

Several research confirming the protective effect of VMMC against HIV infection have been published [30, 31, 33–35]. Baeten et al. [35] conducted an observational study with 1096 African HIV-1 sero-discordant couples in which the index partner (HIV-1 seropositive partner) was male. The sample was drawn from 7 Southern African (Gaborone, Botswana; Cape Town, Orange Farm, and Soweto, South Africa; Kitwe, Lusaka, and Ndola, Zambia) and 7 eastern African Africa (Eldoret, Kisumu, Nairobi and Thika, Kenya; Kigali, Rwanda; Moshi, Tanzania; Kampala, Uganda) sites. The results showed a non-statistically significant decrease in the risk of HIV-1 transmission for circumcised HIV-1 infected men to their female partners in comparison to couples with uncircumcised HIV-1 infected men. This finding adds to a limited body of data relating circumcision status in HIV-1 infected men to the risk of male-to-female HIV-1 transmission, data which may be helpful for programmes working to scale-up male circumcision for HIV-1 prevention. Randomised trials from Kenya, South Africa, and Uganda demonstrated that male circumcision reduces a man's risk of acquiring HIV-1 by approximately 60.0%.

Auvert et al. [33] conducted an experimental trial to test the efficacy of Medical circumcision (MC) as a protecting factor against HIV infection among men. The study was the first randomised control trial, in South Africa, that aimed to test the impact of MC on health. The findings demonstrated MC offers a substantially high level of protection for men against acquiring HIV infection, this protection may be seen as effectiveness as what a vaccine of high efficacy would achieve [33]. Furthermore, Auvert et al. [34] continued to do research on medical male circumcision. They implemented the Bophelo Pele community-based HIV campaign (Orange Farm, South Africa). The campaign included the roll-out of free VMMC. A cross-sectional survey was administered with men aged 15–49 years. The results of the survey suggest that the roll-out of VMMC was associated with a reduction in the incidence and prevalence of HIV among circumcised men as compared to uncircumcised men. Furthermore, the findings also provide an argument that the uptake of VMMC is plausible and may become acceptable in communities that were traditionally non-circumcising communities in South Africa and sub-Saharan Africa [34].

4.1.3.2. Family planning

Many sero-discordant couples have high fertility and both (infected and uninfected) partners often report desires of having children with their partner [36]. Pregnancy is a time of heightened risk of sexual transmission and acquisition of HIV. Technologically advanced options for conception for sero-discordant couples include intrauterine or intravaginal insemination (of semen during the fertile period). Vaginal insemination is regarded as the safer method of conception to circumvent the sexual transmission of HIV [37]. However, it may not be accessible or affordable to all, especially in low to middle income countries [36, 39]. As such preconception services for PLHIV and their partners are prudent, and should be part and parcel of the care package they receive. The purpose of preconception care and counselling (PCC) for PLHIV is to ensure that both partners are optimally healthy, prior to pregnancy, and that the risk of HIV transmission to the partner (sexual transmission) and child (through pregnancy, delivery or breastfeeding) are reduced [38]. Options for safer conception, that are less reliant on technology, for sero-discordant couples include ART for the positive partner, timed unprotected intercourse, and PrEP for the uninfected male partner. ART literature shows that safe conception may be feasible when the infected partner is virally suppressed and on ART. While fully suppressive ART use may significantly reduce the chance of sexual transmission, sexual HIV transmission may still occur [36, 37]. Limited and timed unprotected sex and –natural conception for HIV sero-discordant couples involves limited and timed unprotected sexual intercourse during the fertile periods. Women are advised to track their menstrual and ovulation cycles. Couples are encouraged to minimise their sexual encounters to the fertile period to decrease the number of unprotected sexual encounters while maximising their chance of conception [35–37].

Periconception PrEP—is an option for the HIV negative partner. The benefits for the periconception PrEP is higher adherence and lower costs due to the shorter duration of utilisation. It is important to establish whether periconception PrEP regimen will help lower the risk of couples who have decided to conceive despite known risks of transmission to partner and baby. While there are no trials with a particular focus on the risk of HIV transmission among sero-discordant complies during conception, but data drawn from the safety and efficacy of PrEP in future clinical trials among heterosexuals couples and trials testing drugs for PMTCT can offer insights [36, 38, 39].

5. Barrier and facilitators to achieving 90-90-90 among sero-discordant couples

The possibility of sero-discordant relationships are becoming more common, given the improved quality of life and higher life expectancy for people living with HIV [26]. It is therefore imperative to expand HIV prevention efforts that target sero-discordant couples in the effort to reach the 90-90-90 treatment goals.

In regard to HIV testing and counselling, evidence shows that many of the prevention strategies to reduce the risk of HIV transmission in couples are individual as opposed to couples based. HIV testing and counselling practices, thus far, have only included one partner and encouraged clients to invite their partners to test for HIV. It would be ideal to provide health care services and feasible prevention methods for couples as a unit as opposed to individuals. Furthermore, it is evident that services have been gendered to favour females (e.g. who receive antenatal care) who are perceived to be at greater risk and to whom routine testing is encouraged. It may be important to expand the scope of testing for HIV among men who access health facilities for other health services. It may be suggested that there be more emphasis placed on HIV testing among males and this may speak to a need for male-centred health facilities.

In relation to treatment as prevention for sero-discordance, it was found through various clinical trial in South Africa that adherence to using PrEP was a major barrier [29]. This therefore nullifies the excellence of the approach to safeguard the uninfected partner from the transmission of the virus. Furthermore, some of the pre-exposure prophylaxes technologies are yet to be tested. And therefore it is imperative that we explore strategies to increase adherence for ART for the positive partner, more importantly that we should uncover the barriers to adherence for PrEP utilisation.

There are barriers associated with family planning strategies for sero-discordant couples. These include the affordability and accessibility of intrauterine or intravaginal insemination technologies to aid in safe conception. Couples therefore have to rely on manual methods such as timed unprotected sex during fertile periods. This strategy requires health care workers and couples to be cautious and thorough in their actions, so as to reduce the risk of transmission.

Regardless of the existing literature on sero-discordant couples, there is still a need to conduct further research on treatment as prevention and sexual health services that are tailor-made for such couples.

Author details

Jacqueline Mthembu[1]*, Gadija Khan[1] and Thabile Manengela[2]

*Address all correspondence to: jmthembu@hsrc.ac.za

1 Human Sciences Research Council (HAST), Cape Town, South Africa

2 North West University, Mmabatho, South Africa

References

[1] Kharsany AB, Karim QA. HIV infection and AIDS in sub-Saharan Africa: Current status, challenges and opportunities. The Open AIDS Journal. 2016;**10**:34

[2] Simelela NP, Venter WDF. A brief history of South Africa's response to AIDS. SAMJ: South African Medical Journal. 2014;**104**(3):249-251

[3] Cluver LD, Orkin MF, Yakubovich AR, Sherr L. Combination social protection for reducing HIV-risk behavior amongst adolescents in South Africa. Journal of Acquired Immune Deficiency Syndromes (1999). 2016;**72**(1):96

[4] Shisana O, Rehle T, Simbayi LC, Zuma K, Jooste S, Zungu N, Labadarios D, Onoya D et al. South African National HIV Prevalence, Incidence and Behaviour Survey, 2012. Cape Town: HSRC Press; 2014

[5] Zuma K, Shisana O, Rehle TM, Simbayi LC, Jooste S, Zungu N, et al. New insights into HIV epidemic in South Africa: Key findings from the national HIV prevalence, incidence and behaviour survey, 2012. African Journal of AIDS Research. 2016;**15**(1):67-75

[6] Mashaphu S, Burns JK. Couples-based interventions in the context of HIV discordance. South African Journal of Psychiatry. 2017;**23**:a1009

[7] Kilembe W, Wall KM, Mokgoro M, Mwaanga A, Dissen E, Kamusoko M, et al. Knowledge of HIV serodiscordance, transmission, and prevention among couples in Durban, South Africa. PLoS One. 2015;**10**(4):e0124548

[8] Ndirangu G. Fertility and conception options for HIV-serodiscordant couples in Sub Saharan Africa. Finland: Arcada University of Applied Sciences; 2017

[9] Wilton J. HIV prevention within serodiscordant couples: A changing paradigm. Prevention in Focus. Canada: Spring; 2015. Available: http://www.catie.ca/en/pif/spring-2015/hiv-prevention-within-serodiscordant-couples-changing-paradigm

[10] Guthrie BL, De Bruyn G, Farquhar C. HIV-1-discordant couples in sub-Saharan Africa: Explanations and implications for high rates of discordancy. Current HIV Research. 2007;**5**(4):416-429

[11] Dunkle KL, Stephenson R, Karita E, Chomba E, Kayitenkore K, Vwalika C, et al. New heterosexually transmitted HIV infections in married or cohabiting couples in urban Zambia and Rwanda: An analysis of survey and clinical data. The Lancet. 2008;**371**(9631): 2183-2191

[12] Matthews LT, Crankshaw T, Giddy J, Kaida A, Smit JA, Ware NC, Bangsberg DR. Reproductive decision-making and periconception practices among HIV-positive men and women attending HIV services in Durban, South Africa. AIDS and Behavior. 2013;**17**(2): 461-470

[13] Eyawo O, De Walque D, Ford N, Gakii G, Lester RT, Mills EJ. HIV status in discordant couples in sub-Saharan Africa: A systematic review and meta-analysis. The Lancet Infectious Diseases. 2010;**10**(11):770-777

[14] Patel RC, Stanford-Moore G, Odoyo J, Pyra M, Wakhungu I, Anand K, Brown JM. "Since both of us are using antiretrovirals, we have been supportive to each other": Facilitators and barriers of pre-exposure prophylaxis use in heterosexual HIV serodiscordant couples in Kisumu, Kenya. Journal of the International AIDS Society. 2016;**19**(1):1-10

[15] Mahlangu P, Vearey J, Thomas L, Goudge J. Implementing a multi-sectoral response to

HIV: A case study of AIDS councils in the Mpumalanga Province, South Africa. Global Health Action. 2017;**10**(1):1387411

[16] Johnson LF. Access to antiretroviral treatment in South Africa, 2004-2011. Southern African Journal of HIV Medicine. 2012;**13**(1):22-27

[17] Bain LE, Nkoke C, Noubiap JJN. UNAIDS 90-90-90 targets to end the AIDS epidemic by 2020 are not realistic: Comment on "Can the UNAIDS 90-90-90 target be achieved? A systematic analysis of national HIV treatment cascades". BMJ Global Health. 2017;**2**(2):e000227

[18] South African National AIDS Council (SANAC). Let our Actions Count: National Strategic Plan 2017-2022 [pdf]. 2017

[19] Burton J, Darbes LA, Operario D. Couples-focused behavioral interventions for prevention of HIV: Systematic review of the state of evidence. AIDS and Behavior. 2010;**14**(1):1-10. DOI: 10.1007/s10461-008-9471-4

[20] World Health Organization. Service delivery approaches to HIV testing and counselling (HTC): a strategic policy framework. 2012. Available: http://apps.who.int/iris/bitstream/10665/75206/1/9789241593877_eng.pdf. Accessed March 19, 2018

[21] Desgrées-du-loû A, Orne-gliemann J. Couple-centred testing and counselling for HIV serodiscordant heterosexual couples in sub-Saharan Africa. Reproductive Health Matters. 2008;**8080**:151-161. DOI: 10.1016/S0968-8080(08)32407-0

[22] Jones D, Weiss SM, Arheart K, Cook R, Chitalu N. Implementation of HIV prevention interventions in resource limited settings: The partner project. Journal of Community Health. 2014;**39**(1):151-158

[23] Medley A, Baggaley R, Bachanas P, Cohen M, Shaffer N, Lo YR. Maximizing the impact of HIV prevention efforts: Interventions for couples. AIDS care. 2013;**25**(12):1569-1580

[24] World Health Organization. ARV Guidelines, What Is New in the Guidelines and how Did Markets React, Pierriens J Coordinator, HIV Technology and Commodities HIV Department. Geneva: WHO; 2013

[25] Lasry A, Sansom SL, Wolitski RJ, Green TA, Borkowf CB, Patel P, Mermin J. HIV sexual transmission risk among serodiscordant couples: Assessing the effects of combining prevention strategies. AIDS. 2014;**28**(10):1521-1529

[26] Hallal RC, Raxach JC, Barcellos NT, Maksud I. Strategies to prevent HIV transmission to serodiscordant couples. Revista Brasileira de Epidemiologia. 2015a;**18**(suppl 1):169-182. DOI: 10.1590/1809-4503201500050013

[27] Donnell D, Baeten JM, Kiarie J, Thomas K, Stevens W, Cohen CR, et al. Heterosexual HIV-1 transmission after initiation of antiretroviral therapy: A prospective cohort analysis. Lancet. 2010;**375**(9731):2092-2098. DOI: 10.1016/S0140-6736(10)60705-2

[28] Oldenburg CE, Bärnighausen T, Tanser F, Iwuji CC, Gruttola V, De Iii GRS, Harling G. Antiretroviral therapy to prevent HIV acquisition in serodiscordant couples in a hyperendemic community in Rural South Africa. Clinical Infectious Diseases. 2018;**63**(4):635-643. https://doi.org/10.1093/cid/ciw335

[29] Robyn E, Venter WDF, Rees H. Pre-exposure prophylaxis for HIV prevention: Ready for prime time in South Africa? South African Medical Journal. 2013;**103**(8):515-516. DOI: 10.7196/SAMJ.6937

[30] Manuscript A. NIH Public Access. 2015;**11**(4):434-446. DOI: 10.1007/s11904-014-0225-9

[31] Muessig KE, Cohen MS. Advances in HIV prevention for serodiscordant couples. Current HIV/AIDS Reports. 2014;**11**(4):434-446. DOI: 10.1007/s11904-014-0225-9

[32] Abdool KQ, Abdool Karim SS, Frohlich JA, Grobler AC, Baxter C, Mansoor LE, et al. Effectiveness and safety of tenofovir gel, an antiretroviral microbicide, for the prevention of HIV infection in women. Science. 2010;**329**(2010):1168-1174. DOI: 10.1126/science.1193748

[33] Auvert B, Taljaard D, Lagarde E, Sobngwi-Tambekou J, Sitta R, Puren A. Randomized, controlled intervention trial of male circumcision for reduction of HIV infection risk: The ANRS 1265 trial. PLoS One. 2005;**2**(11):e298. DOI: 10.1371/journal.pmed.0020298

[34] Auvert B, Taljaard D, Rech D, Lissouba P, Singh B, Bouscaillou J, Mahiane G. Association of the ANRS-12126 male circumcision project with HIV levels among men in a south African township : Evaluation of effectiveness using cross-sectional surveys. Pl. 2013; **10**(9):1-12. DOI: 10.1371/journal.pmed.1001509

[35] Baeten JM, Donnell D, Kapiga SH, Ronald A, John- G, Inambao M, et al. Male circumcision and risk of male-to-female HIV-1 transmission: A multinational prospective study in African HIV-1 serodiscordant couples. AIDS. 2011;**24**(5):737-744. DOI: 10.1097/QAD.0b013e32833616e0

[36] Curran K, Baeten JM, Coates TJ, Kurth A, Mugo NR, Celum C. HIV-1 prevention for HIV-1 serodiscordant couples. Current HIV/AIDS Reports. 2012;**9**(2):160-170

[37] Mason J, Medley A, Yeiser S, Nightingale VR, Mani N, Sripipatana T, et al. The role of family planning in achieving safe pregnancy for serodiscordant couples: Commentary from the United States government' s interagency task force on family planning and HIV service integration. Journal of the International AIDS Society. 2017;**20**(1):4-11. DOI: 10.1080/17582652.2017.1278945

[38] Mmeje O, Cohen CR, Cohan D. Evaluating Safer Conception Options for HIV-Serodiscordant Couples (HIV-Infected Female/HIV-Uninfected Male): A Closer Look at Vaginal Insemination. Infectious Diseases in Obstetrics and Gynecology. 2012;**2012**:1-7. Article ID: 587651. https://doi.org/10.1155/2012/587651

[39] Mmeje O, Cohen CR, Murage A, Ong'ech J, Kiarie J, Poel SVD. Promoting Reproductive Options for HIV-Affected Couples in Sub-Saharan Africa. BJOG: An International Journal of Obstetrics & Gynaecology. 2014;**121**(s5):79-86

11

Immune Disorders in HIV-Infected Patients Coinfected with Hepatitis C Virus

Konstantin Shmagel and Evgeniya Saidakova

Abstract

In Russia, more than half of HIV-infected people are coinfected with hepatitis C. Both viruses interact with the immune system compounding the disease course. HIV infection accelerates the onset of hepatitis-mediated liver fibrosis and cirrhosis. Hepatitis C slows down the recovery of CD4+ T-lymphocytes during antiretroviral treatment and fuels the already intense chronic inflammation. In the present review, we discuss coinfection prevalence and reasons for its abundance, provide extensive coverage of the known mechanisms that give rise to the detrimental health effects in HIV/hepatitis C-coinfected patients, and report our own data on the double infection consequences in people with discordant immunologic response to treatment.

Keywords: HIV infection, hepatitis C, HIV/HCV coinfection, innate immunity, adaptive immunity, discordant immunologic response, highly active antiretroviral therapy

1. Introduction

More than any other infectious disease, HIV infection claims to be called "the coinfection illness" [1]. Coinfections can significantly change the illness pattern and the immune activation profile [2–4] and typically lead to the rise in morbidity and mortality [5–7]. The coinfection most often associated with HIV is hepatitis C virus (HCV) infection. This is due to the worldwide prevalence of both illnesses (there are approximately 40 million HIV-infected and about 120 million HCV-infected subjects worldwide) and the overlap in infection transmission routes [8, 9]. In Western Europe and the United States, the proportion of hepatitis C chronically infected patients among HIV-positive people is 25–30% [10], and in Eastern Europe, it is more than 50% [11]. In Russia, the increase in injection drug use has led to a significant rise in the prevalence of HIV/HCV coinfection. Its level among drug users reaches 93% [12]. The problem is complicated by the rise in non-AIDS-defining morbidity and mortality in HIV/HCV-coinfected subjects [13, 14].

There is considerable evidence that HIV infection adversely affects the course of a hepatitis C infection. When HIV/HCV coinfection is compared with HCV monoinfection, a more rapid fibrosis [15, 16] and liver cirrhosis [16, 17] are observed. Coinfected subjects also have an increased risk of hepatocellular carcinoma, which occurs at an earlier age and in a shorter time interval after HCV infection [18–20]. It was found that HIV/HCV-coinfected patients compared to HCV-monoinfected patients were more resistant to interferon therapy. In HIV-seronegative subjects infected with HCV genotype 1, 50–80% can achieve a complete recovery. However, in HIV-seropositive individuals coinfected with the same HCV type, interferon therapy is successful only in 20–35% of patients [21]. This accounts for the increased mortality rate among HIV-/HCV-coinfected patients when compared with HIV-monoinfected patients [22, 23].

Less is known about the effect of hepatitis C on the natural course of HIV infection. Among the negative influences, one can point to direct viral effects, hepatocyte destruction by immunocompetent cells, hepatic cell apoptosis, immune activation, and specific antiviral immune response alterations [24–26]. The complexity of the problem is largely due to the lack of knowledge about the biology of both HIV and HCV. It remains unknown whether the viruses interact with each other and in what ways that interaction might be expressed.

2. Liver fibrosis in HIV/HCV coinfection

Evidence indicates that the HCV viral load is lower in hepatitis C-monoinfected patients when compared to HIV/HCV-coinfected patients [27, 28]. Similar results were obtained when estimating the viral load in hepatic tissue [29]. In addition, multiyear cohort studies state that in patients with hepatitis C the HCV RNA blood level significantly increases after exposure to HIV [30, 31]. HCV replication enhancement in coinfection is attributed to both the development of immunodeficiency and the direct impact of HIV. While attempting to determine the mechanism(s) of these effects, it was shown that inactivated HIV or its component (gp120) can intensify viral replication in HCV-infected hepatoma cells in vitro [32]. This effect of HIV was shown to be due to transforming growth factor-beta 1 (TGF-β1) synthesis (antibodies against the cytokine blocked the HCV replication enhancement). Researchers also noted that HIV engages CCR5 or CXCR4 co-receptors for the related intracellular signal induction. Those data are significant not only for demonstrating the ability of HIV to increase HCV replication (with a monoinfection of hepatitis C, viral load is usually not associated with the disease severity) but also for illuminating the possible pathogenetic mechanism of fibrosis in HIV/HCV coinfection.

In many studies, HIV/HCV-coinfected patients demonstrated an inverse correlation between the CD4+ T-cell count and the HCV viral load [33–37]. Moreover, in those patients, low CD4+ T-lymphocyte quantity was used as a liver fibrosis predictor [34, 38, 39]. This suggests a negative impact of HIV infection on the course of hepatitis C through the development of CD4+ T-cell deficiency. It should be noted that a decrease in the CD4+ T-lymphocyte count is also found in those monoinfected with HCV. Indeed, the majority of HIV-seronegative subjects with liver cirrhosis have a reduced CD4+ T-cell count [40, 41]. Most researchers state that HIV infection, accompanied by a profound depletion in the CD4+ T-lymphocyte pool, is a prominent mediator of the accelerated liver fibrosis development in HIV-/HCV-coinfected people [42–44]. Based on those results and the opinions of leading specialists, the European AIDS Clinical Society recommends the early administration of highly active antiretroviral therapy (ART) to HCV-coinfected patients not only to optimize their hepatitis C management but also to slow down the development of fibrosis [45].

The main cellular element involved in the process of hepatic tissue fibrosis is the liver stellate cell (LSC) [46–49] located around the sinuses and usually not showing high activity until the organ is damaged [50, 51]. However, various destructive processes in the liver are accompanied by the reaction of hepatocytes, endotheliocytes, and Kupffer cells to produce various humoral factors [52]. Of those, TGF-β1 [53, 54] and PDGF (platelet-derived growth factor) have the most pronounced effect on LSC [52, 55]. Both cytokines induce LSC activation and differentiation into myofibroblast-like cells, which actively synthesize extracellular matrix proteins [56]. However, it should be noted that TGF-β1 and PDGF blood concentrations (as opposed to analyzing the hyaluronic acid or hepatocytes' growth factor content) have no high diagnostic value for the detection of fibrosis [57–60]. Moreover, it has recently been established that HIV influences the liver by infecting hepatocytes and liver stellate cells [61].

3. Anti-HCV immunity in HIV/HCV coinfection

Protection against HCV is implemented by various factors with an important role for interferons, natural killer (NK) cells, neutralizing antibodies, and T-lymphocytes. Type I interferons (IFN-α and IFN-β) and type III interferon (IFN-λ) are synthesized in response to the virus and induce interferon-stimulated gene (ISG) expression [62, 63]. In the cytosol, the pathogen's RNA is detected by the RIG-I (retinoic acid-inducible gene I) sensors, protein kinase R, and MDA5 (melanoma differentiation-associated protein 5). The first two mediate the interferon response at the early stages of the disease, and the third one mediates at the later infection phase [64, 65]. In endosomes, the virus is primarily detected by Toll-like receptor 3 (TLR3) that also triggers the IFN production and the ISG expression [66]. In hepatocytes of HCV-infected patients, the viral RNA and ISGs' mRNA are detected simultaneously, which confirms the connection between the cell genetic response and the presence of the pathogen [67]. The result of the activated ISG status in HCV infection leads to viral replication inhibition [68, 69]. However, prolonged ISG expression has a negative effect on the process of HCV spontaneous elimination [70, 71] and on the results of interferon and ribavirin combination therapy [72, 73].

NK cells play an important role in the pathogenesis of an HCV infection. It was found that in the healthy liver they represent the majority of the innate immune cells [74]. In the acute phase of the disease, NK cells affected by the virus are activated, produce IFN-γ, and perform cytotoxic functions [75]. In the chronic infection phase, IFN-γ and tumor necrosis factor (TNF)-α synthesis are reduced [76–78] even though the NK cell cytotoxic potential remains high [79, 80]. Since the protective effect of IFN-γ was demonstrated in HCV-infected hepatoma cells [81] and in experiments with chimpanzees given primary and repeated infections [82], it is believed that reduced IFN-γ production weakens the NK cell's antiviral activity. Thus, in the chronic stage of HCV infection, in spite of being activated and ready to perform cytotoxic functions, the NK lymphocytes are unable to effectively resist HCV due to the failure of IFN-γ production. However, the saved killing function can produce a positive result. NK cells from HCV-infected subjects are capable of killing activated LSC by NKG2D- and tumor necrosis factor-related apoptosis-inducing ligand (TRAIL)-dependent apoptosis, which allows them to be considered as active participants in liver fibrosis suppression [83].

The role of neutralizing antibodies (nAB) in protection against an HCV infection is not yet sufficiently understood. Based on known cases of spontaneous recovery before nAB emerge [84] and based on the ability of some patients with hypogammaglobulinemia to control the infection [85, 86], it could be concluded that the humoral immune response does not determine resistance to the disease. At the same time, there is evidence of a protective function for antibodies directed against HCV surface proteins. HCV envelope glycoprotein E1 and glycoprotein E2 seroconversion is usually observed a few weeks after an infection [87]. The ability of viral envelope-specific antibodies to block the infectious process was demonstrated in chimpanzees [88, 89] and in mice with genetically humanized liver [90, 91]. The emergence of nAB in the acute phase of HCV infection is accompanied by an alteration in the virus and its escape from immune control [92]. The authors also showed that despite the increased virus flexibility, high antibody titers significantly increase the chance for clearance of the infection. The acute-phase nAB titers are usually low in patients subsequently entering the chronic stage of the disease.

As was established in monkeys with induced CD4+ or CD8+ T-cell deficiency [93, 94], T-lymphocytes play an important role in the development of hepatitis C. It should be noted that the HCV-specific T-cell response usually develops 2–3 months after the infection [95, 96], although according to some authors such a "slow" reaction has little effect on the disease outcome [84]. It seems that the quality of the immune response achieved by CD4+ and CD8+ T-cells is a more important factor [97, 98]. It was found that in the acute phase of the infection, patients spontaneously clearing HCV compared to subjects in whom the disease became chronic had a more robust CD4+ T-lymphocyte response, which manifested in more active proliferation and cytokine (IFN-γ, TNF-α, and IL-2) production [99–102]. Later, it was found that the expression of PD-1 (programmed cell death protein 1) and CTLA-4 (cytotoxic T-lymphocyte-associated protein 4) inhibitory molecules was increased on the surface of CD4+ T-cells in patients chronically infected with HCV [103]. Blocking of PD-1 ligand (PD-L1/PD-L2), IL-10, and TGF-β1 in cultured lymphocytes isolated from the blood of these patients increased the virus-specific expansion of CD4+ T-lymphocytes. Neutralization of IL-10 and TGF-β1 enhanced the synthesis of IFN-γ, IL-2, and TNF-α. Further studies revealed that IL-21-producing CD4+ T-lymphocytes are lost in individuals with a chronic hepatitis C infection [104]. It has also been demonstrated that the deficiency of Th17 cells synthesizing IL-21 limits the HCV-specific CD8+ T-lymphocyte function and survival. The inability of CD4+ and CD8+ T-cells to control viral replication leads to their exhaustion. According to the authors, in chronic HCV infection, the increase in regulatory T-cell number and activity is aimed at suppressing an ineffective immune response and reducing inflammation. The other side of that process is fibrosis intensification. Thus, based on the above data, one can conclude that CD4+ T-lymphocytes are the key cells in protection against HCV. Hence, it becomes clear why a low CD4+ T-cell count is a negative predictor for liver fibrosis development in HIV-/HCV-coinfected patients.

4. Detrimental effects of hepatitis C on the course of HIV infection

It is more difficult to assess the effect of hepatitis C on the natural course of HIV infection. One of the parameters characterizing that effect is CD4+ T-cell count reconstitution after the administration of ART. To date, the accumulated data indicate slowing of the CD4+ T-lymphocyte restoration process in HIV-positive subjects coinfected with hepatitis C [35, 105–108]. The rate of CD4+ T-cell counts increases after receiving ART was reduced sevenfold in coinfected individuals compared with HIV-monoinfected patients [35]. The authors also established an association between impaired immunity regeneration and the level of HCV replication. In another study, it was demonstrated that in hepatitis C-positive patients, ineffective ART-mediated restoration affected not only the total CD4+ T-lymphocyte numbers but also their naive subset [106]. However, it should be noted that not all researchers support the idea of the negative effect of HCV coinfection on the treatment-induced CD4+ T-cell response [109, 110]. Still, an extensive multicenter study involving 22,533 patients showed that immune regeneration during ART is slower in coinfected patients, and the lower the nadir CD4+ T-lymphocyte level, the more pronounced the effect [111]. However, as noted in the paper, the differences in the CD4+ T-cell recovery between HIV + HCV+ and HIV + HCV− subjects are canceled by early treatment administration and uninterrupted long-term ART.

HIV infection causes severe devastation in the lymphoid structures of the digestive tract. It is accompanied by intestinal epithelial barrier destruction [112, 113] and the entry of microbes and their products into the bloodstream [114]. The increase in intestinal permeability is due to the direct destructive effect of HIV on the intestinal epithelium [115] followed by the development of inflammation and tissue remodeling [116]. Another cause for the pathological changes to the epithelial barrier is the deficiency of lymphocytes producing IL-17 and IL-22 which are necessary to maintain the epithelial lining integrity [117, 118]. To date, the role of microbial translocation in the immune system activation has been well established [119–121]. In addition, it has been shown that the blood levels of lipopolysaccharide (LPS) and soluble macrophage receptor CD14 (sCD14, capable of binding LPS) in HIV-infected patients can be used to predict disease progression and mortality [122–124]. Recently, in a large cohort of non-treated HIV-infected patients, an association between LPS-dependent immune activation and intestinal damage markers in serum was demonstrated [125]. However, a relationship between the immune system activation and viral load in blood was not found. Other data obtained in a study of bacterial-induced immune activation in patients with suppressed viral load also confirm its independence from the HIV load in blood [121, 126, 127]. It is assumed that the immune activation is mediated through TLRs [128–130].

It is widely accepted that liver cirrhosis compounds microbial translocation from the intestine into the bloodstream. A comparison of sCD14 blood levels in HIV/HCV-coinfected subjects, with varying degrees of liver fibrosis, showed that in patients with higher cirrhosis the soluble receptor concentration was more than in subjects with minimal organ destruction [131–133]. In HIV infection, the role of cirrhosis in the enhancement of the systemic inflammatory process was demonstrated while comparing two variants: compensated and uncompensated inflammations [134]. When uncompensated, a significantly higher level of LPS-binding protein (LBP) was detected in the patients' blood. The increase in the LBP content was accompanied by the rise in sCD14, sTNFR-I, and IL-6 concentrations.

Entry of large amounts of microbial products into the liver can have a negative impact on its function in HIV-infected individuals [135]. Liver cells actively express TLRs [136–139] that can interact with bacterial molecules and cause a marked inflammatory response in liver tissue [140, 141]. However, in experiments, it has been shown that prolonged exposure to LPS leads to a gradual decrease in the hepatocyte's sensitivity and a weakening of its ability to capture the bacterial lipopolysaccharide [142]. This causes a decrease in the detoxification function of the liver in patients monoinfected with HIV. The presence of hepatitis and cirrhosis additionally contributes to the decrease in LPS clearance by hepatocytes [143]. Consequently, in coinfection, microbial products entering the blood should cause strong immune activation. Indeed, the level of immune activation in HIV/HCV coinfection is higher than that in HIV [144, 145] or HCV [146, 147] monoinfection alone.

Activation of CD4+ and CD8+ T-cells is often followed by apoptosis: a phenomenon called "activation-induced cell death" (AICD) [148, 149]. AICD can be achieved through several mechanisms involving T-cell receptor stimulation, CD95, and various cytokines [150]. The role of innate immunity receptors in this phenomenon has also been established. Addition of various TLR ligands to cultured T-lymphocytes from healthy donors induced CD38 expression on CD4+ and CD8+ T-cells in short-term (less than 24 h) cultures [129]. Long-term culture (7 days) with TLR ligands led to a pronounced CD69 expression on CD8+ T-lymphocytes and Ki-67 expression in CD4+ T-cells. In such a case, CD8+ elements retained viability, and cycling CD4+ T-lymphocytes died. The data presented show how CD4+ T-cells, activated by microbial products, can die in HIV/HCV-coinfected patients. It is known that in untreated HIV-infected patients, HCV coinfection increases the apoptosis indices, but that effect is canceled by ART [151]. Later, the same authors found that in HIV/HCV coinfection, CD4+ T-lymphocytes are sensitized to Fas-induced apoptosis [152].

5. HIV/HCV-coinfected immunological nonresponders

A current concern is that as many as 30% of treated HIV-infected patients experience poor CD4+ T-cell restoration despite prolonged suppression of viral replication during ART (discordant immune response). These "immune nonresponders" (INRs) contrast with "immune responders" who recover their CD4+ T-cells to the normal range (>500/μL) while being treated. The discordant immune response is linked to an additional risk of mortality and non-AIDS-defining morbidities [153]. Still, the mechanisms responsible for insufficient CD4+ T-cell recovery during ART have not been fully discerned.

Our own studies have provided some additional information on the negative impact of hepatitis C on the natural course of an HIV infection. In our Russian cohort, we showed that HCV coinfection is a sufficient risk factor for the formation of a discordant CD4+ T-lymphocyte response to ART [154]. At the same time, we found that in coinfected patients when compared with patients monoinfected with HIV the increase in systemic inflammation was associated with liver damage and destruction of the hepatic barrier that protects against microbial products coming from the intestine [155]. INRs have a higher degree of hepatic tissue destruction and express more sclerosing processes [156]. We also found that HIV/HCV-coinfected

INR subjects are characterized not only by a deep CD4+ T-lymphocyte deficiency but also by decreased IL-2 production. Earlier, it was demonstrated [157] that through the secretion of this cytokine, T-cells can stimulate the natural killer cell's antifibrotic activity (realized through the killing of liver stellate cells). Thus, in HIV/HCV-coinfected INR patients, the IL-2 deficiency may be regarded as a liver fibrosis-accelerating factor.

In summary, it can be concluded that HIV/HCV-coinfected INRs are characterized by both a CD4+ T-lymphocyte deficiency and reduced IL-2 production which leads to liver destruction and cirrhosis formation. Under such conditions increased intestinal permeability (due to HIV infection) is supplemented by destruction of the hepatic barrier, accompanied by the entry of microbial products into the bloodstream. As a result, despite the ART-mediated HIV replication suppression, a pronounced systemic inflammation develops, leading to non-AIDS-defining diseases. Therefore, in coinfection, not only HIV infection therapy but also hepatitis C treatment should be actively carried out.

6. Conclusion

In HIV/HCV coinfection, the level of immune activation is higher than in HIV and HCV monoinfections. The transition of immunocompetent cells to the activated state is accompanied not only by their loss through the AICD mechanism but also leads to the development of non-AIDS-defining diseases, especially against the background of ART administration.

It can also be concluded that HIV infection exerts a greater influence on the natural course of a hepatitis C infection than the opposite. The key link in this influence is the depletion of CD4+ T-cells. However, not only CD4+ T-lymphocyte deficiency determines the HIV-negative impact on the development of hepatitis C. Even on the background of ART, HIV infection has a pronounced suppressive effect on NK cell activity against HCV. In HIV/HCV coinfection, a decrease in natural killer cell numbers and their ability to respond to IL-2 is observed. More importantly, the production of IFN-γ by those cells is also significantly impaired [158]. The outcome is the rapid development of liver fibrosis and cirrhosis.

As to changing the course of HIV infection against the background of hepatitis C, many questions remain. It is necessary to identify the main CD4+ and CD8+ T-cell subsets which are affected by HCV infection. In addition, studies of functional changes in T-lymphocytes like exhaustion [159–161], senescence [162–164], and loss of cytokine receptors [165, 166] must occur. It is also important to understand the nature of the immune system activation in HIV/HCV coinfection which is important in predicting the development of non-AIDS-defining diseases. Solving these issues requires further experimental and clinical research.

Acknowledgements

This work was supported by the Russian Foundation for Basic Research (17-54-30006).

Conflict of interest

The authors have no conflicts of interest to disclose.

Author details

Konstantin Shmagel[1,2]* and Evgeniya Saidakova[1,2]

*Address all correspondence to: shmagel@iegm.ru

1 Institute of Ecology and Genetics of Microorganisms, UB RAS, Perm, Russia

2 Perm State University, Perm, Russia

References

[1] Boulougoura A, Sereti I. HIV infection and immune activation: The role of coinfections. Current Opinion in HIV and AIDS. 2016;**11**(2):191-200

[2] Appay V, Kelleher AD. Immune activation and immune aging in HIV infection. Current Opinion in HIV and AIDS. 2016;**11**(2):242-249

[3] Taiwo B, Barcena L, Tressler R. Understanding and controlling chronic immune activation in the HIV-infected patients suppressed on combination antiretroviral therapy. Current HIV/AIDS Reports. 2013;**10**(1):21-32

[4] Masia M, Robledano C, de la Tabla VO, Antequera P, Lumbreras B, Hernandez I, et al. Coinfection with human herpesvirus 8 is associated with persistent inflammation and immune activation in virologically suppressed HIV-infected patients. PLoS One [Internet]. 2014;**9**(8):e105442

[5] Matthews PC, Geretti AM, Goulder PJ, Klenerman P. Epidemiology and impact of HIV coinfection with hepatitis B and hepatitis C viruses in Sub-Saharan Africa. Journal of Clinical Virology. 2014;**61**(1):20-33

[6] Deffur A, Mulder NJ, Wilkinson RJ. Co-infection with *Mycobacterium tuberculosis* and human immunodeficiency virus: An overview and motivation for systems approaches. Pathogens and Disease. 2013;**69**(2):101-113

[7] Effros RB. The silent war of CMV in aging and HIV infection. Mechanisms of Ageing and Development [Internet]. Sep 2016;**158**:46-52. DOI: 10.1016/j.mad.2015.09.003

[8] Webster DP, Klenerman P, Dusheiko GM. Hepatitis C. Lancet. 2015;**385**(9973):1124-1135

[9] Platt L, Easterbrook P, Gower E, McDonald B, Sabin K, McGowan C, et al. Prevalence and burden of HCV co-infection in people living with HIV: A global systematic review and meta-analysis. The Lancet Infectious Diseases. 2016;**16**(7):797-808

[10] Alter MJ. Epidemiology of viral hepatitis and HIV co-infection. Journal of Hepatology. 2006;**44**(1 Suppl):S6-S9

[11] Peters L, Mocroft A, Lundgren J, Grint D, Kirk O, Rockstroh J. HIV and hepatitis C co-infection in Europe, Israel and Argentina: A EuroSIDA perspective. BMC Infectious Diseases [Internet]. 2014;**14**(Suppl. 6):S13

[12] Rhodes T, Platt L, Judd A, Mikhailova LA, Sarang A, Wallis N, et al. Hepatitis C virus infection, HIV co-infection, and associated risk among injecting drug users in Togliatti, Russia. International Journal of STD & AIDS. 2005;**16**(11):749-754

[13] Chen TY, Ding EL, Seage Iii GR, Kim AY. Meta-analysis: Increased mortality associated with hepatitis C in HIV-infected persons is unrelated to HIV disease progression. Clinical Infectious Diseases. 2009;**49**(10):1605-1615

[14] Puoti M, Moioli MC, Travi G, Rossotti R. The burden of liver disease in human immunodeficiency virus-infected patients. Seminars in Liver Disease. 2012;**32**(2):103-113

[15] Macias J, Berenguer J, Japon MA, Giron JA, Rivero A, Lopez-Cortes LF, et al. Fast fibrosis progression between repeated liver biopsies in patients coinfected with human immunodeficiency virus/hepatitis C virus. Hepatology. 2009;**50**(4):1056-1063

[16] Deng LP, Gui XE, Zhang YX, Gao SC, Yang RR. Impact of human immunodeficiency virus infection on the course of hepatitis C virus infection: A meta-analysis. World Journal of Gastroenterology. 2009;**15**(8):996-1003

[17] Hernandez MD, Sherman KE. HIV/hepatitis C coinfection natural history and disease progression. Current Opinion in HIV and AIDS. 2011;**6**(6):478-482

[18] Garcia-Samaniego J, Rodriguez M, Berenguer J, Rodriguez-Rosado R, Carbo J, Asensi V, et al. Hepatocellular carcinoma in HIV-infected patients with chronic hepatitis C. The American Journal of Gastroenterology. 2001;**96**(1):179-183

[19] Puoti M, Bruno R, Soriano V, Donato F, Gaeta GB, Quinzan GP, et al. Hepatocellular carcinoma in HIV-infected patients: Epidemiological features, clinical presentation and outcome. AIDS. 2004;**18**(17):2285-2293

[20] Brau N, Fox RK, Xiao P, Marks K, Naqvi Z, Taylor LE, et al. Presentation and outcome of hepatocellular carcinoma in HIV-infected patients: A U.S.-Canadian multicenter study. Journal of Hepatology. 2007;**47**(4):527-537

[21] Operskalski EA, Kovacs A. HIV/HCV co-infection: Pathogenesis, clinical complications, treatment, and new therapeutic technologies. Current HIV/AIDS Reports. 2011;**8**(1):12-22

[22] Sabin CA, Walker AS, Dunn D. HIV/HCV coinfection, HAART, and liver-related mortality. Lancet. 2004;**364**(9436):757-758 author reply 8

[23] Hernando V, Alejos B, Monge S, Berenguer J, Anta L, Vinuesa D, et al. All-cause mortality in the cohorts of the Spanish AIDS Research Network (RIS) compared with the general population: 1997-2010. BMC Infectious Diseases. 2013;**13**:382

[24] Rotman Y, Liang TJ. Coinfection with hepatitis C virus and human immunodeficiency virus: Virological, immunological, and clinical outcomes. Journal of Virology. 2009;**83**(15):7366-7374

[25] Roe B, Hall WW. Cellular and molecular interactions in coinfection with hepatitis C virus and human immunodeficiency virus. Expert Reviews in Molecular Medicine. 2008;**10**:e30

[26] Kim AY, Chung RT. Coinfection with HIV-1 and HCV—A one-two punch. Gastroenterology. 2009;**137**(3):795-814

[27] Sherman KE, O'Brien J, Gutierrez AG, Harrison S, Urdea M, Neuwald P, et al. Quantitative evaluation of hepatitis C virus RNA in patients with concurrent human immunodeficiency virus infections. Journal of Clinical Microbiology. 1993;**31**(10):2679-2682

[28] Thomas DL, Astemborski J, Vlahov D, Strathdee SA, Ray SC, Nelson KE, et al. Determinants of the quantity of hepatitis C virus RNA. The Journal of Infectious Diseases. 2000;**181**(3):844-851

[29] Bonacini M, Govindarajan S, Blatt LM, Schmid P, Conrad A, Lindsay KL. Patients co-infected with human immunodeficiency virus and hepatitis C virus demonstrate higher levels of hepatic HCV RNA. Journal of Viral Hepatitis. 1999;**6**(3):203-208

[30] Beld M, Penning M, Lukashov V, McMorrow M, Roos M, Pakker N, et al. Evidence that both HIV and HIV-induced immunodeficiency enhance HCV replication among HCV seroconverters. Virology. 1998;**244**(2):504-512

[31] Eyster ME, Fried MW, Di Bisceglie AM, Goedert JJ. Increasing hepatitis C virus RNA levels in hemophiliacs: Relationship to human immunodeficiency virus infection and liver disease. Multicenter Hemophilia Cohort Study. Blood. 1994;**84**(4):1020-1023

[32] Lin W, Weinberg EM, Tai AW, Peng LF, Brockman MA, Kim KA, et al. HIV increases HCV replication in a TGF-beta1-dependent manner. Gastroenterology. 2008;**134**(3):803-811

[33] Martinez-Sierra C, Arizcorreta A, Diaz F, Roldan R, Martin-Herrera L, Perez-Guzman E, et al. Progression of chronic hepatitis C to liver fibrosis and cirrhosis in patients coinfected with hepatitis C virus and human immunodeficiency virus. Clinical Infectious Diseases. 2003;**36**(4):491-498

[34] Benhamou Y, Bochet M, Di Martino V, Charlotte F, Azria F, Coutellier A, et al. Liver fibrosis progression in human immunodeficiency virus and hepatitis C virus coinfected patients. The Multivirc Group. Hepatology. 1999;**30**(4):1054-1058

[35] Potter M, Odueyungbo A, Yang H, Saeed S, Klein MB. Canadian Co-infection Cohort Study I. Impact of hepatitis C viral replication on CD4+ T-lymphocyte progression in HIV-HCV coinfection before and after antiretroviral therapy. AIDS. 2010;**24**(12):1857-1865

[36] Falconer K, Gonzalez VD, Reichard O, Sandberg JK, Alaeus A. Spontaneous HCV clearance in HCV/HIV-1 coinfection associated with normalized CD4 counts, low level of chronic immune activation and high level of T cell function. Journal of Clinical Virology. 2008;**41**(2):160-163

[37] Rohrbach J, Robinson N, Harcourt G, Hammond E, Gaudieri S, Gorgievski M, et al. Cellular immune responses to HCV core increase and HCV RNA levels decrease during successful antiretroviral therapy. Gut. 2010;**59**(9):1252-1258

[38] Reiberger T, Ferlitsch A, Sieghart W, Kreil A, Breitenecker F, Rieger A, et al. HIV-HCV co-infected patients with low CD4+ cell nadirs are at risk for faster fibrosis progression and portal hypertension. Journal of Viral Hepatitis. 2010;**17**(6):400-409

[39] Mohsen AH, Easterbrook PJ, Taylor C, Portmann B, Kulasegaram R, Murad S, et al. Impact of human immunodeficiency virus (HIV) infection on the progression of liver fibrosis in hepatitis C virus infected patients. Gut. 2003;**52**(7):1035-1040

[40] McGovern BH, Golan Y, Lopez M, Pratt D, Lawton A, Moore G, et al. The impact of cirrhosis on CD4+ T cell counts in HIV-seronegative patients. Clinical Infectious Diseases. 2007;**44**(3):431-437

[41] Rashkin S, Rouster S, Goodman ZD, Sherman KE. T-helper cells and liver fibrosis in hepatitis C virus-monoinfected patients. Journal of Viral Hepatitis. 2010;**17**(3):222-226

[42] Mandorfer M, Payer BA, Schwabl P, Steiner S, Ferlitsch A, Aichelburg MC, et al. Revisiting liver disease progression in HIV/HCV-coinfected patients: The influence of vitamin D, insulin resistance, immune status, IL28B and PNPLA3. Liver International. 2015;**35**(3):876-885

[43] Kooij KW, Wit FW, van Zoest RA, Schouten J, Kootstra NA, van Vugt M, et al. Liver fibrosis in HIV-infected individuals on long-term antiretroviral therapy: Associated with immune activation, immunodeficiency and prior use of didanosine. AIDS. 2016;**30**(11):1771-1780

[44] Swanson S, Ma Y, Scherzer R, Huhn G, French AL, Plankey MW, et al. Association of HIV, hepatitis C virus, and liver fibrosis severity with the enhanced liver fibrosis score. The Journal of Infectious Diseases. 2016;**213**(7):1079-1086

[45] Mandorfer M, Schwabl P, Steiner S, Reiberger T, Peck-Radosavljevic M. Advances in the management of HIV/HCV coinfection. Hepatology International. 2016;**10**(3):424-435

[46] Hui AY, Friedman SL. Molecular basis of hepatic fibrosis. Expert Reviews in Molecular Medicine. 2003;**5**(5):1-23

[47] Zhao Q, Qin CY, Zhao ZH, Fan YC, Wang K. Epigenetic modifications in hepatic stellate cells contribute to liver fibrosis. The Tohoku Journal of Experimental Medicine. 2013;**229**(1):35-43

[48] Friedman SL. Hepatic stellate cells: Protean, multifunctional, and enigmatic cells of the liver. Physiological Reviews. 2008;**88**(1):125-172

[49] Lee UE, Friedman SL. Mechanisms of hepatic fibrogenesis. Best Practice & Research. Clinical Gastroenterology. 2011;**25**(2):195-206

[50] Marrone G, Shah VH, Gracia-Sancho J. Sinusoidal communication in liver fibrosis and regeneration. Journal of Hepatology. 2016

[51] Yin C, Evason KJ, Asahina K, Stainier DY. Hepatic stellate cells in liver development, regeneration, and cancer. The Journal of Clinical Investigation. 2013;**123**(5):1902-1910

[52] Greuter T, Shah VH. Hepatic sinusoids in liver injury, inflammation, and fibrosis: New pathophysiological insights. Journal of Gastroenterology. 2016;**51**(6):511-519

[53] Rossmanith W, Schulte-Hermann R. Biology of transforming growth factor beta in hepatocarcinogenesis. Microscopy Research and Technique. 2001;**52**(4):430-436

[54] Matsuzaki K. Modulation of TGF-beta signaling during progression of chronic liver diseases. Frontiers in Bioscience (Landmark Ed). 2009 Jan 1;**14**:2923-2934

[55] Hernandez-Gea V, Friedman SL. Pathogenesis of liver fibrosis. Annual Review of Pathology. 2011;**6**:425-456

[56] Tsukamoto H, Zhu NL, Asahina K, Mann DA, Mann J. Epigenetic cell fate regulation of hepatic stellate cells. Hepatology Research. 2011;**41**(7):675-682

[57] Anatol P, Robert F, Danuta P. Effect of interferon alpha2b plus ribavirin treatment on selected growth factors in respect to inflammation and fibrosis in chronic hepatitis C. World Journal of Gastroenterology. 2005;**11**(12):1854-1858

[58] Jain MK, Adams-Huet B, Terekhova D, Kushner LE, Bedimo R, Li X, et al. Acute and chronic immune biomarker changes during interferon/ribavirin treatment in HIV/HCV co-infected patients. Journal of Viral Hepatitis. 2015;**22**(1):25-36

[59] El-Bassiouni NE, Nosseir MM, Madkour ME, Zoheiry MM, Bekheit IW, Ibrahim RA, et al. Role of fibrogenic markers in chronic hepatitis C and associated hepatocellular carcinoma. Molecular Biology Reports. 2012;**39**(6):6843-6850

[60] Nath NC, Rahman MA, Khan MR, Hasan MS, Bhuiyan TM, Hoque MN, et al. Serum hyaluronic acid as a predictor of fibrosis in chronic hepatitis B and C virus infection. Mymensingh Medical Journal. 2011;**20**(4):614-619

[61] Kong L, Cardona Maya W, Moreno-Fernandez ME, Ma G, Shata MT, Sherman KE, et al. Low-level HIV infection of hepatocytes. Virology Journal. 2012;9:157

[62] Ciccaglione AR, Marcantonio C, Tritarelli E, Tataseo P, Ferraris A, Bruni R, et al. Microarray analysis identifies a common set of cellular genes modulated by different HCV replicon clones. BMC Genomics. 2008;**9**:309

[63] Su AI, Pezacki JP, Wodicka L, Brideau AD, Supekova L, Thimme R, et al. Genomic analysis of the host response to hepatitis C virus infection. Proceedings of the National Academy of Sciences of the United States of America. 2002;**99**(24):15669-15674

[64] Hiet MS, Bauhofer O, Zayas M, Roth H, Tanaka Y, Schirmacher P, et al. Control of temporal activation of hepatitis C virus-induced interferon response by domain 2 of nonstructural protein 5A. Journal of Hepatology. 2015;**63**(4):829-837

[65] Arnaud N, Dabo S, Akazawa D, Fukasawa M, Shinkai-Ouchi F, Hugon J, et al. Hepatitis C virus reveals a novel early control in acute immune response. PLOS Pathogens [Internet]. 2011;**7**(10):e1002289

[66] Li K, Li NL, Wei D, Pfeffer SR, Fan M, Pfeffer LM. Activation of chemokine and inflammatory cytokine response in hepatitis C virus-infected hepatocytes depends on Toll-like receptor 3 sensing of hepatitis C virus double-stranded RNA intermediates. Hepatology. 2012;**55**(3):666-675

[67] Wieland S, Makowska Z, Campana B, Calabrese D, Dill MT, Chung J, et al. Simultaneous detection of hepatitis C virus and interferon stimulated gene expression in infected human liver. Hepatology. 2014;**59**(6):2121-2130

[68] Schoggins JW, Wilson SJ, Panis M, Murphy MY, Jones CT, Bieniasz P, et al. A diverse range of gene products are effectors of the type I interferon antiviral response. Nature. 2011;**472**(7344):481-485

[69] Metz P, Dazert E, Ruggieri A, Mazur J, Kaderali L, Kaul A, et al. Identification of type I and type II interferon-induced effectors controlling hepatitis C virus replication. Hepatology. 2012;**56**(6):2082-2093

[70] Terczynska-Dyla E, Bibert S, Duong FH, Krol I, Jorgensen S, Collinet E, et al. Reduced IFNλ4 activity is associated with improved HCV clearance and reduced expression of interferon-stimulated genes. Nature Communications. 2014;**5**:5699

[71] Scagnolari C, Monteleone K, Cacciotti G, Antonelli G. Role of interferons in chronic hepatitis C infection. Current Drug Targets. 2017;**18**(7):844-850

[72] Dill MT, Duong FH, Vogt JE, Bibert S, Bochud PY, Terracciano L, et al. Interferon-induced gene expression is a stronger predictor of treatment response than IL28B genotype in patients with hepatitis C. Gastroenterology. 2011;**140**(3):1021-1031

[73] Lanford RE, Guerra B, Bigger CB, Lee H, Chavez D, Brasky KM. Lack of response to exogenous interferon-alpha in the liver of chimpanzees chronically infected with hepatitis C virus. Hepatology. 2007;**46**(4):999-1008

[74] Norris S, Collins C, Doherty DG, Smith F, McEntee G, Traynor O, et al. Resident human hepatic lymphocytes are phenotypically different from circulating lymphocytes. Journal of Hepatology. 1998;**28**(1):84-90

[75] Amadei B, Urbani S, Cazaly A, Fisicaro P, Zerbini A, Ahmed P, et al. Activation of natural killer cells during acute infection with hepatitis C virus. Gastroenterology. 2010;**138**(4):1536-1545

[76] Holder KA, Stapleton SN, Gallant ME, Russell RS, Grant MD. Hepatitis C virus-infected cells downregulate NKp30 and inhibit ex vivo NK cell functions. Journal of Immunology. 2013;**191**(6):3308-3318

[77] Yoon JC, Lim JB, Park JH, Lee JM. Cell-to-cell contact with hepatitis C virus-infected cells reduces functional capacity of natural killer cells. Journal of Virology. 2011;**85**(23):12557-12569

[78] Mondelli MU, Oliviero B, Mele D, Mantovani S, Gazzabin C, Varchetta S. Natural killer cell functional dichotomy: A feature of chronic viral hepatitis? Frontiers in Immunology [Internet]. 2012;**3**:351

[79] Oliviero B, Varchetta S, Paudice E, Michelone G, Zaramella M, Mavilio D, et al. Natural killer cell functional dichotomy in chronic hepatitis B and chronic hepatitis C virus infections. Gastroenterology, 60. 2009;**137**(3):1151, 60 e1-7

[80] Ahlenstiel G, Titerence RH, Koh C, Edlich B, Feld JJ, Rotman Y, et al. Natural killer cells

are polarized toward cytotoxicity in chronic hepatitis C in an interferon-alfa-dependent manner. Gastroenterology. 2010;**138**(1):325-335 e1-2

[81] Frese M, Schwarzle V, Barth K, Krieger N, Lohmann V, Mihm S, et al. Interferon-gamma inhibits replication of subgenomic and genomic hepatitis C virus RNAs. Hepatology. 2002;**35**(3):694-703

[82] Major ME, Mihalik K, Puig M, Rehermann B, Nascimbeni M, Rice CM, et al. Previously infected and recovered chimpanzees exhibit rapid responses that control hepatitis C virus replication upon rechallenge. Journal of Virology. 2002;**76**(13):6586-6595

[83] Glässner A, Eisenhardt M, Krämer B, Körner C, Coenen M, Sauerbruch T, et al. NK cells from HCV-infected patients effectively induce apoptosis of activated primary human hepatic stellate cells in a TRAIL-, FasL- and NKG2D-dependent manner. Laboratory Investigation. 2012;**92**(7):967-977

[84] Terilli RR, Cox AL. Immunity and hepatitis C: A review. Current HIV/AIDS Reports. 2013;**10**(1):51-58

[85] Christie JM, Healey CJ, Watson J, Wong VS, Duddridge M, Snowden N, et al. Clinical outcome of hypogammaglobulinaemic patients following outbreak of acute hepatitis C: 2 year follow up. Clinical and Experimental Immunology. 1997;**110**(1):4-8

[86] Semmo N, Lucas M, Krashias G, Lauer G, Chapel H, Klenerman P. Maintenance of HCV-specific T-cell responses in antibody-deficient patients a decade after early therapy. Blood. 2006;**107**(11):4570-4571

[87] Lauer GM, Walker BD. Hepatitis C virus infection. The New England Journal of Medicine. 2001;**345**(1):41-52

[88] Farci P, Shimoda A, Wong D, Cabezon T, De Gioannis D, Strazzera A, et al. Prevention of hepatitis C virus infection in chimpanzees by hyperimmune serum against the hypervariable region 1 of the envelope 2 protein. Proceedings of the National Academy of Sciences of the United States of America. 1996;**93**(26):15394-15399

[89] Morin TJ, Broering TJ, Leav BA, Blair BM, Rowley KJ, Boucher EN, et al. Human monoclonal antibody HCV1 effectively prevents and treats HCV infection in chimpanzees. PLOS Pathogens [Internet]. 2012;**8**(8):e1002895

[90] Law M, Maruyama T, Lewis J, Giang E, Tarr AW, Stamataki Z, et al. Broadly neutralizing antibodies protect against hepatitis C virus quasispecies challenge. Nature Medicine. 2008;**14**(1):25-27

[91] Vanwolleghem T, Bukh J, Meuleman P, Desombere I, Meunier JC, Alter H, et al. Polyclonal immunoglobulins from a chronic hepatitis C virus patient protect human liver-chimeric mice from infection with a homologous hepatitis C virus strain. Hepatology. 2008;**47**(6): 1846-1855

[92] Dowd KA, Netski DM, Wang XH, Cox AL, Ray SC. Selection pressure from neutralizing antibodies drives sequence evolution during acute infection with hepatitis C virus. Gastroenterology. 2009;**136**(7):2377-2386

[93] Grakoui A, Shoukry NH, Woollard DJ, Han JH, Hanson HL, Ghrayeb J, et al. HCV

persistence and immune evasion in the absence of memory T cell help. Science. 2003;**302**(5645):659-662

[94] Shoukry NH, Grakoui A, Houghton M, Chien DY, Ghrayeb J, Reimann KA, et al. Memory CD8+ T cells are required for protection from persistent hepatitis C virus infection. The Journal of Experimental Medicine. 2003;**197**(12):1645-1655

[95] Thimme R, Bukh J, Spangenberg HC, Wieland S, Pemberton J, Steiger C, et al. Viral and immunological determinants of hepatitis C virus clearance, persistence, and disease. Proceedings of the National Academy of Sciences of the United States of America. 2002;**99**(24):15661-15668

[96] Shin EC, Park SH, Demino M, Nascimbeni M, Mihalik K, Major M, et al. Delayed induction, not impaired recruitment, of specific CD8(+) T cells causes the late onset of acute hepatitis C. Gastroenterology. 2011;**141**(2):686-695, 95 e1

[97] Neumann-Haefelin C, Thimme R. Success and failure of virus-specific T cell responses in hepatitis C virus infection. Digestive Diseases. 2011;**29**(4):416-422

[98] Klenerman P, Thimme R. T cell responses in hepatitis C: The good, the bad and the unconventional. Gut. 2012;**61**(8):1226-1234

[99] Diepolder HM, Zachoval R, Hoffmann RM, Wierenga EA, Santantonio T, Jung MC, et al. Possible mechanism involving T-lymphocyte response to non-structural protein 3 in viral clearance in acute hepatitis C virus infection. Lancet. 1995;**346**(8981):1006-1007

[100] Missale G, Bertoni R, Lamonaca V, Valli A, Massari M, Mori C, et al. Different clinical behaviors of acute hepatitis C virus infection are associated with different vigor of the anti-viral cell-mediated immune response. The Journal of Clinical Investigation. 1996;**98**(3):706-714

[101] Smyk-Pearson S, Tester IA, Klarquist J, Palmer BE, Pawlotsky JM, Golden-Mason L, et al. Spontaneous recovery in acute human hepatitis C virus infection: Functional T-cell thresholds and relative importance of CD4 help. Journal of Virology. 2008; **82**(4):1827-1837

[102] Urbani S, Amadei B, Fisicaro P, Tola D, Orlandini A, Sacchelli L, et al. Outcome of acute hepatitis C is related to virus-specific CD4 function and maturation of antiviral memory CD8 responses. Hepatology. 2006;**44**(1):126-139

[103] Raziorrouh B, Ulsenheimer A, Schraut W, Heeg M, Kurktschiev P, Zachoval R, et al. Inhibitory molecules that regulate expansion and restoration of HCV-specific CD4+ T cells in patients with chronic infection. Gastroenterology. 2011;**141**(4):1422-1431, 31 e1-6

[104] Kared H, Fabre T, Bedard N, Bruneau J, Shoukry NH. Galectin-9 and IL-21 mediate cross-regulation between Th17 and Treg cells during acute hepatitis C. PLOS Pathogens [Internet]. 2013;**9**(6):e1003422

[105] Greub G, Ledergerber B, Battegay M, Grob P, Perrin L, Furrer H, et al. Clinical progression, survival, and immune recovery during antiretroviral therapy in patients

with HIV-1 and hepatitis C virus coinfection: The Swiss HIV Cohort Study. Lancet. 2000;**356**(9244):1800-1805

[106] Santin M, Mestre M, Shaw E, Barbera MJ, Casanova A, Niubo J, et al. Impact of hepatitis C virus coinfection on immune restoration during successful antiretroviral therapy in chronic human immunodeficiency virus type 1 disease. European Journal of Clinical Microbiology & Infectious Diseases. 2008;**27**(1):65-73

[107] Taye S, Lakew M. Impact of hepatitis C virus co-infection on HIV patients before and after highly active antiretroviral therapy: An immunological and clinical chemistry observation, Addis Ababa, Ethiopia. BMC Immunology [Internet]. 2013;**14**:23

[108] Weis N, Lindhardt BO, Kronborg G, Hansen AB, Laursen AL, Christensen PB, et al. Impact of hepatitis C virus coinfection on response to highly active antiretroviral therapy and outcome in HIV-infected individuals: A nationwide cohort study. Clinical Infectious Diseases. 2006;**42**(10):1481-1487

[109] Yacisin K, Maida I, Rios MJ, Soriano V, Nunez M. Hepatitis C virus coinfection does not affect CD4 restoration in HIV-infected patients after initiation of antiretroviral therapy. AIDS Research and Human Retroviruses. 2008;**24**(7):935-940

[110] Rockstroh JK, Mocroft A, Soriano V, Tural C, Losso MH, Horban A, et al. Influence of hepatitis C virus infection on HIV-1 disease progression and response to highly active antiretroviral therapy. The Journal of Infectious Diseases. 2005;**192**(6):992-1002

[111] Tsiara CG, Nikolopoulos GK, Dimou NL, Bagos PG, Saroglou G, Velonakis E, et al. Effect of hepatitis C virus on immunological and virological responses in HIV-infected patients initiating highly active antiretroviral therapy: A meta-analysis. Journal of Viral Hepatitis. 2013;**20**(10):715-724

[112] Mohan M, Kaushal D, Aye PP, Alvarez X, Veazey RS, Lackner AA. Focused examination of the intestinal epithelium reveals transcriptional signatures consistent with disturbances in enterocyte maturation and differentiation during the course of SIV infection. PLoS One [Internet]. 2013;**8**(4):e60122

[113] Sharpstone D, Neild P, Crane R, Taylor C, Hodgson C, Sherwood R, et al. Small intestinal transit, absorption, and permeability in patients with AIDS with and without diarrhoea. Gut. 1999;**45**(1):70-76

[114] Klatt NR, Funderburg NT, Brenchley JM. Microbial translocation, immune activation, and HIV disease. Trends in Microbiology. 2013;**21**(1):6-13

[115] Nazli A, Chan O, Dobson-Belaire WN, Ouellet M, Tremblay MJ, Gray-Owen SD, et al. Exposure to HIV-1 directly impairs mucosal epithelial barrier integrity allowing microbial translocation. PLOS Pathogens [Internet]. 2010;**6**(4):e1000852

[116] Smith AJ, Schacker TW, Reilly CS, Haase AT. A role for syndecan-1 and claudin-2 in microbial translocation during HIV-1 infection. JAIDS Journal of Acquired Immune Deficiency Syndromes. 2010;**55**(3):306-315

[117] Gordon SN, Cervasi B, Odorizzi P, Silverman R, Aberra F, Ginsberg G, et al. Disruption

of intestinal CD4+ T cell homeostasis is a key marker of systemic CD4+ T cell activation in HIV-infected individuals. Journal of Immunology. 2010;**185**(9):5169-5179

[118] Klatt NR, Estes JD, Sun X, Ortiz AM, Barber JS, Harris LD, et al. Loss of mucosal CD103+ DCs and IL-17+ and IL-22+ lymphocytes is associated with mucosal damage in SIV infection. Mucosal Immunology. 2012;**5**(6):646-657

[119] Brenchley JM, Price DA, Schacker TW, Asher TE, Silvestri G, Rao S, et al. Microbial translocation is a cause of systemic immune activation in chronic HIV infection. Nature Medicine. 2006;**12**(12):1365-1371

[120] Estes JD, Harris LD, Klatt NR, Tabb B, Pittaluga S, Paiardini M, et al. Damaged intestinal epithelial integrity linked to microbial translocation in pathogenic simian immunodeficiency virus infections. PLOS Pathogens [Internet]. 2010;**6**(8):e1001052

[121] Marchetti G, Bellistri GM, Borghi E, Tincati C, Ferramosca S, La Francesca M, et al. Microbial translocation is associated with sustained failure in CD4+ T-cell reconstitution in HIV-infected patients on long-term highly active antiretroviral therapy. AIDS. 2008;**22**(15):2035-2038

[122] Leon A, Leal L, Torres B, Lucero C, Inciarte A, Arnedo M, et al. Association of microbial translocation biomarkers with clinical outcome in controllers HIV-infected patients. AIDS. 2015;**29**(6):675-681

[123] Marchetti G, Cozzi-Lepri A, Merlini E, Bellistri GM, Castagna A, Galli M, et al. Microbial translocation predicts disease progression of HIV-infected antiretroviral-naive patients with high CD4(+) cell count. AIDS. 2011;**25**(11):1385-1394

[124] Sandler NG, Wand H, Roque A, Law M, Nason MC, Nixon DE, et al. Plasma levels of soluble CD14 independently predict mortality in HIV infection. The Journal of Infectious Diseases. 2011;**203**(6):780-790

[125] Perkins MR, Bartha I, Timmer JK, Liebner JC, Wolinsky D, Gunthard HF, et al. The interplay between host genetic variation, viral replication, and microbial translocation in untreated HIV-infected individuals. The Journal of Infectious Diseases. 2015;**212**(4):578-584

[126] Jiang W, Lederman MM, Hunt P, Sieg SF, Haley K, Rodriguez B, et al. Plasma levels of bacterial DNA correlate with immune activation and the magnitude of immune restoration in persons with antiretroviral-treated HIV infection. The Journal of Infectious Diseases. 2009;**199**(8):1177-1185

[127] Marchetti G, Gori A, Casabianca A, Magnani M, Franzetti F, Clerici M, et al. Comparative analysis of T-cell turnover and homeostatic parameters in HIV-infected patients with discordant immune-virological responses to HAART. AIDS. 2006;**20**(13):1727-1736

[128] Bukh AR, Melchjorsen J, Offersen R, Jensen JMB, Toft L, Stovring H, et al. Endotoxemia is associated with altered innate and adaptive immune responses in untreated HIV-1 infected individuals. PLoS One [Internet]. 2011;**6**(6):e21275

[129] Funderburg N, Luciano AA, Jiang W, Rodriguez B, Sieg SF, Lederman MM. Toll-like receptor ligands induce human T cell activation and death, a model for HIV pathogenesis. PLoS One [Internet]. 2008;**3**(4):e1915

[130] Novati S, Sacchi P, Cima S, Zuccaro V, Columpsi P, Pagani L, et al. General issues on microbial translocation in HIV-infected patients. European Review for Medical and Pharmacological Sciences. 2015;**19**(5):866-878

[131] Sandler NG, Koh C, Roque A, Eccleston JL, Siegel RB, Demino M, et al. Host response to translocated microbial products predicts outcomes of patients with HBV or HCV infection. Gastroenterology. 2011;**141**(4):1220-30, 30 e1-3

[132] Balagopal A, Philp FH, Astemborski J, Block TM, Mehta A, Long R, et al. Human immunodeficiency virus-related microbial translocation and progression of hepatitis C. Gastroenterology. 2008;**135**(1):226-233

[133] Marchetti G, Nasta P, Bai F, Gatti F, Bellistri GM, Tincati C, et al. Circulating sCD14 is associated with virological response to pegylated-interferon-alpha/ribavirin treatment in HIV/HCV co-infected patients. PLoS One [Internet]. 2012;**7**(2):e32028

[134] de Oca Arjona MM, Marquez M, Soto MJ, Rodriguez-Ramos C, Terron A, Vergara A, et al. Bacterial translocation in HIV-infected patients with HCV cirrhosis: Implication in hemodynamic alterations and mortality. Journal of Acquired Immune Deficiency Syndromes. 2011;**56**(5):420-427

[135] Scarpellini E, Valenza V, Gabrielli M, Lauritano EC, Perotti G, Merra G, et al. Intestinal permeability in cirrhotic patients with and without spontaneous bacterial peritonitis: Is the ring closed? The American Journal of Gastroenterology. 2010;**105**(2):323-327

[136] Su GL, Klein RD, Aminlari A, Zhang HY, Steinstraesser L, Alarcon WH, et al. Kupffer cell activation by lipopolysaccharide in rats: Role for lipopolysaccharide binding protein and toll-like receptor 4. Hepatology. 2000;**31**(4):932-936

[137] Jiang W, Sun R, Wei H, Tian Z. Toll-like receptor 3 ligand attenuates LPS-induced liver injury by down-regulation of toll-like receptor 4 expression on macrophages. Proceedings of the National Academy of Sciences of the United States of America. 2005;**102**(47):17077-17082

[138] Guo J, Loke J, Zheng F, Hong F, Yea S, Fukata M, et al. Functional linkage of cirrhosis-predictive single nucleotide polymorphisms of toll-like receptor 4 to hepatic stellate cell responses. Hepatology. 2009;**49**(3):960-968

[139] Nakamoto N, Kanai T. Role of toll-like receptors in immune activation and tolerance in the liver. Frontiers in Immunology [Internet]. 2014;**5**:e221

[140] Paik YH, Schwabe RF, Bataller R, Russo MP, Jobin C, Brenner DA. Toll-like receptor 4 mediates inflammatory signaling by bacterial lipopolysaccharide in human hepatic stellate cells. Hepatology. 2003;**37**(5):1043-1055

[141] Kopydlowski KM, Salkowski CA, Cody MJ, van Rooijen N, Major J, Hamilton TA, et al.

Regulation of macrophage chemokine expression by lipopolysaccharide in vitro and in vivo. Journal of Immunology. 1999;**163**(3):1537-1544

[142] Scott MJ, Liu S, Shapiro RA, Vodovotz Y, Billiar TR. Endotoxin uptake in mouse liver is blocked by endotoxin pretreatment through a suppressor of cytokine signaling-1-dependent mechanism. Hepatology. 2009;**49**(5):1695-1708

[143] Lumsden AB, Henderson JM, Kutner MH. Endotoxin levels measured by a chromogenic assay in portal, hepatic and peripheral venous blood in patients with cirrhosis. Hepatology. 1988;**8**(2):232-236

[144] Kovacs A, Al-Harthi L, Christensen S, Mack W, Cohen M, Landay A. CD8(+) T cell activation in women coinfected with human immunodeficiency virus type 1 and hepatitis C virus. The Journal of Infectious Diseases. 2008;**197**(10):1402-1407

[145] Gonzalez VD, Falconer K, Blom KG, Reichard O, Morn B, Laursen AL, et al. High levels of chronic immune activation in the T-cell compartments of patients coinfected with hepatitis C virus and human immunodeficiency virus type 1 and on highly active antiretroviral therapy are reverted by alpha interferon and ribavirin treatment. Journal of Virology. 2009;**83**(21):11407-11411

[146] Feuth T, Arends JE, Fransen JH, Nanlohy NM, van Erpecum KJ, Siersema PD, et al. Complementary role of HCV and HIV in T-cell activation and exhaustion in HIV/HCV coinfection. PLoS One [Internet]. 2013;**8**(3):e59302

[147] Hodowanec AC, Brady KE, Gao W, Kincaid SL, Plants J, Bahk M, et al. Characterization of CD4(+) T-cell immune activation and interleukin 10 levels among HIV, hepatitis C virus, and HIV/HCV-coinfected patients. Journal of Acquired Immune Deficiency Syndromes. 2013;**64**(3):232-240

[148] Budd RC. Activation-induced cell death. Current Opinion in Immunology. 2001;**13**(3): 356-362

[149] Green DR, Droin N, Pinkoski M. Activation-induced cell death in T cells. Immunological Reviews. 2003;**193**:70-81

[150] Brenner D, Krammer PH, Arnold R. Concepts of activated T cell death. Critical Reviews in Oncology/Hematology. 2008;**66**(1):52-64

[151] Körner C, Krämer B, Schulte D, Coenen M, Mauss S, Fatkenheuer G, et al. Effects of HCV co-infection on apoptosis of CD4+ T-cells in HIV-positive patients. Clinical Science (London, England). 2009;**116**(12):861-870

[152] Körner C, Tolksdorf F, Riesner K, Krämer B, Schulte D, Nattermann J, et al. Hepatitis C coinfection enhances sensitization of CD4(+) T-cells towards Fas-induced apoptosis in viraemic and HAART-controlled HIV-1-positive patients. Antiviral Therapy. 2011;**16**(7):1047-1055

[153] Lederman MM, Calabrese L, Funderburg NT, Clagett B, Medvik K, Bonilla H, et al. Immunologic failure despite suppressive antiretroviral therapy is related to activation and turnover of memory CD4 cells. The Journal of Infectious Diseases. 2011;**204**(8):1217-1226

[154] Shmagel N, Shmagel K, Chereshnev V. Clinical aspects of inefficiency of highly active antiretroviral therapy. Infectious Diseases. 2011;**9**(11):5-10

[155] Shmagel KV, Saidakova EV, Shmagel NG, Korolevskaya LB, Chereshnev VA, Robinson J, et al. Systemic inflammation and liver damage in HIV/hepatitis C virus coinfection. HIV Medicine. 2016 Sep;**17**(8):581-589

[156] Shmagel NG, Shmagel KV, Saidakova EV, Korolevskaya LB, Chereshnev VA. Discordant response of CD4(+) T cells to antiretroviral therapy in HIV-infected patients coinfected with hepatitis C virus is accompanied by increased liver damage. Doklady. Biochemistry and Biophysics. 2015;**465**:358-360

[157] Glassner A, Eisenhardt M, Kokordelis P, Kramer B, Wolter F, Nischalke HD, et al. Impaired CD4(+) T cell stimulation of NK cell anti-fibrotic activity may contribute to accelerated liver fibrosis progression in HIV/HCV patients. Journal of Hepatology. 2013;**59**(3):427-433

[158] Goeser F, Glassner A, Kokordelis P, Wolter F, Lutz P, Kaczmarek DJ, et al. HIV mono-infection is associated with an impaired anti-hepatitis C virus activity of natural killer cells. AIDS. 2016;**30**(3):355-363

[159] Kahan SM, Wherry EJ, Zajac AJ. T cell exhaustion during persistent viral infections. Virology. 2015;**479-480**:180-193

[160] Fuertes Marraco SA, Neubert NJ, Verdeil G, Speiser DE. Inhibitory receptors beyond T cell exhaustion. Frontiers in Immunology. 2015;**6**:310

[161] Bui JK, Mellors JW. Reversal of T-cell exhaustion as a strategy to improve immune control of HIV-1. AIDS. 2015;**29**(15):1911-1915

[162] Aberg JA. Aging, inflammation, and HIV infection. Topics in Antiviral Medicine. 2012;**20**(3):101-105

[163] Chou JP, Effros RB. T cell replicative senescence in human aging. Current Pharmaceutical Design. 2013;**19**(9):1680-1698

[164] Tsoukas C. Immunosenescence and aging in HIV. Current Opinion in HIV and AIDS. 2014;**9**(4):398-404

[165] Bai F, Bellistri GM, Tincati C, Savoldi A, Pandolfo A, Bini T, et al. Reduced CD127 expression on peripheral CD4+ T cells impairs immunological recovery in course of suppressive highly active antiretroviral therapy. AIDS. 2010;**24**(16):2590-2593

[166] Hartling HJ, Jespersen S, Gaardbo JC, Sambleben C, Thorsteinsson K, Gerstoft J, et al. Reduced IL-7R T cell expression and increased plasma sCD127 in late presenting HIV-infected individuals. Journal of Acquired Immune Deficiency Syndromes. 2017 Jan 1;**74**(1):81-90

12

Clinical Presentation, Diagnosis and Management of TB-HIV Comorbidity in Children

Elena Vasilyeva, Marina Lozovskaya,
Lyudmila Klochkova and Yuliya Yarovaya

Abstract

The problem of combination of tuberculosis and human immunodeficiency virus (HIV) infection remains urgent. Ninety percent of women with HIV infection are of childbearing age that results in increasing the number of children with HIV infection in perinatal contact. In Saint Petersburg from 2014 to 2017, about 5000 children were born from a perinatal contact for HIV infection; by 2017, more than 300 children have confirmed HIV infection. The comparative analysis of case histories of 25 children with TB/HIV combination and 50 children with tuberculosis without HIV infection was performed. Analysis of the study results showed that there are cases of late diagnosis of HIV infection. TB is detected clinically more frequently in children with HIV infection than in children without HIV infection (25 and 5%, respectively). More than one-third of the patients with coinfection had negative sensitivity to tuberculin and DST. The prevalence and the severity of TB in children with HIV infection correlates with the degree of immunosuppression. Eight percent of children had immune reconstitution inflammatory syndrome. Treatment of patients with coinfection associated in most cases with the increased period of total treatment course. Four children with HIV infection vaccinated with BCG were diagnosed with generalized tuberculosis.

Keywords: tuberculosis, HIV infection, children, diagnostics, clinic, prevention, treatment

1. Relevance of the problem of TB/HIV in children

It is generally recognized that tuberculosis is one of the main and the most common diseases associated with HIV infection. Under the WHO estimations, about 5 million people on the planet are infected with both *Mycobacterium tuberculosis* (MBT) and human immunodeficiency virus (HIV). In 2017 in Russia at the total tuberculosis incidence of 41.6 per 100,000 of the population, the incidence of coinfection of TB/HIV was 8.4 per 100,000 or 20.2%. HIV infection facilitates the transition of the state of infection with *Mycobacterium tuberculosis* to TB disease because the immune system in people infected with HIV loses the ability to delay MBT growth and spread. The risk of TB among the HIV-infected patients is in 10–15 times higher than among HIV-negative patients [1]. In recent years there has been an increase in the number of young women with tuberculosis and HIV. Changing their reproductive behavior in favor of the maintenance of pregnancy leads to an increase in the number of children with HIV infection in perinatal contact [2]. So, across Russia in 2008, every seventh (14.6%) woman among delivered women was not followed up during pregnancy. In these HIV-positive women, the combination of HIV with tuberculosis, viral hepatitis, and other infectious diseases is possible. Social status of adults with HIV infection (drug addiction, alcoholism, low material level, etc.) increases the risk of children contact with TB-infected persons that leads to the development of the combined TB/HIV infection. In the period from 2012 to 2017 in Russia, there were about 300 cases of TB/HIV combination in children of 0–14 years old. The problem of tuberculosis and HIV coinfection is closely overlapped with the detection of *Mycobacterium tuberculosis* resistance to anti-TB medicines increasing the risk of extremely unfavorable course of tuberculosis.

2. Tuberculosis and HIV infection in children

2.1. Pathogenesis of TB/HIV coinfection

The coinfection TB and HIV may be considered as two interacting diseases. Patients with comorbidities shall be divided into the following groups: Group 1 for TB/HIV with HIV infection being the primary disease, and tuberculosis is associated with HIV (this type of coinfection prevails in children), and Group 2 for TB/HIV where tuberculosis is primary. In tuberculosis development as in HIV, the great role plays immune processes, mainly associated with lymphocytes, macrophages, and monocytes. Moreover, TB causes disturbances in the same part of the immune system that HIV infects.

2.1.1. The impact of HIV infection on TB

The level of CD4 and CD8 lymphocytes, markers of the immune system activation, and pro-inflammatory cytokines play an important role in the immune response in tuberculosis [3, 4]. The decrease in CD4 lymphocytes typical for HIV infection initiates the series of immune disorders and thus complicates tuberculosis course and prognosis. The level of IL-2 and IFN-gamma involved in the cell immunity decreases continuously. Decreased ability of mononuclear cells to migrate from the bloodstream into the lungs and changes in cytokine secretion cause the reduction of local pulmonary immunity and create conditions for active MBT reproduction, dissemination, and generalization of the tuberculous process.

2.1.2. *The impact of TB on HIV infection*

Tuberculosis in turn reducing the level of CD4 lymphocytes enhances HIV replication inside the cells. Mononuclear cells in the peripheral blood of patients with TB/HIV coinfection produce a greater number of tumor necrosis factor (TNF-alpha) than in patients with only TB or only HIV infection [1]. So, the development of active tuberculosis infection associated with HIV infection increases immunological disorders and promotes more rapid HIV replication resulting in impairment of the immunodeficiency and activation of reproduction of both infection pathogens. These infections result in damage and death of alveolar macrophages. While decreasing the level of CD4 lymphocytes in the zone of tuberculous inflammation, tubercles are less common and then disappear; there are no Langhans-Pirogov cells in tubercles, and epithelioid cells greatly reduce. Then, the number of macrophages may be not reduced; however, because of their defects, they are not able to form granulomas. The tissue reaction occurs mainly in the form of caseous necrosis with a large number of MBT that is associated significantly with increasing levels of tumor necrosis factor. Thus, in patients with tuberculosis and HIV infection, tubercle formation is strongly depressed or absent; alteration and exudation and caseous-necrotic changes prevail that in the future may progress and lead to a patient's death due to immune deficiency.

2.1.3. *TB/HIV pathogenesis in children*

Specifics of the development of TB/HIV comorbidity in children depends on infection way of children with HIV that is mainly the transmission of infection from a mother to a fetus during pregnancy and delivery. In the Russian Federation, the ratio of children infected with HIV due to perinatal transmission is 99.4% of the total number of patients with HIV infection of 0–14 years old [2]. Infection of a child from an HIV-infected mother occurs with equal frequency as in the prenatal period and during a delivery. Infection through the mother's breast milk occurs much less likely. If the virus is detected within 48 h after birth, a child is considered as infected in the prenatal period; infection during a delivery may be assumed in the case of changes of the negative results obtained in the first days of life to positive ones between 7 and 90 days of life.

Pathogenesis of HIV infection in children is determined by the peculiarities of HIV interaction with a child's body and, on the other hand, by the set of cofactors. Perinatal HIV infection affects the immature immune system of a fetus; clinical manifestation occurs earlier. Almost in 15% of children, AIDS symptoms are recorded already by the first year of life, and by 4 years old—in 50% of children. In newborns immunosuppression with significant decrease of CD4 cells comes quickly. In young children earlier there is a failure not only of T-cell but also B-cell immunity system. The decrease in the antibody productions determines a high frequency of bacterial infection recurrence [1].

Due to perinatal HIV infection of children, TB/HIV coinfection had some features in comparison with adults: (1) the risk of TB/HIV coinfection from an early age; (2) HIV infection is always primary in relation to tuberculosis (in adults it may be vice versa); (3) more rapid progression of HIV infection associated with perinatal infection; (4) development of severe generalized forms of tuberculosis due to the age failure of the immune system increased by the development of HIV infection; and (5) MBT infection often occurs as a result of family contact with active TB patients.

2.2. Specific aspects in detection and diagnosis of tuberculosis in children with HIV infection

Tuberculosis is the specific infectious disease without pathognomonic symptoms in any location; in this regard, tuberculosis diagnostics remain quite complex and require the comprehensive evaluation of all the results obtained. HIV infection complicates the assessment of the obtained data, because the interpretation of immunological parameters and tuberculin tests may not always be correct in these cases.

The main methods of early detection of TB in children with or without HIV infection are immunodiagnostics, the epidemiological method, the method of work with risk groups, and the clinical method [4].

2.2.1. *Immunodiagnostics*

Immunodiagnostics means performing specific diagnostic tests using antigens of *Mycobacterium tuberculosis* to identify sensitization (infection) of the organism with *Mycobacterium tuberculosis* that cause, under certain conditions, the development of tuberculosis. Diagnostic tests include the conventional Mantoux test, the test with the tuberculous recombinant allergen and immunological and cell tests in vitro.

2.2.1.1. *Conventional tuberculinodiagnosis*

Mantoux intracutaneous test with 2 TU of PPD-L. The medicine—tuberculosis allergen—is purified in standard dilution with 2 TU per 0.1 mL. When intracutaneous introduction of tuberculin causes specific skin allergic reaction of delayed hypersensitivity in the case of MBT infection or in the first years after BCG vaccination, the severity of the reaction may be negative, doubtful (a wheal of 2–4 mm, hyperemia of any size), positive (5 mm or more), and hyperergic (17 mm and more).

2.2.1.2. *Diaskin test*

Diaskin test (the recombinant tuberculosis allergen) is the test for tuberculosis immunodiagnostics developed by Russian scientists on the basis of features of the virulent *Mycobacterium tuberculosis* genome of the BCG vaccine strain [5]. It is the recombinant protein produced by genetically modified *Escherichia coli* containing two specific antigens ESAT-6 and CFP-10 that are present in virulent, actively reproducing *M. tuberculosis* and *M. bovis* but are absent in *M. bovis* BCG and saprophytic mycobacteria. One dose (0.1 mL) of the product contains recombinant protein in the amount of 0.2 μg. When intracutaneous introduction of the tuberculosis recombinant allergen causes the specific skin reaction of delayed hypersensitivity in most persons with active tuberculosis infection in patients vaccinated with BCG and non-infected with MBT, there is no reaction to this test. Diaskin test response may be negative, doubtful (only hyperemia), positive (a wheal up to 14 mm), and hyperergic (a wheal more than 15 mm).

2.2.1.3. *Immunologic cell tests in vitro*

These tests are based on releasing interferon-gamma (IFN-gamma) by T lymphocytes. The QuantiFERON-TB Gold test stimulates the T lymphocytes of a patient's blood with recombinant proteins ESAT-6 and CFP-10 that in the presence of specific sensitization of T lymphocytes produce interferon-gamma measured by the enzyme-linked immunosorbent assay (ELISA) [6].

The T-SPOT.TB test using the ELISpot method determines the number of mononuclear cells of the peripheral blood that produce IFN-gamma in response to stimulation by antigens ESAT-6 and CFP-10.

Detection of immune response to the antigens ESAT-6 and CFP-10 indicates the presence of tuberculosis infection in the body. Thus, the tests QuantiFERON-TB Gold and T-SPOT.TB give positive results both in latent tuberculosis infection and active tuberculosis. Patients with TB/HIV skin tests with tuberculosis allergens and immunological in vitro tests have often false-negative results due to the immunity lack.

2.2.2. *The epidemiological method*

The epidemiological method is based on the number of events among persons in contact with tuberculosis patients and is aimed at early identification of the disease in these children. Prolonged contact with TB patients is dangerous for a child of any age. The risk of developing the disease of parents is particularly enhanced by drug addiction, alcoholism, a stay in a prison, and poor material living conditions that in turn increases the risk of a child's disease in a family of a patient with tuberculosis. The above-specified confounding factors not only increase the risk of developing tuberculosis but also make the measures for TB detection difficult.

Children with HIV infection in contact with TB patients are at an increased risk, because human immunodeficiency virus negatively impacts the immune-competent cells responsible for TB immunity. In this regard, all contacting children are registered in TB dispensaries. The frequency of control examinations of children from centers of high epidemiological risk is one time every 3–4 months, from less dangerous areas—one time per 6 months.

2.2.3. *Work with risk groups*

TB risk groups include children with newly positive hyperergic sensitivity to tuberculin, increase of tuberculin reactions, and no BCG vaccination, children with chronic diseases of different organs and systems, and children with HIV infection. These children have immunodiagnostics two times a year. At the same time, children infected with MBT with undetermined HIV infection but with a history of frequent recurrent pneumonia and bronchitis, with confirmed cytomegalovirus, herpes infection, hepatitis B and C, lymphoid interstitial pneumonia, cardiomyopathy, recurrent bacterial infections, and long-lasting low-grade fever, shall be tested not only for tuberculosis but also for HIV.

2.2.4. Clinical method

In some children TB develops with severe clinical symptoms. The symptoms may be similar to other diseases—tuberculosis "masking." The change in a child's condition is not improved for a long period but is persistent and forced to go to the hospital. Clinical, laboratory, and radiological data suggest a local form of tuberculosis. This method of detection is the most relevant in the group of children of early age, when often there are mild reactions to tuberculin, not allowing to suspect tuberculosis; also, some children with HIV infection may not always indicate the presence or absence of MBT infection due to sensitivity to tuberculin in this category of patients.

We analyzed the medical records of 75 children with TB and hospitalized in the TB department of Children Infectious Hospital No. 3 of Saint Petersburg since 2010 till 2017. The age of children is from 1 to 14 years old. Patients were divided into two groups:

Group 1 is the main group with 25 children with TB and HIV combination (TB/HIV).

Group 2 is the comparison group with 50 children with tuberculosis without HIV infection (TB).

All children in the hospital underwent complex clinical and laboratory examination using intracutaneous tests with tuberculosis allergens, X-ray examination, and MSCT, the bacteriological study.

According to our research data, in the group of children with tuberculosis and HIV infection, local forms of tuberculosis were detected with the change of the sensitivity to tuberculin in 44% of cases (11 patients); in the group of patients without HIV infection, tuberculosis was detected by the method of tuberculinodiagnosis in 56% of cases (28 children) ($p = 0.1$). The disease was detected during examination associated with the contact in the group of children with TB/HIV coinfection in 28% (7 children), while in the children without HIV in 40% of cases (20 children) ($p = 0.1$). However, in patients with HIV infection, tuberculosis was detected more frequently than in children without HIV when visiting a doctor with clinical complaints. So, in Group 1 TB was detected by the clinical method in 28% of cases (7 children), whereas in Group 2, in 4% of cases (2 children) ($p = 0.04$).

During the study, we also analyzed the terms of HIV infection detection in patients. Thus, of the 25 children with TB/HIV, 24 ones had confirmed perinatal HIV infection contact; for 1 child HIV infection of the mother was not determined. HIV infection in 11 children (44%) was confirmed in the first months of life, and later in 14 children (56%) among them in the first 3 years, in 9 patients, at the age of 6–13 years old, in 5 children. It should be noted that in four children (7, 8, 9, and 13 years old), HIV infection was detected under the diagnostic examination for tuberculosis. HIV infection diagnostics in children in the later periods may be associated with a long seronegative period in the development of HIV infection and insufficient control of examination of pregnant women from risk groups.

2.2.5. Tuberculosis diagnostics in children with HIV infection

Diagnostics is carried out only in specialized tuberculosis facilities. When suspecting TB in children with HIV infection, the complex of diagnostic measures is applied, including the thorough history, the physical examination, and laboratory tests of blood and urine; the chest plane X-ray examination, the chest and the abdomen MSCT, bronchoscopy, and abdominal ultrasound examination; sputum, urine, epithelial lining fluid MBT test (microscopy, solid medium inoculation, BACTEC, PCR), and immunodiagnostics.

2.2.6. History

Collecting the anamnesis, a physician shall identify factors that could contribute to the development of both HIV infection and tuberculosis. The great attention shall be paid to a perinatal history: diseases of the mother prior and during pregnancy, especially the presence of a hepatitis B and C, HIV, drug addiction, alcoholism, gestation course, parents' lifestyle, and social status. The above factors place a child at the high risk of infection not only with HIV and hepatitis B and C but also with MBT. The analysis of the socio-epidemiological factors in groups of our patients demonstrated that the deprived social background was observed in 100% patients of Group 1 and in 60% of children of Group 2 ($p < 0.01$). Family and relative contacts with tuberculosis patients were more often detected in children with TB without HIV infection in 71% of cases, whereas in the group of children with TB/HIV, in 50% of patients. HIV infection is detected in mothers of children of Group 2 in 18% of cases and in patients of Group 1, in 96% of cases ($p = 0.01$) (for one child HIV infection of the mother was not determined). Parents' drug addiction and alcoholism were detected in the majority in the group of children with tuberculosis and HIV infection (85%), while in the group of children without HIV infection, in 22% of cases ($p = 0.02$).

It should be find a child's endured diseases and concomitant pathology, the presence of cytomegalovirus, herpes infections, the frequency of respiratory infections, the presence of chronic diseases, allergic reactions, etc.

A phthisiatrician shall always obtain information about vaccination, especially BCG vaccination and revaccination, and the history of Mantoux tests. Due to the absence of BCG vaccination in children with HIV, the presence of suspicious or positive reaction to tuberculin is the indication for the enhanced examination as such a result may not be indicative of postvaccination allergy.

2.2.7. Physical examination

In children with TB/HIV coinfection, there is more evident asthenization; in some cases, there may be failure to physical development.

Children usually have pale grayish skin and "shadows" under the eyes. There is no postvaccinal scar on the skin of the shoulder in children with HIV infection due to medical exemption from BCG vaccination. Children with TB/HIV have dry skin, decreasing the subcutaneous fat tissue, long-term course of the disease, and the decrease in tissue tension. There are palpable peripheral lymph nodes more than six to seven groups (cervical group, supra- and sub-clavicular, axillary, thoracic, cubital, inguinal ones) enlarged up to 1 cm or more. Under palpation of the abdomen, the liver and the spleen are moderately enlarged. In rare cases, there are enlarged mesenteric lymph nodes.

Percussion and auscultation changes depend on the form of tuberculosis, the lesion volume, the extent of the process, the presence of complications, and a child's age. At the various local forms, it is possible to determine the zone of percussion sound shortening in the lung tissue, regions of hyperresonant resonance. There are no commonly distinct symptoms with limited forms by auscultation. With more severe lesions of the lung tissue, the type of breathing may change, and rattling appears. More often, these symptoms appear in children of early age with the complicated course, particularly in bronchopulmonary lesions.

2.2.8. Radiology diagnostics

Sectional roentgenography remains the leading method in the diagnostics of tuberculosis in children with and without HIV infection. X-ray diagnostics uses digital or analogue chest X-ray, linear tomography, multislice computed tomography, and ultrasound. During the initial examination of a child, the attention shall be paid to the presence of lesions and foci in the pulmonary tissue, dimensions, and structuredness of the lung roots. In recent years, the method for multislice computed tomography has the greatest diagnostic value. This method is more informative and more clearly demonstrates the location, the extent of the process, the structure of the lymph nodes, the presence of small foci, and the calcifications in areas that are poorly visualized under standard X-ray examinations. Chest ultrasound examination is used when suspecting the presence of liquid in the pleural cavity, for the differential diagnosis of fibrosing aortic ligament and calcifications of the intrathoracic nodes in this area.

2.2.9. Bronchoscopy

This study helps to assess the condition of the bronchial tree in children, to identify specific lesions of the bronchi, the presence of indirect signs of the intrathoracic lymph node enlargement. During bronchoscopy the material is sampled for bacteriological, immunological, and cytological tests. In the cases of tuberculosis and HIV coinfection, this method has an important diagnostic value.

2.2.10. Abdominal ultrasound examination

In children with TB with or without HIV infection, enlargement of the liver and the spleen, changes in the organ tissue structure, the presence of the lymph nodes at the gate of the liver and the spleen, hyperechogenic inclusions in the spleen, calcifications, abnormal changes in the kidneys, and enlarged mesenteric lymph nodes are found.

2.2.11. Immunodiagnostics

The analysis of tuberculin test and DST results in our patients demonstrated the following findings. Under the Mantoux test with 2 TU, the positive results are detected in the group of patients with TB/HIV in 10 children (40%), and in the group of patients with TB without HIV infection, in 34 children (68%) ($p = 0.05$). Hyperergic reactions were in 5 children with TB/HIV (20%) and in 16 children with TB and with or without HIV infection (32%). Negative sensitivity was detected only in patients of Group 2, 10 cases (40%) ($p = 0.03$), that correspond to the literature data [7]. According to the results of DST, the positive results were more often detected in children without HIV infection in 34 children (68%), and in patients with TB/HIV, the positive sensitivity to Diaskin test was observed in eight children (32%) ($p = 0.04$). Hyperergic reactions was observed in 8 children of Group 2 (16%) and 3 children of Group 1 (12%) ($p = 0.09$), while the negative results were detected with greater frequency in the group of children with TB/HIV, in 14 children (56%), than in the group of children with TB without HIV infection—in 8 children (16%) ($p = 0.04$).

2.2.12. *Laboratory diagnostics*

The severity of hemogram changes depends on the form, the phase, and the presence of process complications. Children with tuberculosis and HIV infection have long-lasting anemia, thrombocytopenia, and a more evident and persistent increase of ESR. A smaller part of children with TB with or without HIV infection may have moderate proteinuria and erythrocyturia. Biochemical blood count in children with TB and HIV shows a sharper increase of beta-lipoproteins and gamma globulins, reducing the overall level of albumins. Such values of biochemical parameters may indicate the activity of tuberculous process and the immune system disorder in a child with HIV.

The complex examination of children with suspected tuberculosis (without HIV) mandatorily includes the blood test for HIV; hepatitis A, B, and C; and under indications—for cytomegalovirus, herpes virus, etc. If HIV is found, a child shall be examined and then constantly followed up in an infectious disease center.

2.2.13. *Bacteriological study*

To verify the TB diagnosis, the following shall be studied: sputum, pleural liquid, urine, cerebrospinal fluid, the lymph nodes, punctates, etc. For children the gastric lavage study is optimal. Smear microscopy and culture study (solid and liquid medium inoculation) are performed. Molecular and genetic study methods are used. The most widely used method is the polymerase chain reaction with the specific MBT primer. Among our patients with TB/HIV coinfection in only one case, MBT was extracted by solid medium inoculation; in other children the results of bacteriological studies were negative. So, in connection with the difficulties of diagnostics of tuberculosis in children with HIV infection, one cannot rely on the clinical minimum used for tuberculosis in children without comorbidities. For children with HIV infection, all obtained results shall be comprehensively evaluated.

2.3. Clinical forms and progression of tuberculosis in children with HIV infection

Clinical signs of tuberculosis in all age groups depend on the stage of HIV infection. The structure of clinical forms, clinical signs, frequency of bacterial excretion, and the effectiveness of treatment in patients with indicators of CD4 close to the norm do not differ from those in the group of HIV-negative patients. At lower CD4 tuberculous inflammation gradually loses classic features and is characterized by an atypical course. In the structure of clinical forms, the disseminated forms begin to prevail creating extrapulmonary lesions in the lymph nodes, the intestines, the liver, the spleen, and the meninges.

HIV infection depending on the stage and the condition of the cell immunity may also impact on the clinical signs of tuberculosis in children. A child's age, the duration of contact with TB patients, the lesion form and area, and the presence of complications affect the course and symptoms of tuberculosis.

In the structure of clinical forms of our patients both in the group of children with tuberculosis and HIV infection and in the group of children with tuberculosis without HIV infection, tuberculosis of the intrathoracic lymph nodes prevails—in 56 and 78%, respectively ($p = 0.8$). At the same time, in the group of children with TB/HIV coinfection, primary tuberculosis complex was detected with greater frequency in six cases (24%) and generalized tuberculosis in 20% of cases (five children), whereas in the group of children without HIV, primary complex was diagnosed in six children (13%) and generalized forms in two children (4.1%) ($p = 0.05$). Our studies demonstrated the dependence of the TB form on the severity of immunodeficiency and viral load. So, severe generalized forms of tuberculosis were diagnosed in children with severe immunodeficiency—CD4 from 2 to 9% and high viral load from 675,000 to 1 million cop/mL. At low viral load, from 65,000 to 480,000 cop/mL, and moderate immunosuppression, CD4 from 15 to 34%, children had tuberculosis of the intrathoracic lymphatic nodes or primary tuberculous complex in the phase of infiltration, induration, or calcification.

2.3.1. Tuberculosis of the intrathoracic lymph nodes and primary tuberculosis complex in children with HIV infection

In clinical signs of primary forms of tuberculosis in children with HIV infection, in most cases evident intoxication syndrome prevails; in the majority there are evident such as emotional lability, mood swings, depression, and sometimes negativity and unmotivated aggression toward others.

The intoxication syndrome appears in the form of decreased body weight, periorbital cyanosis, the evident pale grayish skin, and reduced tissue tension. Under studying clinical symptoms and laboratory indicators, we found that the decrease in the body weight was observed in the group of children with TB/HIV coinfection in 52% of children. Low-grade fever was detected in the majority (85%) of patients with HIV infection. Hepatosplenomegaly by palpation and under abdominal ultrasound examination and enlargement of the liver and the spleen in 1 cm and more against normal age-related indicators are found. So, the enlarged liver and spleen were observed in 68% of patients. The constant symptom accompanying the primary forms of tuberculosis and HIV infection in 100% of cases is peripheral polyadenopathy. In such children the palpable multiple peripheral lymph nodes (more than six in groups) with polymorphism are seen: from small and dense to large ones with periadenitis; enlarged cervical, supra- and sub-clavicular, thoracic, cubital, and inguinal groups of the lymph nodes are also seen. Typically, in primary forms of tuberculosis, percussion symptoms prevail in the chest. In primary tuberculous complex, especially with significant lung affect (that is observed in children of early age), there is shortening of the percussion sound over the affected area. In primary tuberculous complex, hard breathing and also weakened breathing over the lesion may be detected by auscultation; sometimes, there is rattling. A hemogram of children with primary forms of tuberculosis and HIV infection shows hypo- or normochromic anemia (according to our data in 40% of children), moderate leukocytosis, and lymphopenia at the early stages with subsequent lymphocytosis. These children have significant ESR increase: from 20 to 60 mm/h. Most children with the comorbidity had recorded PLT decrease associated with HIV infection. The above changes of blood parameters retained in children with TB/HIV for more periods of term with slower normalization even against the combined therapy (for up to 6 months). Under biochemical parameter study (according to our studies) in children with TB and the initial signs of HIV infection, there is less increase of gamma globulin fractions; more often in these children, there is a decrease of concentrations of gamma globulins and increased alpha-2 globulins. At the same time, children at the later HIV stages (severe immunodeficiency) have the sharp increase of gamma globulins (up to 30–42%). Under X-ray exam in the presence of the enlarged intrathoracic lymph nodes, the mediastinum shadow is expanded with changes in the shadow outlines. Due to periadenitis the nodes are merged into packages with polycyclic boundaries. Some children had calcium inclusions in the thoracic lymph nodes (20% of cases). In primary tuberculosis complex, radiologically, there is a focus of different sizes located mainly in the upper regions, less in the lower segments. There is the lymph path from the primary affect to the enlarged regional lymph nodes of the root. In children of early age, the pulmonary component usually is located in the root zone, often in the lower sections. When detecting the disease at the later stages, calcium inclusions may be visualized in the area of primary affect and in the lung root.

2.3.2. *Tuberculosis complications*

The course of the tuberculosis process in studied children with HIV is characterized by a tendency to a prolonged course, slow regression, complications of the process (bronchopulmonary lesions, seeding in the lung tissue when affecting the intrathoracic lymph nodes), and frequent outcomes with the calcification formation. Complicated course of tuberculosis in children with HIV infection according to our observations was diagnosed in ten children (40.2%), five of them (20%) have the generalized form of tuberculosis. Complicated course presents the development of atelectasis in one child, bronchopulmonary lesion in two children, and seeding in the lung tissue in two children. Tuberculous process relapse was observed in two children, and recurrence in 2 years after the end of TB treatment was developed in one child of a younger age. The reasons for the complicated course are the late detection of tuberculosis in children with HIV infection, late onset of therapy, and the negative impact of HIV on the course of tuberculosis. TB acute condition or relapse was caused in all cases by cessation of antiretroviral therapy (due to the negative attitude toward the treatment of the parents) that resulted in a decrease of the immunity and, as a consequence, the relapse of the tuberculous process.

2.3.3. *Generalized tuberculosis in children with HIV*

The development of such severe form in children with HIV infection may be associated with the late detection of tuberculosis due to negative sensitivity to tuberculin under the planned tuberculinodiagnosis in HIV-infected children; according to some authors, the lack of BCG vaccination at birth and vaccination later than in 18 months; long closed contact with TB patients against adverse social conditions [4].

The disease begins acutely in children of early age and in older children begins gradually with condition worsening to severe. The temperature rises to 39–40°C, intoxication symptoms and weakness are strongly evident. Some children have short breathing, cyanosis, and dry cough. Children with TB/HIV may have symptoms of herpes infection and candidiasis. At the same time, the absence of evident objective changes against the general severe condition of a child is conspicuous. There are multiple palpable lymph nodes in seven to nine groups; the liver and spleen are enlarged significantly. There is hyperresonant sound resonance over all lung fields by percussion, decreased breath by auscultation, and mild moist rale auscultated better in the paravertebral areas.

In the blood of children with HIV infection, there is more evident increase of ESR (up to 60 mm/h), anemia, and thrombocytopenia. Tuberculin sensitivity in the cases of generalized tuberculosis in children with HIV infection almost in all cases is negative. In the absence of typical clinical and laboratory findings inherent to the generalized forms of tuberculosis, the X-ray method remains determinant. In the early period (the first week of the disease), there is weakening of the lung pattern and unusual ripple; in 7–10 days, there is evident dissemination of clear uniform lesions in the lung tissue in the form of event rashes with a diameter of 2–3 mm. At the same time, as a rule, in children enlarged intrathoracic lymph nodes are found, because they are the source of dissemination; the cases of disseminated processes with the lung tissue degradation are described. When detecting dissemination, the study of other organs and systems shall be performed (ophthalmologist examination, abdominal ultrasound, and CT studies). In all our patients with generalized tuberculosis (five children) along with affection of the lungs and the intrathoracic lymph nodes, the affected peripheral lymph nodes, the mesenteric lymph nodes, and the spleen nodes were seen; two children had tuberculous meningoencephalitis.

Bacteriological study usually does not show positive results. Diagnostically significant method in these cases may be the molecular genetic diagnostics (PCR).

2.3.4. *Comorbidity*

We analyzed the frequency and the nature of comorbidity in patients with TB/HIV. So, chronic recurrent herpes infection in children with tuberculosis and HIV infection was diagnosed in 17 patients (68%). Signs of allergic dermatitis were observed in 10 (40%) children with TB/HIV; candidiasis was diagnosed in five patients (20%). In the group of children with TB/HIV, there is one case of thrombocytopenic purpura (4%). Viral hepatitis B was observed in two children with TB/HIV (8%), viral hepatitis C in three patients in this group (12%), and toxoplasmosis and cytomegalovirus infection in one child (4%).

2.4. Difficulties in the treatment of tuberculosis in children with HIV infection

In the treatment of tuberculosis in children with or without HIV infection, the main principles of therapy shall be met [8]. For children with HIV infection, the important point is the joint follow-up of such patient by a phtisiologist and an infectiologist, because a patient receives simultaneously two kinds of therapy. The antituberculous and antiretroviral medicines have mutual con-founding toxic effects moreover, in children, HIV may be associated with secondary diseases (cytomegalovirus, herpes infection, etc.). TB chemotherapy includes two phases—the intensive phase (the maximum number of TB drugs to achieve significant effect) and the continuation phase. The treatment is performed in accordance with therapy regimens using TB medicines of the primary and alternative series. Indications for initiation of antiretroviral therapy in patients with comorbidity do not differ from the indications for treatment of patients with HIV infection without tuberculosis. Currently, there is no conclusive evidence that prolongation of TB therapy for over 6 months in patients with HIV infection improves treatment results. At the same time, the prolonged treatment (up to 8–9 months) is still more preferable in these patients due to reducing relapses compared with short-term chemotherapy. When detecting drug-resistant tuberculosis or at the high risk of tuberculosis with multidrug resistance of the pathogen (TB), children with HIV infection receive alternative medicines under life-saving indications. Antiretroviral therapy (ARVT) shall be indicated for children with tuberculosis regardless of the level of immunosuppression in 2 weeks after starting TB treatment to prevent the development of immune reconstitution inflammatory syndrome. Immune reconstitution inflammatory syndrome occurred in two children (8%) with HIV infection detected at once with tuberculosis, with severe immunodeficiency. Immune reconstitution inflammatory syndrome appeared in the form of impairment of the clinical condition of children and the progression of dissemination in the lung tissue in one case and increase of infiltrative changes and size of the intrathoracic lymph nodes in the second case. Most patients in both groups received therapy under regimen I, but children of Group 1 in most cases required an individual approach due to ARVT and the presence of comorbidities. According to our research data, the intensive phase of treatment with four TB drugs for children with TB/HIV was performed in 31% of cases, and the remaining 69% received three chemotherapy medicines. The duration of the intensive phase of chemotherapy in 43% of children with TB/HIV was more than 6 months, only in one-third of cases up to 3 months, the rest 3–6 months. The total duration of treatment was 9–12 months only in 50% of the patients; in one-third of cases, the therapy lasted 18–24 months. Cancel of antituberculosis drugs was required by 26% of children in this group due to intolerance symptoms. We established the relationship between the level of immunosuppression and the duration of the intensive phase of chemotherapy. All children with the severe immunosuppression received the treatment in the intensive phase for 6–9 months that exceeds the recommended duration of the therapy. A longer treatment of children with tuberculosis and HIV infection coinfection is caused by the evident toxic effect both of TB and antiretroviral medicines, also due to the addition of secondary disorders and intercurrent diseases required by the treatment.

2.5. Features of tuberculosis prevention in children with HIV infection

2.5.1. BCG vaccination

Now, tuberculosis immunization is one of the main and most effective methods of tuberculosis prevention among children. BCG vaccination of children born by HIV-infected mothers is ambiguous, since the administration of live vaccines against the immunodeficiency may not only cause severe postvaccination complications but the progression of HIV infection. In Russia until 2010, BCG vaccination was allowed after the complete exclusion of HIV infection in a child of 18 months of age [9].

Currently, due to the implementation of prevention of HIV transmission from a mother during gestation and delivery, the frequency of children infection was reduced from 40 to 2%. Considering this fact, the prohibition to administer the BCG vaccine to children born from HIV-infected mothers was lifted in the absence of a child's immunodeficiency and after a three-stage prevention of HIV infection.

According to our data, among 25 children with subsequent TB/HIV, 17 children (68%) were vaccinated with BCG vaccine. However, 10 children of 17 vaccinated ones (58.8%) were immunized in a maternity hospital, the remaining eight children—at a later time—in 6 months to 2 years old. Subsequently, generalized forms of tuberculosis were diagnosed in four children vaccinated earlier with BCG; two of them had suspected generalized BCG infection. Thus, in the presence of immunodeficiency, immunization with the BCG vaccine increases the risk of a transient increase of HIV replication and the development of postvaccination complications with the generalization of BCG infection.

2.5.2. *Preventive treatment and chemoprophylaxis of tuberculosis*

When prescribing the preventive treatment and the chemoprophylaxis, the additional TB risk factors shall be considered:

the lack of BCG vaccination (BCG-M), in contact with a TB patient, the age of children between 3 years old and adolescence, and chronic nonspecific diseases of different organs and systems, immunodeficiency, drug abuse, low material level, migration, and homelessness among children and adolescents.

Children and adolescents for the preventive treatment shall be selected by a phtisiologist, if necessary together with a specialist in HIV infection.

Preventive treatment is performed for children: due to contact with a tuberculosis patient, with latent tuberculosis infection (in the case of positive results of DST and tests with tuberculous antigens in vitro), hyperergic reaction to tuberculin, the enhancing reaction to tuberculin, MBT in combination with nonspecific risk factors, and in the presence of the immunodeficiency.

The preventive treatment of tuberculosis for children with HIV infection is carried out depending on the level of the immunodeficiency. In the absence of immunodeficiency at the early stages of HIV infection, the preventive treatment is carried out under the general rules. The duration of the preventive treatment with doubtful and positive reaction to Diaskin test is not less than 6 months with two TB medicines. In the presence of immunodeficiency, the chemoprophylaxis shall be prescribed individually. With a moderate immunodeficiency and negative results of immunodiagnostics, the preventive treatment is prescribed for 3–6 months with two TB medicines. For significant and severe immunodeficiency, the preventive treatment is indicated regardless of the results of immunodiagnostics with two TB medicines to increase CD4 over the criteria of the evident immunodeficiency, but not less than 6 months.

The basic medicines for the preventive treatment are isoniazid and pyrazinamide (ethambutol, less rifampicin are used).

According to our data, among all patients with TB/HIV, the preventive treatment was prescribed only to four children (16%). In this case, only one child received the complete treatment; the others received incomplete courses. Incomplete coverage of these patients with the preventive treatment may be associated with tuberculosis detection prior to diagnosis of HIV infection in some children, with antisocial behavior of parents and non-compliance of the recommendations and refusal from the preventive treatment.

3. Conclusion

Thus, tuberculosis and HIV infection in children are the serious problems of the modern medicine. There is the tendency to increasing the number of children with tuberculosis and HIV infection due to the increase in the number of patients with HIV and tuberculosis among young women, in most cases, with antisocial lifestyle. The presence of immunodeficiency of varying severity in children with HIV infection makes early detection and diagnosis of tuberculosis by conventional methods difficult and requires the use of a wide range of diagnostic procedures and the use of new diagnostic methods.

The treatment of children with TB/HIV coinfection due to the late TB detection also has certain features. These children shall be followed up jointly by a phtisiologist, an infectiologist, and a pediatrician. BCG vaccination, chemoprophylaxis, and preventive treatment of these children require a differentiated approach in each case. Promotion of the healthy lifestyle, the fight against drug addiction, and improving health literacy, especially among young persons and women of reproductive age, are important for the prevention of the development of tuberculosis and HIV in children.

Author details

Elena Vasilyeva*, Marina Lozovskaya, Lyudmila Klochkova and Yuliya Yarovaya

*Address all correspondence to: helenchern27@mail.ru

St. Petersburg State Pediatric Medical University, Saint Petersburg, Russia

References

[1] HIV infection and AIDS. In: Pokrovsky VV, editor. National Guideline. GEOTAR—Media; 2014. 528 p. ISBN 978-5-9704-2891-7

[2] Levanovitch VV, Timchenko VN, Arkhipova YA, et al. HIV infection at the turn of the century: Manual for physicians of all specialities. In: Levanovitch VV, Timchenko VN, editors. SPb.: Publishing House N-L; 2012. 496 p. ISBN 978-5-94869-154-1

[3] Belozyorov ES, Zmushko EI. HIV Infection. 2nd ed. SPb: Piter; 2003. 368 p. (Series Quick Guide). ISBN 5-272-00374-8

[4] Vasilyeva EB. Tuberculosis and HIV Infection in Children. Guidance Manual. Edition of SPbGPMU; 2014. 44 p

[5] Lozovskaya ME, Belushkov VB, Gurina OP, et al. The comparative evaluation of innovative tests in the diagnostics of latent and active tuberculosis infection in children. Pediatrics. 2014;**5**(3):46-50. ISSN 2079-7850

[6] Mordovskaya LI, Vladimirsky MA, Aksyonova VA, Efremov EE, Ignashenkova GI, Vlasik TN. The induction of interferon-gamma in whole blood samples in vitro—The test for the determination of tuberculosis infection in children and adolescents. Problems of Tuberculosis and Lung Diseases. 2009;**6**:19-24. ISSN 2075-1230

[7] Perez J, Portu J, Aldamiz M, et al. Mantoux test in HIV infection. In: 5th European Conference on Clinical Aspects and Treatment of HIV-1 Infection; Copenhagen; 1995. p. 73

[8] Federal Clinical Guidelines for Prevention, Diagnostics and Treatment of Tuberculosis in Patients with HIV-infection. Moscow: ROF; 2016. 41 p

[9] Clevno NI, Aksyonova VA, Levi DT. Problems of TB vaccination of HIV-positive children. In: TB Today: Materials of the VIII Russian Congress of phthisiatricians. 2007. pp. 276-277

13

Artificial Epitope-Based Immunogens in HIV-Vaccine Design

Larisa I. Karpenko, Sergei I. Bazhan,
Alexey M. Eroshkin, Denis V. Antonets,
Anton N. Chikaev and Alexander A. Ilyichev

Abstract

One of the promising approaches for designing HIV vaccines is construction of synthetic polyepitope HIV-1 immunogen using a wide range of conservative T- and B-cell epitopes of the main virus antigens. In theory this approach helps cope with HIV-1 antigenic variability, focuses immune responses on protective determinants and enables to exclude from the vaccine compound adverse regions of viral proteins that can induce autoantibodies or antibodies enhancing infectivity of virus. The paper presents the experience of our team in development of artificial polyepitope HIV-1 immunogens, which can induce both a humoral response, and responses of cytotoxic (CD8 + CTL) and helpers (CD4 + Th) T-cells. The design of HIV-immunogens has been done using our original software, TEpredict and PolyCTLDesigner. We describe development of the candidate HIV-1/AIDS vaccine – CombiHIVvac, which included two artificial polyepitope immunogens TBI and TCI for stimulating humoral and cellular responses. The results of the specific activity and safety of CombiHIVvac vaccine, obtained during preclinical and clinical trials, are presented.

Keywords: HIV-1 vaccine, artificial polyepitope T- and B-cell immunogens, rational design, preclinical and clinical trials

1. Introduction

For over 200 years a vaccine development effort was to isolate microbes or viruses and prepare a killed or attenuated pathogen vaccine. For many self-limiting bacterial and viral infections the vaccine strategy is to mimic the infectious process and natural immunity against a particular pathogen. However, for HIV-1 and for many other chronic viral, bacterial, fungal and parasitic infections, and cancer natural immunity is insufficient for protection [1, 2]. Novel and effective approaches in polyepitope HIV-vaccine development are needed today [3, 4].

Problems that retard development of HIV-1 vaccine are well-known. Firstly, HIV-1 has a high rate of escape mutations with the result that the virus can change the antigenic structure quicker than the immune system is switched to new antigenic variants. Secondly, it is still unclear which type of immune response is more significant when preventing infection: induction of HIV neutralizing antibodies (in systemic vs. mucosal compartments), CD4+ T-helper cells, cytotoxic CD8+ T-cells (both potent high avidity CD8+ T-effector/memory responses and central memory responses), innate immunity, or all factors together. However, recent publications demonstrate that a humoral response to vaccine may be critical to prevent acquisition of HIV, while CD8+ T-cells may be required to control viral replication in vaccinated individual. Thirdly, virus proteins include regions with pathogenic properties due to molecular mimicry of physiologically significant functions or induction of autoimmune responses that might contribute to immunodeficiency. Finally, when studying HIV-infection, experimental models are very limited [1, 5–7].

Well-known HIV-1 vaccine design strategies are based on the use of different forms of viral antigen including inactivated virus, modified or attenuated virus, native and genetically engineered proteins, and peptides [5]. The first generation candidate vaccines (such as AIDSVAX B/B and AIDSVAX B/E) were constructed for inducing humoral immunity, to elicit virus-neutralizing antibodies. Development of such vaccines was based on the use of full-length proteins of HIV envelope or their fragments [8]. The second generation vaccines (e.g. Merck Ad5 gag/pol/nef of B subtype) were aimed to mediate protection by inducing HIV-specific cytotoxic T-lymphocytes (CTLs) capable to recognize and eliminate HIV-infected cells [9]. Many candidates were tested in human or animals; however, none of them has demonstrated efficacy in phase II-III trials [10].

The first promising and statistically significant results were obtained in clinical trials of RV144 vaccine stimulating both humoral and cellular immunity. It is a combination of two previously developed vaccines ALVAC-HIV (Sanofi Pasteur) and AIDSVAX B/E gp120 (VAXGEN) [11]. Despite rather low protective efficacy (31.2%), RV144 clinical trials made it possible to draw several weighty conclusions, i.e. (1) HIV-1 vaccine is not a myth but a reality; (2) efficient vaccine should induce both humoral and cell immune responses against HIV-1, and (3) new approaches are needed to increase vaccine efficacy [2, 3, 12].

One of them includes construction of completely artificial polyepitope (mosaic) anti-HIV-1 immunogens comprising a broad range of protective T- and B-cell epitopes based on the main viral antigens capable of inducing production of neutralizing antibodies and responses of cytotoxic (CD8+ CTL) and helper (CD4+ Th) T-lymphocytes. This approach seems to be rather promising when developing new generation HIV-vaccines. In theory, it makes it possible to overcome HIV-1 antigenic variability, focus immune responses on protective epitopes and allows to exclude undesirable determinants from a vaccine compound capable of inducing autoantibodies or antibodies increasing virus infectivity [3, 4, 13]. This paper discusses our experience in designing artificial polyepitope antigens – HIV-1 candidate vaccines.

2. Artificial TBI and TCI immunogens

The first immunogen designed in our project, short for T- and B-cell epitopes containing Immunogen (TBI), was constructed with the use of conservative epitopes from Env and Gag HIV-1 based on a well-known protein space motif, i.e. four helix bundle (**Figure 1**). When designing immunogen, four Th-cell epitopes (amphipathic α-helix) and five B-cell epitopes (regions with flexible hydrophilic loops) were used as blocks [14, 15]. The rationale for TBI design was that combining T- and B-cell epitopes in one construct will stimulate both proper B-cell and T-cell responses and the necessary interplay between B- and T-cells. Recombinant protein TBI has a CD spectra similar to ones in α-helical proteins and was able to form crystals - that was demonstrated for artificial protein with a predicted tertiary structure for the first time [16]. Based on its ability to crystallize we assumed that TBI protein structure is similar to that of the natural proteins.

Mice and Macaque rhesus immunized with TBI formed both cell and humoral responses to HIV-1. TBI-induced antibodies showed virus-neutralizing activity to HIV-1 [17].

The second artificial polyepitope immunogen we developed was TCI (short for T-Cell Immunogen) aimed at stimulation of T-cell immunity [18]. When constructing immunogen, we selected highly conservative T-cell epitopes among three main HIV-1 subtypes (A, B, and C) (**Figure 2**). TCI comprises more than 80 T-cell epitopes (both CD8+ CTL and CD4+ Th) from Env, Gag, Pol, and Nef proteins [18]. We analyzed CTL-epitopes that were together restricted with 10 different optimally selected alleles of human MHC class I. As known, it is sufficient to cover genetic diversity of MHC class I antigens in population from almost all geographic regions. Since antigen processing and presentation through MHC class I pathway were found to be the most efficient for proteins synthesized inside the cell, the target vaccine construct was designed in the form of DNA-vaccine via cloning a gene encoding TCI protein into vector plasmid pcDNA3.1 [18].

The obtained DNA-vaccine pcDNA-TCI was used for genetic immunization; we showed that the vaccine is capable of inducing both specific T-cell responses and specific antibodies in immunized BALB/c mice [18–20].

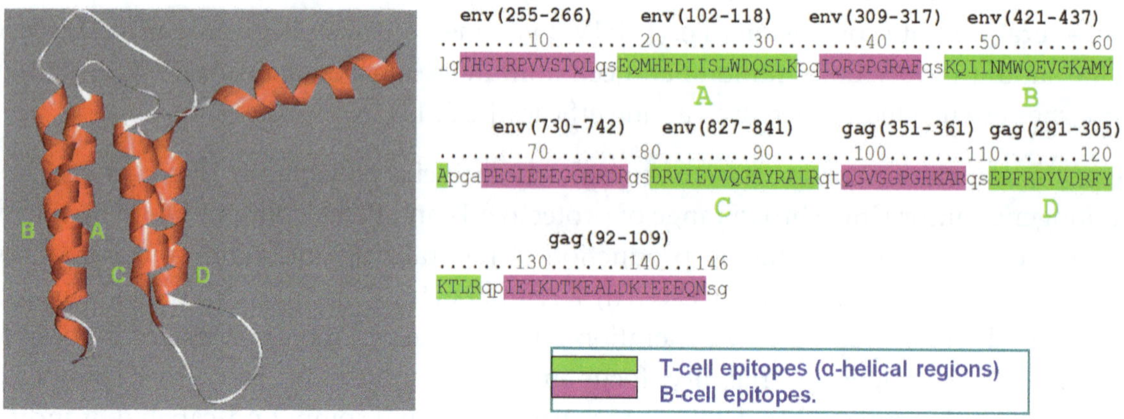

Figure 1. A model of TBI protein tertiary structure. T-cell epitopes are located in the region of α-helices, B-cell epitopes are located at loop sites and N- and C-terminuses.

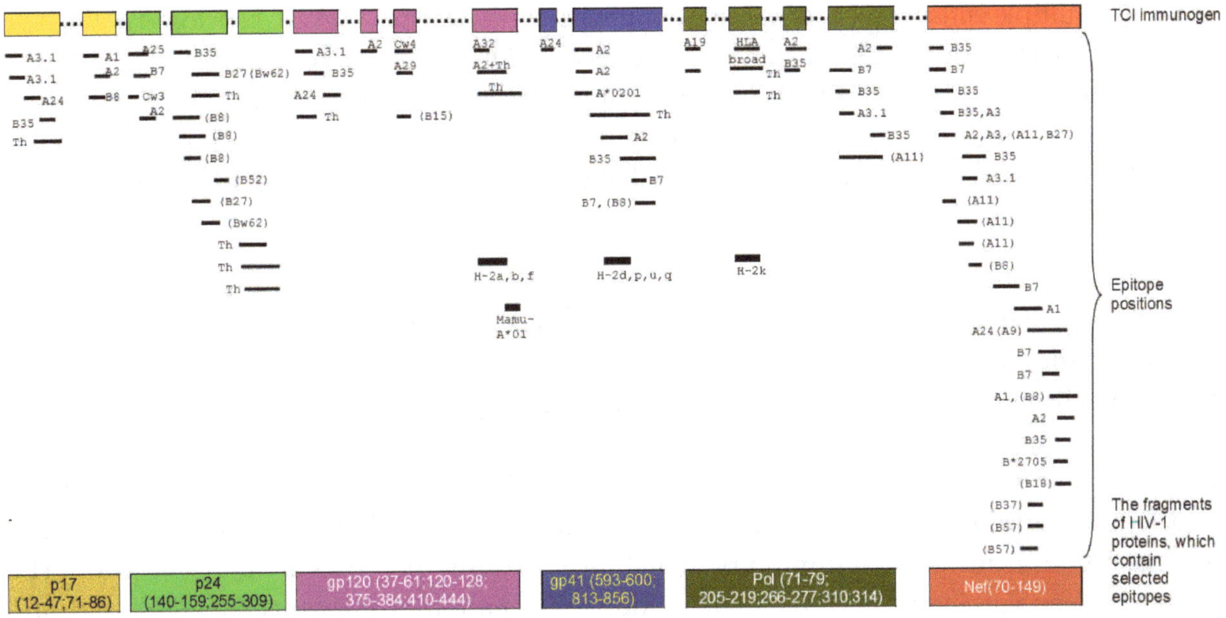

Figure 2. Design of the CTL immunogen, a candidate for the in HIV-1 vaccine: a general schematic. The bar patterns indicate the polyepitope CTL immunogen and the origin of the sequences. The positions of individual epitopes and their MHC restrictions (HLA-A, B, Cw – human; H-2a, b, d, f, k, p, u, q – mouse; Mamu-A*01 – *Macaca mulatta*) are depicted as lines below the CTL immunogen. Th stands for helper epitopes.

In the following, recombinant protein TBI and plasmid pcDNA-TCI were used for the development of CombiHIVvac vaccine [21].

3. CombiHIVvac: a combined vaccine containing two immunogens in a single construct. Preclinical and clinical trials

Since an effective immunoprophylactic vaccine against HIV-infection must induce specific humoral and T-cell immune responses [2, 3, 12], we constructed CombiHIVvac vaccine comprising both above mentioned immunogens, i.e. TBI and TCI [21].

CombiHIVvac was constructed in the form of micelle-like particles based on the original technique combining two different immunogens in a single construct, i.e. polyepitope TBI protein and DNA-vaccine pcDNA-TCI encoding polyepitope protein TCI [19, 21] (**Figure 3**).

TBI protein is conjugated to dextran and mixed with DNA, which leads to formation of microparticles presenting TBI on the surface and containing the DNA inside. Positively charged spermidine provides the binding of the conjugate dextran/protein TBI with negatively charged DNA-vaccine promoting formation of particles on the self-assembly principle (50–250 nm in diameter) [22].

We have previously shown that by combining two immunogens (TBI and TCI) in one construct significant enhancement HIV-specific B cell response was observed [23]. In our opinion, the formation of such particles plays a critical role in the registered effect. CombiHIVvac particles enable more effective absorption by antigen-presenting cells (APCs) compared to individual immunogens. Since TBI protein is fixed on the particle surface and is represented in multiple copies, this provides multiple enhancement of vaccine antigenicity. Besides, pcDNA-TCI enclosed in the vaccine structure is more protected against degradation by DNase I than free pcDNA-TCI, as it was previously demonstrated, resulting in prolongation of DNA-vaccine presence in an organism. Finally, the presence of CD4+ T-helper epitopes in the protein TCI may be the main reason underlying the increased synthesis of antibodies to TBI protein due to a CD4-mediated stimulation of B-cell proliferation and differentiation.

To carry out CombiHIVvac preclinical and clinical trials, we produced experimental series of vaccine of the standard quality according to WHO recommendations. Preclinical studies indicating the safety of the vaccine in tests with animals have been performed, namely, the acute and chronic toxicity has been studied in mice and guinea pigs and the absence of deviations in the vital organs of animals, as well as no changes in hematological and morphological parameters and no immunotoxicity and allergenic activity, have been shown for both single and tenfold administration of vaccine. Specific activity was evaluated based on the parameters of humoral and cellular immunity in BALB/c mice after their twofold immunization. The CombiHIVvac vaccine has been shown to induce formation of HIV-specific antibodies and CTLs [19, 21, 24, 25]. The vaccine did not cause any pyrogenic reaction in rabbits and did not affect the central nervous system and the detoxification liver function in mice. The duration of vaccine persistence in the organisms of laboratory animals has also been estimated and it has been shown that such vaccine component as the plasmid DNA completely eliminated from the organs and tissues of mice for 2 months after vaccination [21]. Thus, preclinical studies showed that CombiHIVvac is safe in animal trials.

Phase I clinical trials were carried out in healthy volunteers to study reactogenicity, safety, and immune activity of CombiHIVvac. The results of clinical trials published in [26]

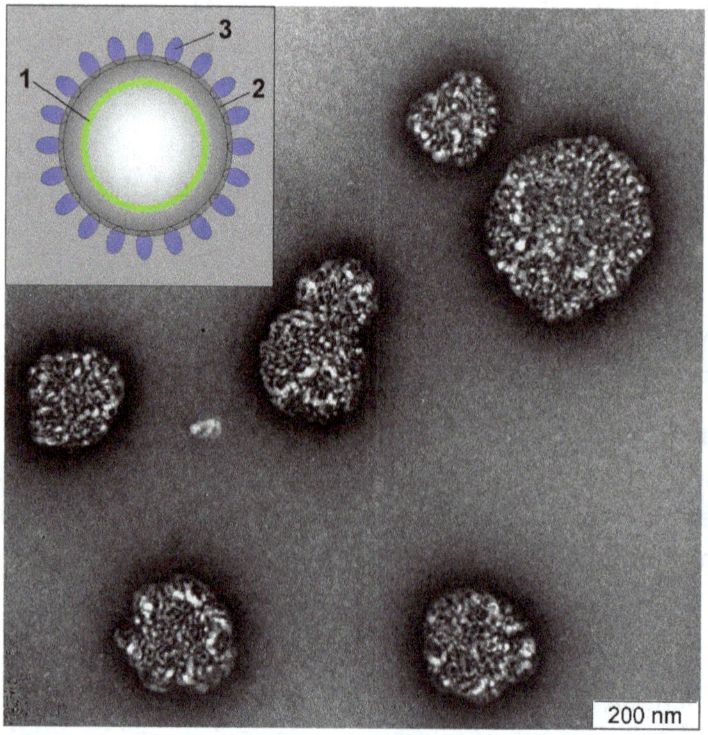

Figure 3. TEM images of CombiHIVvac microparticles with different magnification. A – scale bar 1000 nm, the insert in the left upper corner is a scheme of a CombiHIVvac particle (1 – pcDNA-TCI, 2 – spermidine/dextran, 3 – TBI).

demonstrated that CombiHIVvac is well-tolerated and safe. Neither single nor twofold (with 28-days interval) intramuscular vaccine administration induced significant changes in biochemical and physiological indicators as compared to the baseline values. Local reactions to vaccine administration were absent. There were no pathological changes in volunteers for all observation time. The mean values of the examined biochemical and clinical parameters were within the physiological ranges or near their limits. We failed to detect any regularity in changes of indicators depending on the time from the date of immunization. All studied indicators of immune status came back to the baseline level registered before the vaccination [26].

When carrying out Phase I clinical trials, we assessed CombiHIVvac specific activity in addition to its safety. The obtained results revealed that CombiHIVvac induces both humoral and cell HIV-specific immune responses. It was was confirmed by several methods including immunoblotting, ELISA, env-pseudotyped virus neutralization assay, IFN-γ ELISpot and peptide-MHC-pentamers.

The specific immune response was detected via ELISA 14 days after the first immunization; the second immunization led to enhance the immune response. The maximum immune response is observed by ELISA on the 14th day after the second vaccine administration. Up to the end of observation time (1 year) we detected antibodies in 29% of volunteers.

To confirm antibody production capable of recognizing native HIV-1 during CombiHIVvac administration, we used a kit "New Lav blot" (Bio Rad) on which strips of separate proteins

Analysis		**Percentage of vaccinated volunteers with positive responses**							
		Time after the first vaccination, days		**Time after the second vaccination, days**					
		14	**28**	**14**	**28**	**90**	**180**	**270**	**360**
Neutralization of virus[a]	B/SF162	—	—	71	71	71	64	57	0
	B/PVO4	—	—	36	36	29	29	15	0
	A/392	—	—	86	86	86	71	57	0
	A/SP2010	—	—	79	79	79	64	7	0
IFN-γ ELISpot[b]		71	79	100	93	86	79	50	43
MHC pentamers[c]		100	100	100	100	80	100	80	60

[a]The neutralization of virus was evaluated as IC^{50} value obtained by neutralizing the clones of pseudoviruses of subtypes A (SP-2010 and SP-392) and B (SF162 and PVO4) with blood sera of volunteers vaccinated with CombiHIVvac. The reaction was considered as positive if the neutralization titer was greater than or equal to 1: 100. The neutralizing activities of sera on the 14th and 28th days after immunization were lower than 1: 100.

[b]The ELISpot responses were considered as positive if the number of IFN-γ-producing cells in the vaccinated volunteers was two times larger than the control value.

[c]The results of determination of HIV-specific CD8+ T-lymphocytes in HLA-A*0201-positive volunteers repeatedly vaccinated with CombiHIVvac obtained with the use of MHC pentamers in a complex with Env peptide (KLTPLCVTL) of HIV-1 are given.

Table 1. Evaluation of the response of HIV-specific T-lymphocytes and the activity of virus-neutralizing antibodies in repeatedly vaccinated volunteers.

of virus lysate were sorbed. Using immunoblot analysis, we demonstrated the presence of antibodies to HIV-1 proteins p17, p24, p55, p68, and gp120, i.e. to those proteins which epitopes compose B-cell vaccine component – TBI protein. The response rates differed among volunteers within the same group. Furthermore, during 1 year after the second immunization we registered antibodies at least to one of those proteins in 100% of volunteers.

The results of the study of T-cell response via the IFN-γ ELISpot in repeatedly vaccinated volunteers (**Table 1**) show the HIV-specific response of T-lymphocytes in all volunteers (100%) on the 14th day after the first vaccination, remaining sufficiently strong for 6 months after the second vaccination. Using MHC pentamers in a complex with Env peptide (KLTPLCVTL, gp120 aa 120–128) of HIV-1, it was demonstrated that KLTPLCVTL CD8 T lymphocytes occur in all volunteers (100%) up to the sixth month after the second vaccination (**Table 1**).

Thus, the performed clinical trials showed that the CombiHIVvac vaccine is well tolerated and safe (does not induce any significant changes in biochemical and physiological parameters in comparison to the background values), characterized by low reactogenicity (local reactions to the vaccine are absent) and most importantly capable of inducing the specific humoral and cellular immunity.

Based on the obtained results, the Ministry of Health and Social Development of the Russian Federation has recommended the vaccine for advanced (Phase II) clinical trials.

4. Possible development of CombiHIVvac vaccine platform

Preclinical and clinical trials of CombiHIVvac demonstrated that a combination of two completely artificial polyepitope T- and B-cell antigens is capable of inducing HIV-specific CTLs and antibodies in laboratory animals and human. Furthermore, TCI protein expressed in cells as part of pcDNA-TCI plasmid fulfills a double function: (1) induces specific CD8+ CTL responses and (2) acts as an adjuvant synergistically effecting on synthesis of antibodies to TBI protein with virus-neutralizing activity at least to two HIV-1 subtypes (A and B) [23, 26].

The obtained results imply that CombiHIVvac is actually an original platform for the development and further improvement of combined DNA-protein HIV-vaccines using a broad range of conservative T- and B-cell epitopes based on virus antigens. Providing that TBI and TCI immunogens in CombiHIVvac composition were developed more than 15 year ago concurrently with clinical trials of CombiHIVvac, we carried out works on enhancement of immunogenic and protective properties of artificial polyepitope antigens utilizing new data on the structural-functional organization and immunology of HIV-1.

4.1. B-cell epitopes to HIV-1 generating broadly neutralizing antibodies (bNAbs)

At present when developing efficient B-cell immunogens, researchers mainly rely on epitopes recognized by antibodies neutralizing a broad spectrum of HIV-1 strains (bNAbs). In recent years dozens of B-cell HIV epitopes recognized by bNAbs have been detected [27].

It was shown that many of these antibodies can prevent infection, and some can suppress active infection in hu-mice or macaques [28–32]. Recently results of Phase I clinical trials of mAbs VRC01 were published [33]. It is shown that they are safe and well tolerated after multiple intravenous or subcutaneous administrations in humans, in addition VRC01 from participants' sera were found to avidly capture HIV virions and to mediate antibody-dependent cellular phagocytosis [33].

Exceptional features of bNAbs inspire many researches to develop immunogen capable of their producing (induction). One of the evolving research areas focusing on the design of such immunogens is based on the development of HIV-1 envelope (Env) trimers [6, 34–36]. Despite substantial progress in this area, (a number of questions must be addressed). Firstly, although trimers are rather stable in solution, they produce conformational conditions that fail to provide binding and induction of bNAbs. Secondly, trimers expose undesired immunodominant non-protective HIV epitopes that could prevent adaptive immune response from recognizing neutralizing epitopes, block protective immunity and/or induce increased HIV-infection [4, 36].

An alternative approach to solving this problem includes constructing completely artificial polyepitope anti-HIV-1 immunogens comprising a set of protective epitopes assembled in a single mosaic (polyepitope) construct. Unfortunately, the most bNAbs recognize conformational epitopes and considerably more rarely linear epitopes [37–39]. Furthermore, conformational B-cell epitopes are frequently formed in HIV by lipids and glycans or their combinations [37–40]. It complicates the design of immunogens capable of inducing sufficient B-cell response. Phage peptide libraries offer the unique possibility to obtain mimics of such epitopes [41–46].

Using phage peptide library we can select peptides mimicking epitopes recognized by bnAbs, that make it possible to construct mosaic immunogen on their base to simultaneously induce several neutralizing antibodies [43, 47–52]. **Figure 4** depicts general working scheme.

In our study we used a number of bNAbs against HIV-1, i.e. 2G12, 2F5, IgG1b12, Z13e1, VRC-01, VRC-03, and 697-30D to obtain peptide-mimics. The last five bNAbs were kindly furnished upon NIH AIDS Reagent Program, USA. Each monoclonal antibody was used to perform biopanning using phage peptide libraries (New England Biolabs, USA) [20, 47, 48, 53].

After biopanning of phage libraries using monoclonal antibody 2G12 (recognizes conformational epitope) and 2F5 (recognizes linear epitope), we isolated peptide-mimics that have another amino acid sequences compared to natural epitopes, but able to elicit antibodies in laboratory animals capable to compete with initial bNAbs and neutralizing the virus.

As a result we obtained a collection of phagotops carrying on their surface peptide-mimics of epitopes recognized by above mentioned bNAbs. Specific activity of selected peptides was studied both free and in the compound of phage particles. We carried out chemical synthesis of 134 free peptides. Evaluation of their capacity to compete with HIV-1 epitope for binding to monoclonal antibodies VRC-01, VRC-03, and IgG1b12 was carried out using pseudovirus particles in virus-neutralization assay. To study peptides immunogenicity in the compound of phage particles, the latter were produced in preparative amount using bacterial cells. We used the obtained samples to immunize laboratory animals from which we sampled sera to study their virus-neutralizing activity. It was shown that sera of rabbits immunized with a mix of bacteriophages are able to neutralize pseudotyped viruses obtained on the base of

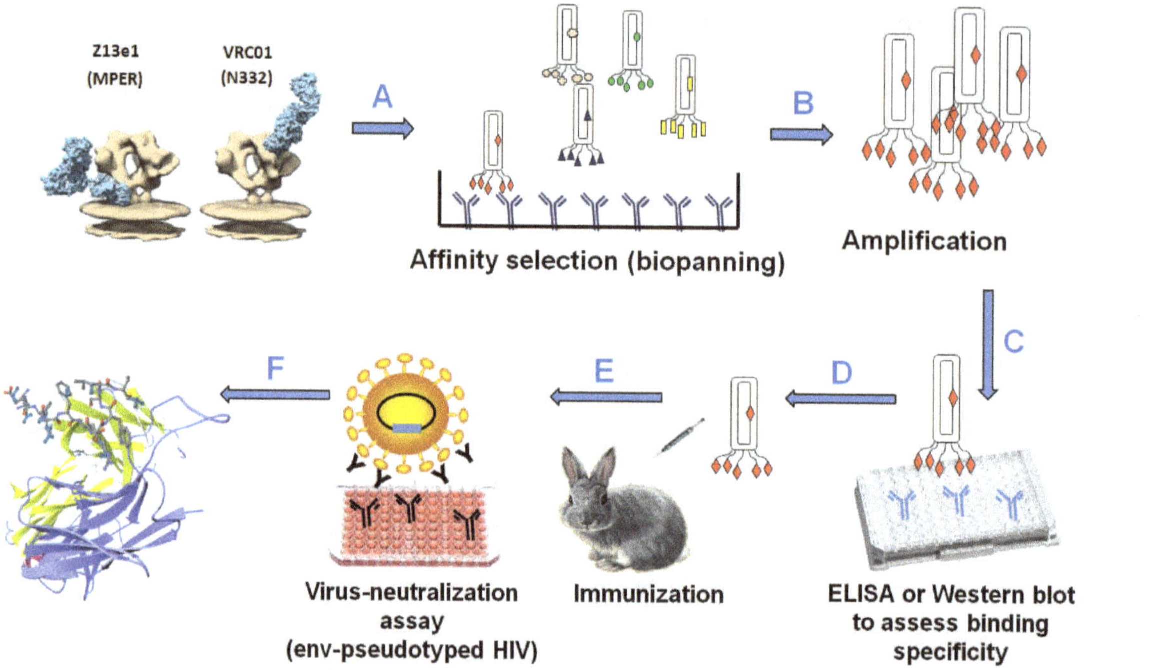

Figure 4. Phage display applications for artificial immunogen design. (A) Randomized peptide library are used to map the residues forming the epitope(s) recognized by monoclonal antibodies immobilized on a solid support; (B) amplification of selected phages; (C) ELISA assay or western blot to determine specificity of selected phages binding; (D) phage particles are used to presentation isolated peptides-mimotopes to the immune system; (E) virus-neutralization assay of immune serum, selection of the most promising mimotope; (F) artificial immunogen design.

HIV-1 subtypes A, B, and AG [20, 47, 48, 53]. Consequently, we succeeded to demonstrate immunologic imitation of conformational antigenic determinants, i.e. HIV-1 epitopes, by linear peptides. Obtained peptide-mimics are material that can serve as a basis for the development of immunoprophylactic HIV-1 vaccine. Besides, peptides can be used when designing diagnostic systems for the detection of antibodies to HIV-1.

4.2. Design of polyepitope T-cell antigens

The progress in identification of T-cell epitopes as well as understanding mechanisms of processing and presentation of antigens through MHC class I and II pathway make it possible to rational design artificial polyepitope vaccines [13, 54].

It is known that CTL recognizes viral protein-antigens synthesized inside the cell not as full-length molecules but as short peptides (8–10 amino acid residues) in complex with MHC class I molecules. These short antigenic epitopes emerge from endogenously synthesized proteins due to proteasome-mediated processing and then are transported to the lumen of endoplasmic reticulum (ER) using transport proteins TAP (transporter associated with antigen processing) where they bind to emerging MHC class I molecules [55, 56]. Since antigen must be synthesized in a cell to induce response of CTL, target T-cell vaccine should be designed as DNA-vaccine because it is the most natural way of presenting CTL-epitopes to CD8+ T-lymphocytes through MHC class I pathway [57].

As opposed to stimulation of CTL, when inducing CD4+ T-lymphocyte-helpers response, antigen should be presented to these cells in a complex with MHC class II molecules. Usually processing and presentation of antigen take place for extracellular antigens which are delivered in cells via endocytosis and phagocytosis. In this case antigen processing occurs in lysosome.

Thus, when designing polyepitope T-cell immunogens capable of inducing high levels of CD4+ and CD8+ T-lymphocyte responses to all epitopes in its compound, one should provide efficient proteasome- and/or lysosome-mediated processing of expression product of target gene through MHC class I and II pathway. For the purpose the following strategies are appropriate:

1. To design poly-CTL-epitope construct one may use spacer sequences dividing epitopes that comprise sites of proteasomal cleavage [58–60] and/or motif for binding to TAP [61–63] to provide polyepitope processing and transport of released peptides (epitopes) into ER.
2. To induce T helper lymphocytes response fragments with T-helper epitopes can be combined with the use of motif [KR][KR] which is a cleavage site for a number of lysosomal cathepsins participating in antigen processing [64, 65].
3. To target polyepitope immunogen into proteasome and presentation of CTL-epitopes to CD8+ T-lymphocytes through MHC class I pathway, researchers typically use genetic attachment of ubiquitin sequence to its N- or C-termini [66].
4. To degrade polyepitope immunogen and present released Th-epitopes to CD4+ T-lymphocytes through MHC class II pathway, researchers typically use a genetic attachment of the sequence of LAMP-1 protein tyrosine motif (Lysosomal-associated membrane protein 1) to its C-terminus to direct the polyepitope immunogen from the secretory pathway to the lysosome [67–70].

To evaluate which of these strategies provide a rational approach to constructing T-cell antigens, we designed a set of polyepitope constructs covering a range of possible structural variants.

To assess the influence of ubiquitin and spacer sequences flanking epitopes on immunogenicity of the polyepitope construct, we designed a set of polyepitope immunogens considering different strategies of processing and presentation of the target antigens. The designed constructs comprised similar set from 10 HLA-A2-restricted CTL-epitopes of the main HIV-1 antigens Env, Gag, Pol, Nef, and Vpr, but differed in a number of structural properties, namely (i) the presence or absence of spacers; (ii) the structure of spacer sequences, and (iii) the presence of N- or C-terminal sequence of ubiquitin. Genes encoding the designed antigens were cloned into plasmid vector and vaccinia virus.

Immunogenicity of the designed immunogens were evaluated after 3-fold prime-boost immunization of HLA-A2 transgenic mice with the obtained recombinant plasmids and recombinant vaccinia virus (rVV). It was demonstrated that the vaccine construct inducing the majority of complexes [peptide/MHC class I] *in vitro* was also the most immunogenic during animal vaccination. This construct comprises N-terminal ubiquitin to target the polyepitope on proteasome. Besides, in the compound of this construct epitopes are divided by spacer sequences comprising sites of proteasomal cleavage of the polyepitope and motifs for TAP-dependent transport of the released peptides into ER where they bind to MHC class I molecules [54].

The obtained results became the basis for the development of original software TEpredict and PolyCTLDesigner that we consider as a universal platform for rational design of polyepitope immunogens – candidate DNA vaccines for induction of T-cell immunity both against infectious and oncological diseases [71, 72] (**Figure 5**).

PolyCTLDesigner enables the user to select a minimal set of epitopes with known or predicted specificity to different allelic variants of MHC class I molecules. This set covers selected repertoire of HLA alleles with the given degree of redundancy. After that PolyCTLDesigner uses the model by Peters et al. [73] to predict binding affinity to TAP for the selected set of known or predicted epitopes. According to this model, the main contribution into peptide binding to TAP is provided by the first three N-terminal amino acid peptide residues and the last C-terminal residue. Considering that epitope C-terminus must be unchanged since C-terminus should contain the site of proteasomal cleavage [74], only N-terminus of antigenic peptide can be extended (if necessary) for optimization of interaction with heterodimer TAP1/TAP2.

Then PolyCTLDesigner analyzes all possible matching of the selected peptides and detects an optimal spacer sequence for each pair providing adequate cleavage of epitopes with release of C-terminus of proximal peptide. To predict proteasomal and/or immunoproteasomal cleavage, PolyCTLDesigner uses models developed by Toes et al. [75].

When analyzing epitopes matching, PolyCTLDesigner creates a directed graph with nodes corresponding to epitopes and edges corresponding to acceptable matching. Each edge has relevant weight vector characterized by the efficiency of proteasomal cleavage, spacer length

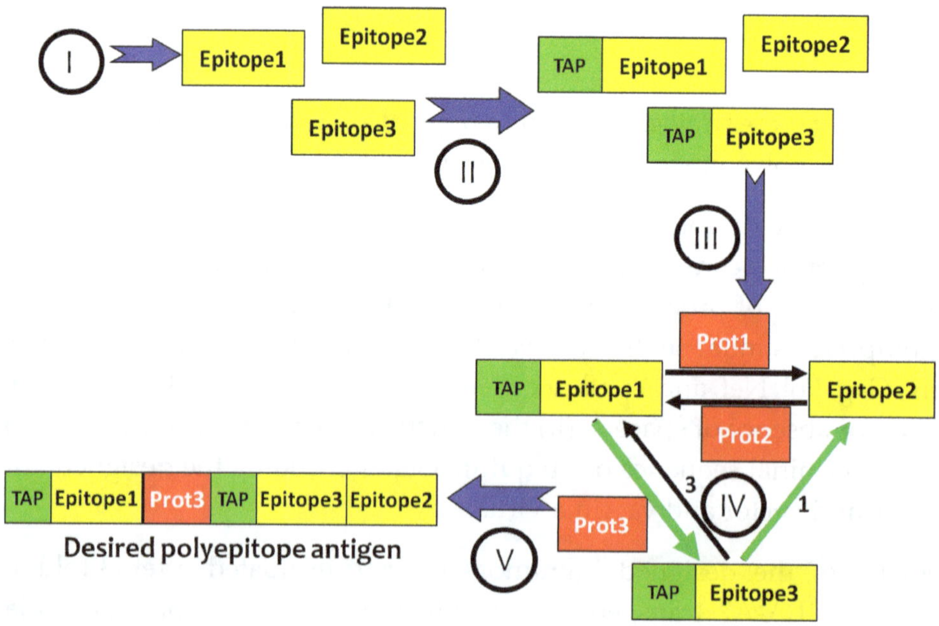

Figure 5. PolyCTLDesigner operation algorithm. I – Selection of minimal set of CD8+ T cell epitopes with the known or predicted specificity towards various allelic variants of MHC class I molecules; II – Prediction of binding affinity of peptides to TAP and, if necessary, addition of N-terminal flanking residues to optimize this binding; III – Prediction of optimal spacer sequences for each pair of peptides; IV – Creating weighted graph, where the nodes are the target epitopes, and the edges are possible variants of their association. Each edge is a weight vector whose attributes are: efficiency of proteasomal cleavage, length of the spacer, and number of predicted non-target epitopes at junction; V – Designing polyepitope immunogen sequence. Resulting sequence is defined as the longest simple path in the graph that has the lowest weight; Prot1, Prot2, Prot3 – proteasomal cleavage sites.

and number of predicted non-target epitopes at the junction. Finally, the software designs an optimal polyepitope immunogen sequence that is calculated as a complete simple way in the constructed graph with the least length (weight).

Besides, PolyCTLDesigner makes it possible to construct a sequence of the epitope fragment comprising T-helper epitopes. In the compound of the selected antigens software predicts peptide fragments with the length of 20–40 amino acid residues with the majority of overlapping T-helper epitopes restricted by the widest possible repertoire of HLA class II allomorphs. Then five C- and N-terminal amino acid residues from the initial antigen sequence are added to each of the selected fragments since it was shown that they can play significant role in binding to T-cell receptors of CD4+ T-lymphocytes [76, 77]. Fragments with T-helper epitopes are combined using [KR][KR] motif which is a cleavage site for a number of lysosomal cathepsins involved in antigen processing.

More detailed information on PolyCTLDesigner software is available at http://tepredict.sourceforge.net/PolyCTLDesigner.html.

We used the developed software when designing new polyepitope constructs – candidate DNA-vaccines against HIV-1. Particularly, when evaluating the influence of proteasome-dependent and lysosome-dependent degradation of polyepitopes on immunogenicity of the target polyepitope construct, we designed three polyepitope HIV-1 immunogens, i.e. TCI-N1, TCI-N2, and TCI-N3 using cytotoxic and helper T-cell epitopes of HIV-1 [78].

All three polyepitope immunogens are based on the same core sequence of polyE, while differences between immunogens lie in the use of different terminal signal sequences (**Figure 6**). Immunogen TCI-N1 comprises only the core sequence polyE. Sequence polyE of TCI-N2 immunogen includes

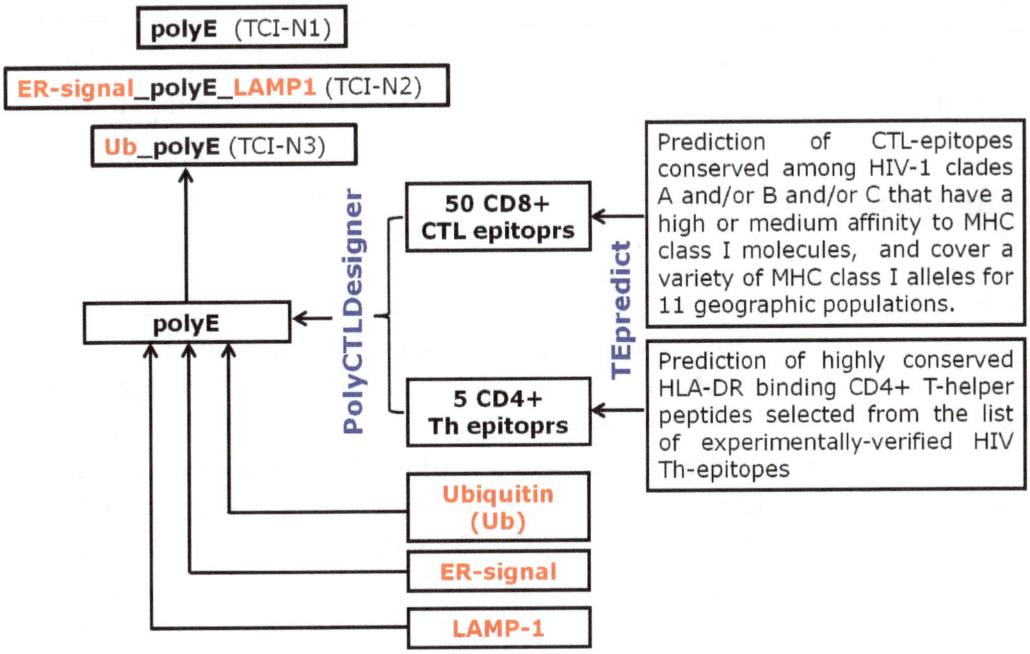

Figure 6. Design of T-cell polyepitope immunogens. polyE – common for all antigens sequence polyE designed using cytotoxic and helper T-cell epitopes of HIV-1; ER-signal – N-terminal signal peptide (in our case MRYMILGLLALAAVCSAA – the signal sequence of the adenovirus protein E3/gp19K); LAMP1 – C-terminal tyrosine-based motif of LAMP-1 glycoprotein (RKRSHAGYQTI); Ub – N-terminal ubiquitin with substitution of the C-terminal Gly to Val to prevent liberation of Ub cleavage by Ub hydrolases.

N-terminal signal peptide and C-terminal tyrosine motif of LAMP-1 protein. N-terminal signal peptides are believed to provide delivery of immunogen in ER, while LAMP-1 protein motif directs immunogen from the secretory pathway to the lysosome and presents epitopes released after the cleavage to CD4+ T-lymphocytes through MHC class II pathway. The sequence polyE of TCI-N3 comprises N-terminal ubiquitin for its delivery into proteasome and presentation of epitopes released after the cleavage to CD8+ T-lymphocytes through MHC class I pathway.

Immunogenicity of the obtained DNA-vaccine constructs was studied in BALB/c mice according to capacity of CD4+ and CD8+ T-cells to produce IL-2 and IFNγ in ELISpot. The obtained results revealed that DNA-vaccine constructs encoding TCI-N2 and TCI-N3 immunogens induce responses of HIV-specific CD4+ and CD8+ T-lymphocytes that are significantly higher than that of the negative control the group of animals immunized with vector plasmid pcDNA3.1 as well as of group of mice that received a construct encoding core immunogen TCI-N1 with no additional signal sequences. At the same time DNA-vaccine construct encoding TCI-N3 immunogen comprising N-terminal ubiquitin induces the highest statistically significant level ($P \leq 0.05$) of CD4+ and CD8+ T-lymphocytes as compared with two other immunogens.

Thus, the obtained results point to a regular correlation between the structure of polyepitope construct and its antigenic and immunogenic properties:

- it is possible to significantly increase the immunogenic potential of the target polyepitope vaccine via optimization of the immunogen structure using the spacer sequences comprising motifs for binding to TAP and the sites of proteasomal and lysosomal cleavage flanking CTL- and Th-epitopes in the compound of the polyepitope construct;
- ubiquitin-dependent targeting of polyepitope at proteasome is the most efficient strategy to induce specific T-cell immune response as compared to LAMP-dependent targeting at lysosome.

Our findings support the concept of vaccine rational design based on existing knowledge on mechanism of presentation of T-cell antigens through MHC class I and II pathway.

5. Conclusions

We did not set ourselves the task of covering all challenges facing designers of HIV-1 vaccine. The paper presents our experience on designing artificial polyepitope HIV-1 immunogens constructed using a broad spectrum of conservative T- and B-cell epitopes. This approach is believed to be promising for the design of new generation HIV-vaccines. In theory, it makes it possible to overcome HIV-1 antigenic variability, focuses immune responses on protective determinants, and allows to exclude from vaccine composition undesired determinants capable of inducing autoantibodies or antibodies increasing virus infectivity. The results demonstrate that completely artificial molecules designed with the use of bioinformatic and combinatorial biology methods are able to induce production of broad-spectrum neutralizing antibodies and responses of cytotoxic (CD8+ CTL) and helper (CD4+ Th) T-lymphocytes in laboratory animals and human.

It is our belief that the proposed approach can play an important and positive role in the development of HIV-1 vaccine.

Acknowledgments

This work was presented on the international conference "Vaccines & Vaccination", Moscow, September 27-October 1, 2017 http://www.onlinereg.ru/VAC&VAC2017 sponsored by Russian Science Fund 15_15_30039, and received the award for the best oral presentation. Authors acknowledge Scientific Committee and Conference organizers for support of the publication.

Conflict of interest

None.

Author details

Larisa I. Karpenko[1*], Sergei I. Bazhan[1], Alexey M. Eroshkin[2], Denis V. Antonets[1], Anton N. Chikaev[3] and Alexander A. Ilyichev[1]

*Address all correspondence to: karpenko@vector.nsc.ru

1 State Research Center of Virology and Biotechnology Vector, Koltsovo, Novosibirsk, Russian Federation

2 Bioinformatics Core, Sanford Burnham Prebys Medical Discovery Institute, La Jolla, CA, USA

3 Institute of Molecular and Cellular Biology of the Siberian Branch of the Russian Academy of Sciences, Novosibirsk, Russian Federation

References

[1] Van Regenmortel MHV. Development of a preventive HIV vaccine requires solving inverse problems which is unattainable by rational vaccine design. Frontiers in Immunology. 2017;**8**:2009. DOI: 10.3389/fimmu.2017.02009

[2] Eisinger RW, Fauci AS. Ending the HIV/AIDS pandemic. Emerging Infectious Diseases. 2018;**3**:413-416. DOI: 10.3201/eid2403.171797

[3] McMichael AJ, Haynes BF. Lessons learned from HIV-1 vaccine trials: New priorities and directions. Nature Immunology. 2012;**5**:423-427. DOI: 10.1038/ni.2264

[4] Sahay B, Nguyen CQ, Yamamoto JK. Conserved HIV epitopes for an effective HIV vaccine. Journal of Clinical and Cellular Immunology. 2017;**8**(4):518. DOI: 10.4172/2155-9899.1000518

[5] Esparza J. A brief history of the global effort to develop a preventive HIV vaccine. Vaccine. 2013;**35**:3502-3518. DOI: 10.1016/j.vaccine.2013.05.018

[6] Haynes BF, Burton DR. Developing an HIV vaccine. Science. 2017;**6330**:1129-1130. DOI: 10.1126/science.aan0662

[7] Corey L, Gilbert PB, Tomaras GD, Haynes BF, Pantaleo G, Fauci AS. Immune correlates of vaccine protection against HIV-1 acquisition. Science Translational Medicine. 2015;**310**:310rv7-310rv7. DOI: 10.1126/scitranslmed.aac7732

[8] Billich A. AIDSVAX (VaxGen). Current Opinion in Investigational Drugs. 2004;**2**:214-221

[9] O'Connell RJ, Kim JH, Corey L, Michael NL. Human immunodeficiency virus vaccine trials. Cold Spring Harbor Perspectives in Medicine. 2012;**12**:a007351. DOI: 10.1101/cshperspect.a007351

[10] Haynes BF. New approaches to HIV vaccine development. Current Opinion in Immunology. 2015;**35**:39-47. DOI: 10.1016/j.coi.2015.05.007

[11] Rerks-Ngarm S, Pitisuttithum P, Nitayaphan S, Kaewkungwal J, Chiu J, Paris R, Premsri N, Namwat C, De Souza M, Adams E, Benenson M, Gurunathan S, Tartaglia J, McNeil JG, Francis DP, Stablein D, Birx DL, Chunsuttiwat S, Khamboonruang C, Thongcharoen P, Robb ML, Michael NL, Kunasol P, Kim JH. Vaccination with ALVAC and AIDSVAX to prevent HIV-1 infection in Thailand. New England Journal of Medicine. 2009;**23**:2209-2220. DOI: 10.1056/NEJMoa0908492

[12] Hsu DC, O'Connell RJ. Progress in HIV vaccine development. Human Vaccines and Immunotherapeutics. 2017;**5**:1018-1030. DOI: 10.1080/21645515.2016.1276138

[13] Karpenko LI, Bazhan SI, Antonets DV, Belyakov IM. Novel approaches in polyepitope T-cell vaccine development against HIV-1. Expert Review of Vaccines. 2014;**1**:155-173. DOI: 10.1586/14760584.2014.861748

[14] Eroshkin AM, Zhilkin PA, Shamin VV, Korolev S, Fedorov BB. Artificial protein vaccines with predetermined tertiary structure: Application to anti-HTV-1 vaccine design. Protein Engineering, Design and Selection. 1993;**8**:997-1001. DOI: 10.1093/protein/6.8.997

[15] Eroshkin AM, Karginova EA, Gileva IP, Lomakin AS, Lebedev LR, Kamyinina TP, Pereboev AV, Ignat'ev GM. Design of four-helix bundle protein as a candidate for HIV vaccine. Protein Engineering, Design and Selection. 1995;**2**:167-173. DOI: 10.1093/protein/8.2.167

[16] Mikhailov AM, Loktev VB, Lebedev LR, Eroshkin AM, Kornev AN, Kornilov VV, Vainshtein BK. Crystallization and X-ray study of the artificial TBI protein, an experimental multiple-epitope vaccine against type 1 human immunodeficiency virus. Crystallography Reports. 1999;**5**:868-870

[17] Loktev VB, Ilyichev AA, Eroshkin AM, Karpenko LI, Pokrovsky AG, Pereboev AV, Svyatchenko VA, Ignat'ev GM, Smolina MI, Melamed NV, Lebedeva CD, Sandakhchiev LS. Design of immunogens as components of a new generation of molecular vaccines. Journal of Biotechnology. 1996;**1-3**:129-137. DOI: 10.1016/0168-1656(95)00089-5

[18] Bazhan SI, Belavin PA, Seregin SV, Danilyuk NK, Babkina IN, Karpenko LI, Nekrasova

NA, Lebedev LR, Ignatyev GM, Agafonov AP, Poryvaeva VA, Aborneva IV, Ilyichev AA. Designing and engineering of DNA-vaccine construction encoding multiple CTL-epitopes of major HIV-1 antigens. Vaccine. 2004;**13-14**:1672-1682. DOI: 10.1016/j.vaccine.2003.09.048

[19] Karpenko LI, Nekrasova NA, Ilyichev AA, Lebedev LR, Ignatyev GM, Agafonov AP, Zaitsev BN, Belavin PA, Seregin SV, Danilyuk NK, Babkina IN, Bazhan SI. Comparative analysis using a mouse model of the immunogenicity of artificial VLP and attenuated Salmonella strain carrying a DNA-vaccine encoding HIV-1 polyepitope CTL-immunogen. Vaccine. 2004;**13-14**:1692-1699. DOI: 10.1016/j.vaccine.2003.09.050

[20] Karpenko LI, Danilenko AV, Bazhan SI, Danilenko ED, Sysoeva GM, Kaplina ON, Volkova OY, Oreshkova SF, Ilyichev AA. Attenuated *Salmonella enteritidis* E23 as a vehicle for the rectal delivery of DNA vaccine coding for HIV-1 polyepitope CTL immunogen. Microbial Biotechnology. 2012;**2**:241-250. DOI: 10.1111/j.1751-7915.2011.00291.x

[21] Karpenko LI, Ilyichev AA, Eroshkin AM, Lebedev LR, Uzhachenko RV, Nekrasova NA, Plyasunova OA, Belavin PA, Seregin SV, Danilyuk NK, Zaitsev BN, Danilenko ED, Masycheva VI, Bazhan SI. Combined virus-like particle-based polyepitope DNA/protein HIV-1 vaccine. Design, immunogenicity and toxicity studies. Vaccine. 2007;**21**:4312-4323. DOI: 10.1016/j.vaccine.2007.02.058

[22] Karpenko LI, Lebedev LR, Bazhan SI, Korneev DV, Zaitsev BB, Ilyichev AA. Visualization of CombiHIVvac vaccine particles using Electron microscopy. Aids Research and Human Retroviruses. 2017;**4**:323-324. DOI: 10.1089/aid.2016.0140

[23] Bazhan SI, Karpenko LI, Lebedev LR, Uzhachenko RV, Belavin PA, Eroshkin AM, Llyichev AA. A synergistic effect of a combined bivalent DNA-protein anti-HIV-I vaccine containing multiple T- and B-cell epitopes of HIV-1 proteins. Molecular Immunology. 2008;**3**:661-669. DOI: 10.1016/j.molimm.2007.07.016

[24] Karpenko LI, Bazhan SI, Eroshkin AM, Lebedev LR, Uzhachenko RV, Nekrasova NA, Plyasunova OA, Belavin PA, Seregin SV, Danilyuk NK, Danilenko ED, Zaitsev BN, Masicheva VI, Ilyichev AA, Sandakhchiev LS. CombiHIVvac vaccine which contains polyepitope B-and T-cell immunogens of HIV-1. Doklady Biochemistry and Biophysics. 2007;**1**:65-67. DOI: 10.1134/S160767290702007X

[25] Reguzova AY, Karpenko LI, Mechetina LV, Belyakov IM. Peptide-MHC multimer-based monitoring of CD8 T-cells in HIV-1 infection and AIDS vaccine development. Expert Review of Vaccines. 2015;**1**:69-84. DOI: 10.1586/14760584.2015.962520

[26] Karpenko LI, Bazhan SI, Bogryantseva MP, Ryndyuk NN, Ginko ZI, Kuzubov VI, Lebedev LR, Kaplina ON, Reguzova AY, Ryzhikov AB, Usova SV, Oreshkova SF, Nechaeva EA, Danilenko ED, Ilyichev AA. Results of phase I clinical trials of a combined vaccine against HIV-1 based on synthetic polyepitope immunogens. Russian Journal of Bioorganic Chemistry. 2016;**2**:170-182. DOI: 10.1134/s1068162016020060

[27] Shcherbakov DN, Bakulina AY, Karpenko LI, Ilyichev AA. Broadly neutralizing antibodies against HIV-1 as a novel aspect of the immune response. Acta Naturae. 2015;**4**:11-21

[28] Klein F, Halper-Stromberg A, Horwitz JA, Gruell H, Scheid JF, Bournazos S, Mouquet H, Spatz LA, Diskin R, Abadir A, Zang T, Dorner M, Billerbeck E, Labitt RN, Gaebler C, Marcovecchio PM, Incesu RB, Eisenreich TR, Bieniasz PD, Seaman MS, Bjorkman PJ, Ravetch JV, Ploss A, Nussenzweig MC. HIV therapy by a combination of broadly neutralizing antibodies in humanized mice. Nature. 2012;**7427**:118-122. DOI: 10.1038/nature11604

[29] Horwitz JA, Halper-Stromberg A, Mouquet H, Gitlin AD, Tretiakova A, Eisenreich TR, Malbec M, Gravemann S, Billerbeck E, Dorner M, Büning H, Schwartz O, Knops E, Kaiser R, Seaman MS, Wilson JM, Rice CM, Ploss A, Bjorkman PJ, Klein F, Nussenzweig MC. HIV-1 suppression and durable control by combining single broadly neutralizing antibodies and antiretroviral drugs in humanized mice. Proceedings of the National Academy of Sciences of the United States of America. 2013;**41**:16538-16543. DOI: 10.1073/pnas.1315295110

[30] Hessell AJ, Jaworski JP, Epson E, Matsuda K, Pandey S, Kahl C, Reed J, Sutton WF, Hammond KB, Cheever TA, Barnette PT, Legasse AW, Planer S, Stanton JJ, Pegu A, Chen X, Wang K, Siess D, Burke D, Park BS, Axthelm MK, Lewis A, Hirsch VM, Graham BS, Mascola JR, Sacha JB, Haigwood NL. Early short-term treatment with neutralizing human monoclonal antibodies halts SHIV infection in infant macaques. Nature Medicine. 2016;**4**:362-368. DOI: 10.1038/nm.4063

[31] Barouch DH, Whitney JB, Moldt B, Klein F, Oliveira TY, Liu J, Stephenson KE, Chang HW, Shekhar K, Gupta S, Nkolola JP, Seaman MS, Smith KM, Borducchi EN, Cabral C, Smith JY, Blackmore S, Sanisetty S, Perry JR, Beck M, Lewis MG, Rinaldi W, Chakraborty AK, Poignard P, Nussenzweig MC, Burton DR. Therapeutic efficacy of potent neutralizing HIV-1-specific monoclonal antibodies in SHIV-infected rhesus monkeys. Nature. 2013;**7475**:224-228. DOI: 10.1038/nature12744

[32] Shingai M, Nishimura Y, Klein F, Mouquet H, Donau OK, Plishka R, Buckler-White A, Seaman M, Piatak M Jr, Lifson JD, Dimitrov D, Nussenzweig MC, Martin MA. Antibody-mediated immunotherapy of macaques chronically infected with SHIV suppresses viraemia. Nature. 2013;**7475**:277-280. DOI: 10.1038/nature12746

[33] Mayer KH, Seaton KE, Huang Y, Grunenberg N, Isaacs A, Allen M, Ledgerwood JE, Frank I, Sobieszczyk ME, Baden LR, Rodriguez B, Van Tieu H, Tomaras GD, Deal A, Goodman D, Bailer RT, Ferrari G, Jensen R, Hural J, Graham BS, Mascola JR, Corey L, Montefiori DC. Safety, pharmacokinetics, and immunological activities of multiple intravenous or subcutaneous doses of an anti-HIV monoclonal antibody, VRC01, administered to HIV-uninfected adults: Results of a phase 1 randomized trial. PLoS Medicine. 2017;**14**(11):e1002435. DOI: 10.1371/journal.pmed.1002435

[34] Dey AK, Cupo A, Ozorowski G, Sharma VK, Behrens AJ, Go EP, Ketas TJ, Yasmeen A, Klasse PJ, Sayeed E, Desaire H, Crispin M, Wilson IA, Sanders RW, Hassell T, Ward AB, Moore JP. cGMP production and analysis of BG505 SOSIP.664, an extensively glycosylated, trimeric HIV-1 envelope glycoprotein vaccine candidate. Biotechnology and Bioengineering. 2018;**4**:885-899. DOI: 10.1002/bit.26498

[35] Briney B, Sok D, Jardine JG, Kulp DW, Skog P, Menis S, Jacak R, Kalyuzhniy O, de Val N, Sesterhenn F, Le KM, Ramos A, Jones M, Saye-Francisco KL, Blane TR, Spencer S, Georgeson E, Hu X, Ozorowski G, Adachi Y, Kubitz M, Sarkar A, Wilson IA, Ward AB,

Nemazee D, Burton DR, Schief WR. Tailored Immunogens direct affinity maturation toward HIV neutralizing antibodies. Cell. 2016;**6**:1459-1470.e11. DOI: 10.1016/j.cell.2016.08.005

[36] Medina-Ramírez M, Sanders RW, Sattentau QJ. Stabilized HIV-1 envelope glycoprotein trimers for vaccine use. Current Opinion in HIV and AIDS. 2017;**3**:241-249. DOI: 10.1097/COH.0000000000000363

[37] Wu X, Kong X-P. Antigenic landscape of the HIV-1 envelope and new immunological concepts defined by HIV-1 broadly neutralizing antibodies. Current Opinion in Immunology. 2016:56-64. DOI: 10.1016/j.coi.2016.05.013

[38] McCoy LE, Burton DR. Identification and specificity of broadly neutralizing antibodies against HIV. Immunological Reviews. 2017;**1**:11-20. DOI: 10.1111/imr.12484

[39] Korber B, Hraber P, Wagh K, Hahn BH. Polyvalent vaccine approaches to combat HIV-1 diversity. Immunological Reviews. 2017;**1**:230-244. DOI: 10.1111/imr.12516

[40] Cerutti N, Loredo-Varela JL, Caillat C, Weissenhorn W. Antigp41 membrane proximal external region antibodies and the art of using the membrane for neutralization. Current Opinion in HIV and AIDS. 2017;**3**:250-256. DOI: 10.1097/COH.0000000000000364

[41] Smith GP. Surface presentation of protein epitopes using bacteriophage expression systems. Current Opinion in Biotechnology. 1991;**5**:668-673. DOI: 10.1016/0958-1669(91)90032-Z

[42] Ilyichev AA, Minenkova OO, Kishchenko GP, Tat'kov SI, Karpishev NN, Eroshkin AM, Ofitzerov VI, Akimenko ZA, Petrenko VA, Sandakhchiev LS. Inserting foreign peptides into the major coat protein of bacteriophage M13. FEBS Letters. 1992;**3**:322-324. DOI: 10.1016/0014-5793(92)80267-K

[43] Zolla-Pazner S. Identifying epitopes of HIV-1 that induce protective antibodies. Nature Reviews Immunology. 2004;**3**:199-210

[44] Delhalle S, Schmit JC, Chevigné A. Phages and HIV-1: From display to interplay. International Journal of Molecular Sciences. 2012;**4**:4727-4794. DOI: 10.3390/ijms13044727

[45] Zhang X, Han X, Dai D, Bao M, Zhang Z, Zhang M, Bice T, Zhao M, Cao Y, Shang H. Mimotopes selected by biopanning with high-titer HIV-neutralizing antibodies in plasma from Chinese slow progressors. Brazilian Journal of Infectious Diseases. 2012;**6**:510-516. DOI: 10.1016/j.bjid.2012.07.003

[46] Gokhale AS, Satyanarayanajois S. Peptides and peptidomimetics as immunomodulators. Immunotherapy. 2014;**6**:755-774. DOI: 10.2217/imt.14.37

[47] Tumanova OY, Kuvshinov VN, Il'ichev AA, Nekrasov BG, Ivanisenko VA, Kozlov AP, Sandakhchiev LS. Localization of the HIV-1 gp120 conformational epitope recognized by virus-neutralizing monoclonal antibodies 2G12. Molecular Biology. 2002;**4**:517-521. DOI: 10.1023/A:1019804511163

[48] Tumanova O, Kuvshinov VN, Orlovskaia IA, Proniaeva TR, Pokrovskii AG, Il'ichev AA,

Sandakhchiev LS. Immunogenetic properties of peptides mimicking a human immunodeficiency virus gp41 (HIV-1) epitope recognized by virus-neutralizing antibody 2F5. Molekuliarnaia Biologiia (Mosk) 2003;**3**:556-560

[49] Gazarian KG, Palacios-Rodríguez Y, Gazarian TG, Huerta L. HIV-1 V3 loop crown epitope-focused mimotope selection by patient serum from random phage display libraries: Implications for the epitope structural features. Molecular Immunology. 2013;**2**:148-156. DOI: 10.1016/j.molimm.2012.11.016

[50] Zwick MB, Bonnycastle LLC, Menendez A, Irving MB, Barbas Iii CF, Parren PWHI, Burton DR, Scott JK. Identification and characterization of a peptide that specifically binds the human, broadly neutralizing anti-human immunodeficiency virus type 1 antibody b12. Journal of Virology. 2001;**14**:6692-6699. DOI: 10.1128/JVI.75.14.6692-6699.2001

[51] Menendez A, Calarese DA, Stanfield RL, Chow KC, Scanlan CN, Kunert R, Katinger H, Burton DR, Wilson IA, Scott JK. A peptide inhibitor of HIV-1 neutralizing antibody 2G12 is not a structural mimic of the natural carbohydrate epitope on gp120. FASEB Journal. 2008;**5**:1380-1392. DOI: 10.1096/fj.07-8983com

[52] Zhu Z, Qin HR, Chen W, Zhao Q, Shen X, Schutte R, Wang Y, Ofek G, Streaker E, Prabakaran P, Fouda GG, Liao HX, Owens J, Louder M, Yang Y, Klaric KA, Moody MA, Mascola JR, Scott JK, Kwong PD, Montefiori D, Haynes BF, Dimitrov GDT. Cross-reactive hiv-1-neutralizing human monoclonal antibodies identified from a patient with 2f5-like antibodies. Journal of Virology. 2011;**21**:11401-11408. DOI: 10.1128/JVI.05312-11

[53] Chikaev AN, Bakulina AY, Burdick RC, Karpenko LI, Pathak VK, Ilyichev AA. Selection of peptide mimics of HIV-1 epitope recognized by neutralizing antibody VRC01. PLoS One. 2015;**3**:e0120847. DOI: 10.1371/journal.pone.0120847

[54] Bazhan SI, Karpenko LI, Ilyicheva TN, Belavin PA, Seregin SV, Danilyuk NK, Antonets DV, Ilyichev AA. Rational design based synthetic polyepitope DNA vaccine for eliciting HIV-specific CD8+ T cell responses. Molecular Immunology. 2010;**7-8**:1507-1515. DOI: 10.1016/j.molimm.2010.01.020

[55] van de Weijer ML, Luteijn RD, Wiertz EJHJ. Viral immune evasion: Lessons in MHC class I antigen presentation. Seminars in Immunology. 2015;**2**:125-137. DOI: 10.1016/j.smim.2015.03.010

[56] Yewdell JW. DRiPs solidify: Progress in understanding endogenous MHC class I antigen processing. Trends in Immunology. 2011;**11**:548-558. DOI: 10.1016/j.it.2011.08.001

[57] Kutzler MA, Weiner DB. DNA vaccines: Ready for prime time? Nature Reviews Genetics. 2008;**10**:776-788. DOI: 10.1038/nrg2432

[58] Livingston BD, Newman M, Crimi C, McKinney D, Chesnut R, Sette A. Optimization of epitope processing enhances immunogenicity of multiepitope DNA vaccines. Vaccine. 2001;**32**:4652-4660. DOI: 10.1016/S0264-410X(01)00233-X

[59] Depla E, Van Der Aa A, Livingston BD, Crimi C, Allosery K, De Brabandere V, Krakover J, Murthy S, Huang M, Power S, Babé L, Dahlberg C, McKinney D, Sette A, Southwood S,

Philip R, Newman MJ, Meheus L. Rational design of a multiepitope vaccine encoding T-lymphocyte epitopes for treatment of chronic hepatitis B virus infections. Journal of Virology. 2008;**1**:435-450. DOI: 10.1128/JVI.01505-07

[60] Schubert B, Kohlbacher O. Designing string-of-beads vaccines with optimal spacers. Genome Medicine. 2016;**8**:9. DOI: 10.1186/s13073-016-0263-6

[61] Uebel S, Wiesmüller KH, Jung G, Tampé R. Peptide Libraries in Cellular Immune Recognition. In: Famulok M, Winnacker EL, Wong CH, editors. Combinatorial Chemistry in Biology. Current Topics in Microbiology and Immunology. Berlin: Heidelberg: Springer; 1999;**243**. DOI: 10.1007/978-3-642-60142-2_1

[62] Peters B, Bulik S, Tampe R, Van Endert PM, Holzhütter HG. Identifying MHC class I epitopes by predicting the TAP transport efficiency of epitope precursors. Journal of Immunology. 2003;**4**:1741-1749. DOI: 10.4049/jimmunol.171.4.1741

[63] Cardinaud S, Bouziat R, Rohrlich PS, Tourdot S, Weiss L, Langlade-Demoyen P, Burgevin A, Fiorentino S, Van Endert P, Lemonnier FA. Design of a HIV-1-derived HLA-B07.02-restricted polyepitope construct. AIDS. 2009;**15**:1945-1954. DOI: 10.1097/QAD.0b013e32832fae88

[64] Zhu H, Liu K, Cerny J, Imoto T, Moudgil KD. Insertion of the dibasic motif in the flanking region of a cryptic self-determinant leads to activation of the epitope-specific T cells. Journal of Immunology. 2005;**4**:2252-2260. DOI: 10.4049/jimmunol.175.4.2252

[65] Schneider SC, Ohmen J, Fosdick L, Gladstone B, Guo J, Ametani A, Sercarz EE, Deng H. Cutting edge: Introduction of an endopeptidase cleavage motif into a determinant flanking region of hen egg lysozyme results in enhanced T cell determinant display. Journal of Immunology. 2000;**1**:20-23. DOI: 10.4049/jimmunol.165.1.20

[66] Varshavsky A, Turner G, Du F, Xie Y. The ubiquitin system and the N-end rule pathway. Biological Chemistry. 2000;**9-10**:779-789

[67] Rowell JF, Ruff AL, Guarnieri FG, Staveley-O'Carroll K, Lin X, Tang J, Thomas August J, Siliciano RF. Lysosome-associated membrane protein-1-mediated targeting of the HIV-1 envelope protein to an endosomal/lysosomal compartment enhances its presentation to MHC class II-restricted T cells. Journal of Immunology. 1995;**4**:1818-1828

[68] Ruff AL, Guarnieri FG, Staveley-O'Carroll K, Siliciano RF, August JT. The enhanced immune response to the HIV gp160/LAMP chimeric gene product targeted to the lysosome membrane protein trafficking pathway. Journal of Biological Chemistry. 1997;**13**:8671-8678. DOI: 10.1074/jbc.272.13.8671

[69] Wu TC, Guarnieri FG, Staveley-O'Carroll KF, Viscidi RP, Levitsky HI, Hedrick L, Cho KR, August JT, Pardoll DM. Engineering an intracellular pathway for major histocompatibility complex class II presentation of antigens. Proceedings of the National Academy of Sciences of the United States of America. 1995;**25**:11671-11675. DOI: 10.1073/pnas.92.25.11671

[70] Guarnieri FG, Arterburn LM, Penno MB, Cha Y, August JT. The motif Tyr-X-X-

hydrophobic residue mediates lysosomal membrane targeting of lysosome-associated membrane protein 1. Journal of Biological Chemistry. 1993;**3**:1941-1946

[71] Antonets DV, Bazhan SI. PolyCTLDesigner: A computational tool for constructing poly-epitope T-cell antigens. BMC Research Notes. 2013;**6**:407. DOI: 10.1186/1756-0500-6-407

[72] Antonets DV, Maksyutov AZ. TEpredict: Software for T-cell epitope prediction. Molecular Biology. 2010;**1**:119-127. DOI: 10.1134/S0026893310010152

[73] Peters B, Tong W, Sidney J, Sette A, Weng Z. Examining the independent binding assumption for binding of peptide epitopes to MHC-I molecules. Bioinformatics. 2003;**14**:1765-1772. DOI: 10.1093/bioinformatics/btg247

[74] Neefjes J, Jongsma MLM, Paul P, Bakke O. Towards a systems understanding of MHC class i and MHC class II antigen presentation. Nature Reviews Immunology. 2011;**12**:823-836. DOI: 10.1038/nri3084

[75] Toes REM, Nussbaum AK, Degermann S, Schirle M, Emmerich NPN, Kraft M, Laplace C, Zwinderman A, Dick TP, Müller J, Schönfisch B, Schmid C, Fehling HJ, Stevanovic S, Rammensee HG, Schild H. Discrete cleavage motifs of constitutive and immunoproteasomes revealed by quantitative analysis of cleavage products. Journal of Experimental Medicine. 2001;**1**:1-12. DOI: 10.1084/jem.194.1.1

[76] Lafuente EM, Reche PA. Prediction of MHC-peptide binding: A systematic and comprehensive overview. Current Pharmaceutical Design. 2009;**28**:3209-3220. DOI: 10.2174/138161209789105162

[77] Liao WWP, Arthur JW. Predicting peptide binding to major histocompatibility complex molecules. Autoimmunity Reviews. 2011;**8**:469-473. DOI: 10.1016/j.autrev.2011.02.003

[78] Reguzova A, Antonets D, Karpenko L, Ilyichev A, Maksyutov R, Bazhan S. Design and evaluation of optimized artificial HIV-1 poly-T cell-epitope Immunogens. PLoS One. 2015;**3**:e0116412. DOI: 10.1371/journal.pone.0116412

Permissions

All chapters in this book were first published in AHIV&AIDSC, by InTech Open; hereby published with permission under the Creative Commons Attribution License or equivalent. Every chapter published in this book has been scrutinized by our experts. Their significance has been extensively debated. The topics covered herein carry significant findings which will fuel the growth of the discipline. They may even be implemented as practical applications or may be referred to as a beginning point for another development.

The contributors of this book come from diverse backgrounds, making this book a truly international effort. This book will bring forth new frontiers with its revolutionizing research information and detailed analysis of the nascent developments around the world.

We would like to thank all the contributing authors for lending their expertise to make the book truly unique. They have played a crucial role in the development of this book. Without their invaluable contributions this book wouldn't have been possible. They have made vital efforts to compile up to date information on the varied aspects of this subject to make this book a valuable addition to the collection of many professionals and students.

This book was conceptualized with the vision of imparting up-to-date information and advanced data in this field. To ensure the same, a matchless editorial board was set up. Every individual on the board went through rigorous rounds of assessment to prove their worth. After which they invested a large part of their time researching and compiling the most relevant data for our readers.

The editorial board has been involved in producing this book since its inception. They have spent rigorous hours researching and exploring the diverse topics which have resulted in the successful publishing of this book. They have passed on their knowledge of decades through this book. To expedite this challenging task, the publisher supported the team at every step. A small team of assistant editors was also appointed to further simplify the editing procedure and attain best results for the readers.

Apart from the editorial board, the designing team has also invested a significant amount of their time in understanding the subject and creating the most relevant covers. They scrutinized every image to scout for the most suitable representation of the subject and create an appropriate cover for the book.

The publishing team has been an ardent support to the editorial, designing and production team. Their endless efforts to recruit the best for this project, has resulted in the accomplishment of this book. They are a veteran in the field of academics and their pool of knowledge is as vast as their experience in printing. Their expertise and guidance has proved useful at every step. Their uncompromising quality standards have made this book an exceptional effort. Their encouragement from time to time has been an inspiration for everyone.

The publisher and the editorial board hope that this book will prove to be a valuable piece of knowledge for researchers, students, practitioners and scholars across the globe.

List of Contributors

Kelly Cristine Tarquinio Marinho, Elcio Magdalena Giovani, Camila Correia dos Santos and Rodolfo Georgevich Neto
Paulista University, São Paulo, SP, Brazil

María-Dolores Veiga-Ochoa, Roberto Ruiz-Caro, Raúl Cazorla-Luna, Araceli Martín-Illana and Fernando Notario-Pérez
Department of Pharmaceutical Technology and Food Technology, Faculty of Pharmacy, Complutense University of Madrid, Madrid, Spain

Rajneesh Thakur and Vangal Krishnaswamy Sashindran
Armed Forces Medical College, Pune, India

Marimuthu Ragavan Rameshkumar
Infectious Diseases Laboratory, Y.R. Gaitonde Centre for AIDS Research and Education, Voluntary Health Service Hospital, Chennai, India

Narasingam Arunagirinathan
Department of Microbiology, Presidency College (Autonomous), Chennai, India
Faculty of Humanities and Science, Meenakshi Academy of Higher Education and Research, Chennai, India

Ariagor Manuel Almanza Avendaño and Anel Hortensia Gómez San Luis
Universidad Autónoma de Baja California, Mexicali, Baja California, Mexico

Martha Patricia Romero Mendoza
Instituto Nacional de Psiquiatría "Ramón de la Fuente Muñiz", Ciudad de México, Mexico

Maryline Santerre
Molecular Studies of Neurodegenerative Diseases Lab, Fels Institute for Cancer Research and Molecular Biology, Lewis Katz School of Medicine, Temple University, Philadelphia, PA, USA

Bassel Sawaya
Molecular Studies of Neurodegenerative Diseases Lab, Fels Institute for Cancer Research and Molecular Biology, Lewis Katz School of Medicine, Temple University, Philadelphia, PA, USA
Department of Neurology, Lewis Katz School of Medicine, Temple University, Philadelphia, PA, USA

Berthold Bivigou-Mboumba
Centre International de Recherches Médicales de Franceville (CIRMF), Libreville, Gabon

Girish Modi, Andre Mochan and Mala Modi
Division of Neurology, Department of Neurosciences, School of Clinical Medicine, Faculty of Health Sciences, University of the Witwatersrand, Johannesburg, South Africa

Hadil Saad and Ntobeko A.B. Ntusi
Department of Medicine., Faculty of Health Sciences, University of Cape Town, Cape Town, South Africa

Jacqueline Mthembu and Gadija Khan
Human Sciences Research Council (HAST), Cape Town, South Africa

Thabile Manengela
North West University, Mmabatho, South Africa

Konstantin Shmagel and Evgeniya Saidakova
Institute of Ecology and Genetics of Microorganisms, UB RAS, Perm, Russia
Perm State University, Perm, Russia

Elena Vasilyeva, Marina Lozovskaya, Lyudmila Klochkova and Yuliya Yarovaya
St Petersburg State Pediatric Medical University, Saint Petersburg, Russia

Larisa I. Karpenko, Sergei I. Bazhan, Denis V. Antonets and Alexander A. Ilyichev
State Research Center of Virology and Biotechnology Vector, Koltsovo, Novosibirsk, Russian Federation

Alexey M. Eroshkin
Bioinformatics Core, Sanford Burnham Prebys Medical Discovery Institute, La Jolla, CA, USA

Anton N. Chikaev
Institute of Molecular and Cellular Biology of the Siberian Branch of the Russian Academy of Sciences, Novosibirsk, Russian Federation

www.ingramcontent.com/pod-product-compliance
Lightning Source LLC
LaVergne TN
LVHW060540210926
848485LV00005B/1232